Mental Health Law

Mental Health Law

a practical guide

second edition

Basant K. Puri MA, PhD, MB BChir, BSc (Hons) MathSci, FRCPsych, DipStat, PG Dip Maths, MMath.
Hammersmith Hospital
Imperial College London and University of Limerick

Robert A. Brown MA Applied Social Studies
Director of Edge Training and Consultancy Ltd. Social Worker. Visiting Fellow
Bournemouth University, Bournemouth, UK

Heather J. McKee MB, ChB, BAO, MRCPsych, LLM
Consultant Neuropsychiatrist, Royal Hospital for Neurodisability, West Hill, Putney, London, UK

Ian H. Treasaden MB, BS, LRCP, MRCS, FRCPsych, LLM
Consultant Forensic Psychiatrist, Three Bridges Medium Secure Unit, West London Mental Health NHS Trust, London; and Honorary Clinical Senior Lecturer in Forensic Psychiatry, Imperial College, London, UK

CRC Press
Taylor & Francis Group
Boca Raton London New York

CRC Press is an imprint of the
Taylor & Francis Group, an **informa** business

CRC Press
Taylor & Francis Group
6000 Broken Sound Parkway NW, Suite 300
Boca Raton, FL 33487-2742

First issued in hardback 2017

ISBN-13: 978-1-4441-1714-1 (pbk)
ISBN-13: 978-1-138-44515-4 (hbk)

Visit the Taylor & Francis Web site at
http://www.taylorandfrancis.com

and the CRC Press Web site at
http://www.crcpress.com

Contents

	Contributors	vii
	Legal advisors	viii
	Preface	ix
1.	History of mental health legislation	1
2.	Definitions used in mental health legislation	13
3.	Professional roles	25
4.	Safeguards for patients under the Mental Health Act	37
5.	Compulsory Admission to Hospital: (Sections 2, 3 and 4 of the Mental Health Act)	43
6.	Consent to Treatment Provisions under the Mental Health Act	53
7.	Community Treatment Orders, Leave of Absence and After-care	57
8.	Guardianship (Sections 7 or 37 of the Mental Health Act)	63
9.	Patients concerned in criminal proceedings or under sentence	73
10.	Mental Health Tribunals	97
11.	Hospital Managers	103
12.	Cross-border arrangements	109
13.	The Mental Health Act Code of Practice and the Reference Guide	115
14.	The Care Quality Commission	123
15.	Consent and Capacity	129
16.	The Mental Capacity Act 2005: Principles	139
17.	Mental Capacity Act 2005: Provisions	143
18.	Assessment of Capacity	155
19.	Safeguards under the Mental Capacity Act 2005	161
20.	The Mental Capacity Act Codes of Practice	167
21.	Human Rights Act 1998 in mental health legislation in the UK	173
22.	Mental health, medication and the law	177
23.	Research ethics	187
24.	Child mental health law	191
25.	Race, culture and mental health	207
26.	Suicidal patients	211
27.	Assessment of risk of violence	217
28.	International comparison of mental health legislation	237
Appendix I	Legal cases	248
Appendix II	Summary of civil treatment codes	263
Appendix III	Summary of civil compulsion sections	265

Appendix IV Flowchart of decisions involving consent to treatment 266
Appendix V Sample forms 267

Index 275

Contributors

Paul Barber BA Oxon

Solicitor and Former Partner, Bevan Brittan Solicitors
Freelance Lecturer and Trainer in Mental Health, Incapacity and Human Rights Law, UK

Sharon Davies BA MBBS MRCPsych

Consultant Adolescent Forensic Psychiatrist, West London Mental Health NHS Trust, London, UK

Claire Dimond BSc MBBS MRCPsych

Consultant Adolescent Forensic Psychiatrist, Adolescent Forensic Directorate, WLMHT

Christine Dixon MRPharmS

Principal Pharmacist
S.W. London Elective Orthopaedic Centre, Epsom, Surrey, UK

Legal advisors

Sections of the manuscript related to mental health law and to criminal law were reviewed by the following advisors, who made suggestions and recommendations to the authors on the basis of their specialised experience and knowledge on current law and legal practice. Their help is much appreciated. The final version of the text is the work of the authors, incorporating those suggestions and recommendations as the authors have judged best:

Nick Hopkins and Rebecca Hill

Solicitors, Needham Poulier & Partners, London, UK

Helen Kingston

Solicitor and Principal Lecturer in Law, Northumbria University, Newcastle upon Tyne, UK

Preface

The preparation of a second edition of this book has given us the opportunity to cover the major developments in mental health legislation since the publication of the previous edition. These have included the new **Mental Health Act 2007**, the **Mental Capacity Act 2005** together with its two Codes (one general and one covering the Deprivation of Liberty Safeguards), the revised **Mental Health Act Code of Practice** published in 2008 and changes in legislation related to research involving the mentally disordered.

Once again, we have sought to strike a balance between the need to provide the reader with a relatively short and portable handbook containing practical advice and the desire to be over-inclusive with detailed considerations of the ramifications of legal argument. While the usual cautionary legal principle is that the reader should always refer to the latest primary legislation, this is rarely realistic in day-to-day practice. However, it is hoped that the new edition of this mental health law handbook will continue to live up to its name and provide helpful practical medico-legal advice.

We wish to thank all those who reviewed the first edition and the draft second edition and we are grateful for the feedback we received.

We are very sorry to relate that Dr Paul Laking, the author of the excellent chapter on child mental health law in the first edition, has died. We valued his contribution greatly and extend our sympathies to his family.

1 History of mental health legislation

In the ancient world, various safeguards were implemented in respect of those suffering from mental illness at the time of committing an offence.

For ancient Israel, the Torah established cities of refuge for those who had accidentally killed someone (Devarim/Deuteronomy Chapter 19). On entering such a city of refuge, a person guilty of manslaughter would be safe from the revenge of relatives of the victim. There is a tradition to take mental illness very seriously within traditional 'orthodox' Judaism; even the usual Shabbat restrictions may be suspended to secure the safety of a person with a mental disorder that could lead to loss of life or serious injury.

In ancient Egypt, Imhotep (Greek Imouthes) combined the roles of priest, statesman, scientist and physician to the second king of the third dynasty, Djoser, who reigned from 2630 to 2611 BCE. The temple of Imhotep became a medical school offering various therapies to patients, such as sleep therapy, occupational therapy, narcotherapy and art therapy.

Aristotle argued that a person was morally responsible for his crime only if guilt was present, with the perpetrator deliberately choosing to commit the act.

Offenders were tried in the forum in the ancient Roman world, whence our term forensic. The Romans took the view that those who were mad were punished enough by their madness and should not be additionally punished (*satis furore punitor*). Under Roman law, the insane were exempt from the usual punishments for causing injury to others: 'An insane person, as well as an infant, are legally incapable of malicious intent and the power to insult, and therefore the action for injuries cannot be brought against them.' (The opinions of Julius Paulus. Book VIII. Title IV: Concerning Injuries; cited in Formigoni 1996.)

That allowance was made in sentencing mentally disordered offenders in England after the fall of the Roman Empire is illustrated by the fact that, during the reign of King Alfred, a judge who hanged a madman, was himself hanged. However, in the UK, up until the nineteenth century, 'lunatics' who committed crimes were sent to gaols or houses of correction, where they were grossly neglected, objects of derision and sources of entertainment and amusement for the public.

Within the UK, there are three separate systems of legislation, for England and Wales, Scotland and Northern Ireland, and therefore three different Mental Health Acts. The Republic of Ireland (Eire), itself, also has separate legislation.

One of the earliest references to legal practice in the UK dealing with the mentally ill was in 1285, when a verdict of misadventure was returned by jurors following the killing of one of the brothers at a hospital in Beverley, Yorkshire, on the grounds that the offender acted at 'the instigation of the devil', as a result of which he had become 'frantic and mad'.

An early distinction in common law between 'the idiot', with significant or severe learning difficulties, and the 'lunatic', who was mentally ill, was made.

Subsequently, these two groups were dealt with at times separately and sometimes together in mental health legislation.

The **Royal Prerogative** (*De Praerogativa Regis*) in 1334 entitled the Crown to the rents and profits of the estates of idiots, subject to the expense of their maintenance and that of their dependent family. The care of an idiot was often entrusted by the Crown to someone who shared the profits of the estate with the Crown ('begging a man for a fool'). In the case of lunatics, however, any income greater than the expense of their maintenance was held in a trust for their recovery or, if they died, for the benefit of their soul.

The Bethlem Hospital was founded in 1247 as the Priory of the Order of St. Mary of Bethlehem. By 1329, it was described as a hospice or hospital. It first took in 'lunatics' in 1377. It remained the only specialised placement for the mentally ill until the seventeenth century.

Overall, in the sixteenth and seventeenth centuries in England, more concern was taken with men who became insane than women who did so. From this time dates the description of Mad Tom, a beggar with tattered clothes and little better than a beast.

The **Poor Law Act 1601** required each parish to take responsibility for the old and the sick, including 'idiots' and 'lunatics'. Overseers could arrange for the poor to be placed in workhouses which were known for their very poor conditions. Mentally disordered patients were among those so housed. By 1770, some workhouses were refusing to take 'lunatics'.

The **1713 and 1744 Vagrancy Acts** allowed for the detention of 'Lunaticks or mad persons'.

The **1713 Vagrancy Act**, 'the Act for ... the more effectual punishing such as Rogues, Vagabonds, Sturdy beggars and Vagrants and Sending them Whither They Ought to be sent', came into operation in 1714. It allowed two or more Justices of the Peace to order the arrest of any person 'furiously mad and dangerous' and for such persons 'to be safely locked up in some secure place' for as long as the 'lunacy or madness shall continue'. Secure places included the workhouse, private mad houses, gaols and Bridewell (a house of correction). 'Lunatics', unlike other vagrants, were excluded from whipping.

In the 1730s, the Bethlem Hospital made provision for incurables and in 1739 stated they would give priority to dangerous rather than harmless incurables.

The **1744 Vagrancy Act** amended the 1713 Act by specifying that 'those who by Lunacy or otherwise are furiously mad or so far disordered in their Senses that they may be dangerous to be permitted to go abroad' could be apprehended by a constable, church warden or overseer of the poor at the authorisation of two or more Justices of the Peace 'and be safely locked in some secure place ... and if necessary) to be there chained ... for and during such time only as the lunacy or madness shall continue'.

In 1760, Laurence, the fourth Earl Ferrers, committed an act of murder for which he was tried by his fellow peers before the House of Lords. The murder having been easily proved to have been committed by him, as part of his defence, Earl Ferrers called several witnesses in order to try to demonstrate that he had been of unsound mind at the time of the index offence. This included the first appearance of a physician at a trial as an expert witness to address the issue of the mental state of a defendant at the time of the offence. (His lordship commented on the fact that he had been reduced to the necessity of attempting to prove himself a lunatic, that he might not be deemed a murderer.) This defence failed and Earl Ferrers was sentenced to death; his petition to be beheaded also failed, and he was duly hanged on 5th May 1760.

Medical certification for insanity was introduced by The **Act for Regulating Private Madhouses 1774** and provided for a fine of £100 unless the proprietor of the private madhouse received an individual under 'an Order in Writing under the Hand and Seal of some Physician, Surgeon or Apothecary, that such person is properly received into such house or Place as a Lunatick'. This followed two cases of habeas corpus (Clark in 1718 and Turlington in 1761) and the parliamentary investigation of London madhouses in 1763.

Ticehurst opened in 1792 and rapidly attracted the aristocracy and became the most expensive private asylum in England. The Retreat in York was founded by William Tuke and the Society of Friends in 1792.

In 1800, James Hadfield, an ex-soldier who had brain damage from a sword wound to the head, believed he had to sacrifice his life to save the world but, feeling unable to commit suicide, he unsuccessfully tried to kill the then King George III whom he shot in an attempt to ensure his own execution. He was acquitted of attempted murder, owing mainly to his lawyer, Erskine, and sent to the Bethlem Hospital. Erskine had emphasised to the court to good effect the exposed head wound with visible throbbing blood vessels of Hadfield. This was the first example of a mentally abnormal offender being sent to a mental hospital by a court. This decision reflected the then sympathy for the mentally ill, as George III suffered from mental illness, probably as a result of the inherited biochemical disorder of haemoglobin, porphyria. The court's decision about Hadfield led in the same year to The **Act for the Safe Custody of Insane Persons Charged with Offences 1800.** This was retrospective legislation providing for the special verdict of not guilty by reason of insanity. Insanity was, however, undefined. The return of this verdict led to the accused being detained in 'strict custody' in the county gaol during His Majesty's pleasure. During the first five years of its operation, 37 people were so detained, which led to the complaint that 'to confine such persons in a common gaol is equally destructive for the recovery of the insane and for the security and comfort of other prisoners'.

By 1807 there were 45 private madhouses in the country. The **Act for the Better Care and Maintenance of Pauper and Criminal Lunatics 1808** allowed for insane offenders to be admitted to asylums at the expense of the responsible parish. The **Lunacy Asylum Enabling Act 1808** authorised counties to raise rates to build asylums, although few responded initially; some psychiatric hospitals today were developed as a result of this Act. They tended to be built in rural areas away from towns, but this may also have reflected the fact that rural areas were where most of the population then lived. This Act is sometimes referred to as the **County Asylums Act 1808.** Conditions in asylums remained poor. For example, in 1814 Godfrey Higgins, a governor and Yorkshire magistrate, discovered at the York Lunatic Asylum 13 women to a cell 12 feet × 7 feet 10 inches and he claimed 144 deaths had been covered up. A subsequent official investigation by Higgins and the Tukes found evidence of murder and rape, widespread use of chains, huge embezzlement and physical neglect. In 1814, James (William) Norris was discovered in the Bethlem Hospital, where he had been an inpatient for 9 to 14 years, in a specially constructed iron restraint encasing his body from the neck down and attached to a short chain running from the ceiling to the floor, which allowed him only to lie on his back and move 12 inches away from the bar. While he had a history of past violence, he was found to be rational.

The **Care and Maintenance Lunacy Act 1815** required overseers of the poor to return lists of idiots and lunatics within parishes together with certificates from medical practitioners.

The **Madhouse Act 1828** repealed the 1774 Act. It also increased the number of Metropolitan Commissioners to 15 (including five medical practitioners who received token payments; the rest gave their services free of charge), and gave them the power to release individuals detained improperly and to remove a private madhouse proprietor's licence if conditions were unsatisfactory. This Act also introduced the first legal requirement for medical attendance at least once a week, including signing a weekly register. A medical superintendent had to be employed where an asylum contained more than 100 patients.

The **County Asylums Act 1828** required magistrates to send annual returns of admissions, discharges and deaths to the Home Office. The Act also allowed the Secretary of State to send a visitor to any county asylum, although the visitor had no power to intervene in the administration of that asylum.

The **Poor Law Amendment Act 1834** restricted the period of detention of any dangerous 'lunatic' or insane person or 'idiot' in any workhouse to 14 days, which resulted in dangerous 'lunatics' being admitted to the county asylums with the workhouses retaining the non-dangerous pauper 'lunatics', although workhouse placement of the latter, if curable, was considered unsatisfactory by the Poor Law Commissioners.

Northampton General Lunatic Asylum, a charitable hospital (now St Andrew's Hospital, an independent psychiatric hospital), opened in 1838, taking all county paupers and patients on a contractual basis, including the poet John Clare in 1841.

The **Insane Prisoners Act 1840** gave the Home Secretary the power to transfer from prison to an asylum any individual awaiting trial or serving a sentence of imprisonment. This required a certificate of insanity signed by two Justices of the Peace and two doctors.

In 1841, the Association of Medical Officers of Asylums and Hospitals for the Insane was formed, the forerunner of the Royal College of Psychiatrists, and they began publishing the *Asylum Journal* in 1853.

In 1843, McNaughton, while deluded, attempted to shoot the Prime Minister, Sir Robert Peel. McNaughton missed, and shot Peel's secretary instead. McNaughton was acquitted on account of his insanity at the time of the offence. The outcry, including from Queen Victoria, at this acquittal led to the law lords issuing guidance known as the McNaughton Rules, from which the defendant may argue that at the time of the index offence he was not guilty by reason of insanity. Further details of the McNaughton Rules are given in Chapter 9.

The **Lunatics Act 1845** introduced detailed certification processes with increased safeguards against the wrongful detention of patients in both public and private facilities. All asylums were ordered to keep a Medical Visitation Book and a record of medical treatment for each patient in a Medical Casebook. This allowed a person who signed an order for admission of a private patient to discharge that patient, although this could be barred by the medical person in charge of the house or a registered medical attendant by certifying that such an individual was 'dangerous and unfit to be at large', which in turn could be overruled by the written consent of the Commissioners in Lunacy. It was also this 1845 Act that introduced the concept of person of unsound mind.

The **Lunatics Asylum Act 1845** required all boroughs and counties to provide, within three years, adequate asylum accommodation for its pauper lunatics at public expense. Counties were also authorised, but not instructed, to erect less costly buildings for chronic lunatics. The subsequent development of county asylums is reflected by the fact that of the 52 counties, in 1944, 15 had made provision for the insane, by 1847, 36, and by 1854, 41.

The **Lunatics Act 1853** required medical officers to record in the medical journal of patients the means, duration and the reasons for restraint and seclusion, or otherwise face a £20 fine. The rules of every asylum had to be formally given to the Home Secretary for approval, although approval was, in fact, undertaken by the Lunacy Commission. The rules were to be 'printed, abided by and observed'. The Bethlem Hospital was also brought under the control of the Lunacy Commission by this Act.

In 1854, the hypodermic syringe was invented.

The **Medical Registration Act 1858** united the medical profession, which had been previously separated into physicians, surgeons and apothecaries.

The Select Committee on Lunacy 1859–60 extended the requirement for an order from a magistrate to detain a lunatic to private, and not just pauper, cases to protect 'the liberty of the subject' and to check on the medical opinion. It also recommended Emergency Certification and the 'terminalability of orders' to reduce the population of asylums.

Although the Bethlem Hospital had been given cash to take mentally disordered offenders, the resulting stigma felt by that hospital led to the **Criminal Lunatic Asylum Act 1860,** under which such offenders were to be placed in a new state criminal lunatic asylum which opened in 1863 and which was later renamed Broadmoor Hospital, the first of the Special Hospitals.

An **Act to Amend the Law relating to Lunatics 1862** resulted in the cost of caring for 'lunatics' being chargeable upon a common fund of the union of parishes instead of upon an individual parish.

The Annual Report of the Lunacy Commission in 1862 indicated that mechanical restraint was used in very few places and on very few occasions by this time. Seclusion was, however, noted to be used in most asylums.

In 1882, paraldehyde was developed.

The **Idiots Act 1886** was the first time legislation had specifically addressed the needs of those with learning disability. They had previously been admitted to workhouses, lunatic asylums and prisons. This Act led to the admission of such individuals to specialised asylums such as the previously established 'asylum for idiots' at Park House, Highgate, later known as Earlswood Asylum, and to the regulation and inspection of such asylums. This legislation introduced separate provisions for 'idiots' and 'imbeciles'.

The distinction between idiots and imbeciles was, however, ignored by the **Lunacy (Consolidation) Act 1890,** which favoured public over private provision and provided for four routes of admission:

- *Summary reception order*: pauper patients were usually received under this order following a Justice of the Peace being petitioned by a police officer or a Poor Law relieving officer with a medical certificate. In an emergency, a wandering lunatic could be detained in a workhouse for up to three days by one of these officers.
- *Reception order*: non-pauper patients were usually admitted under this order. For this, a magistrates' or county court judge was petitioned to order admission by a relative, preferably husband or wife, supported by two medical certificates, one of which, if practical, should be from the individual's usual medical

attendant. The relative was legally required to visit the patient at least once every six months.

- *Urgency order*: private patients could be admitted following a petition from a relative to the asylum authorities in an emergency for up to seven days under this order, following which a reception order was to be obtained, otherwise the patient would be discharged.
- *Chancery lunatics*: such patients could be admitted by a process of application for admission following inquisition.

Reception orders lasted up to one year, but were renewable if the manager of the institution provided a special report and a certificate to the Lunacy Commission, which, if it accepted the opinion of the report, renewed the order for a further year, thereafter for two and then three years, and then for successive periods of five years. If not satisfied, the Lunacy Commission retained the power directly to discharge such patients from asylums. Indeed, one medical and one legal commissioner together could discharge a patient from any hospital or licence house after one visit.

Also under the **Lunacy Act 1890**, with permission of the Lunacy Commission or the licensing justices, managers of licensed houses could receive as boarders 'any person who is desirous of voluntarily submitting to treatment', but they too had to be produced to the Lunacy Commission and the justices on their visits. Such voluntary patients could leave after giving 24 hours' notice. Detention beyond this rendered the proprietor liable to a daily £10 fine. However, the consent of the commissioners and licensing justices was still required and boarders were largely confined to licensed houses.

In 1895, Josef Breuer and Sigmund Freud published their Studies on Hysteria (Studien über Hysterie) detailing their cathartic model of treatment.

In 1896, The National Association for the Care of the Feeble Minded was founded.

In 1900, Freud's *The Interpretation of Dreams* was published, with its topographical model of unconscious, pre-conscious and conscious levels of the mind.

In 1912, the new Rampton State Asylum opened as a criminal lunatic asylum in the village of Woodbeck, North Nottinghamshire. Initially, all patients were transferred from Broadmoor Hospital. It later also took those with learning disability requiring a special hospital placement. It remains as a maximum secure special hospital.The **Mental Deficiency Act 1913** followed the by then current opinion favouring the segregation of 'mental defectives' into four legal classes:

- *Idiots*, who were unable to guard themselves against common physical dangers such as fire, water or traffic.
- *Imbeciles,* who could guard against physical dangers, but were incapable of managing themselves or their affairs.
- *The feeble-minded*, who needed care or control for the protection of self or others.
- *Moral defectives*, who had vicious or criminal propensities. This category was also used to include and detain many poor women with illegitimate or unsupported babies.

This Act also founded a Board of Control and placed on local government the responsibility for the supervision and protection of such individuals, both in institutions and in the community. Also under this Act, local authorities were given statutory responsibility for providing occupation and training for 'mental defectives'.

The **Ministry of Health Act 1919** transferred responsibility for the Board of Control from the Home Office to the newly formed Ministry of Health.

In 1923, Freud's *The Ego and the Id* was published, with its structural model of the mind involving id, ego and superego, together with eros, the life instinct, and thanatos, the death instinct.

In 1926, the Report of the Royal Commission on Lunacy and Mental Disorder (Macmillan) recommended that madness be defined in medical terms. It commented that compulsion was becoming less appropriate. In the same year, the annual report of the Board of Control saw the first official use of the term 'community care'.

The **Mental Deficiency Act 1927** gave more emphasis to care outside the institutions. Mental deficiency was defined as 'a condition of arrested or incomplete development of mind existing before the age of 18 years whether arising from inherent causes or induced by disease or injury'.

The **Mental Treatment Act 1930** allowed for informal voluntary admission and represented the turning point from legal to medical control of psychiatric admissions. 'Lunatics' became 'persons of unsound mind' and asylums became 'mental hospitals'. Voluntary admission was by written application to the person in charge of the hospital, but magistrates continued to be involved in overseeing compulsory hospital admissions. The Act also allowed local authorities to establish psychiatric outpatient clinics in both general and mental hospitals and organise after-care for discharged patients, but services remained centred on the mental hospital.

Insulin coma therapy was invented by the Austrian psychiatrist Manfred Joshua Sakel in 1935. Psycho-surgery (leucotomy) as a treatment of mental illness was established by Egas Moniz in Portugal in 1935, being first used in the UK in Bristol in 1940. In 1934, convulsive therapy by drugs, e.g. camphor, was introduced in Hungary by Ladislas von Meduna and reached the UK in 1937. Electrically induced convulsion (electroconvulsive therapy, ECT) was first undertaken in 1938 by two Italians, Hugo Cerletti and Lucio Beni, on a mute man who suffered from schizophrenia (in contrast to its main use now for severe depression). The patient's first words after his initial treatment were 'You are killing me', but the treatments were continued and the man's mental state improved. ECT was first used in the UK the following year. Also in the late 1930s, amphetamines were used to treat depression. The psychiatric wards started to become unlocked in the UK in the 1930s and 1940s.

The **National Health Service Act 1946** ended the distinction between paying and non-paying patients.

Also in 1946, Judy Fryd, a mother of a child with a learning disability, formed the National Association of Parents of Backward Children. This association changed its name to the National Society for Mentally Handicapped Children in 1956, and then to Mencap in the 1960s.

The **National Assistance Act 1948** made provisions for those in need.

D-Lysergic acid diethylamide (LSD) was used for a therapeutic trial in 1952 when Sandoz supplied Powick Hospital in Worcestershire with this drug. (LSD-25 had been synthesised in 1938 by Albert Hofmann, a chemist working for Sandoz. The first (accidental) human experience of the effects of this chemical was by Hofmann in 1943; he reported seeing 'an uninterrupted stream of fantastic pictures'.

Chlorpromazine (sold as Largactil in the UK and as Thorazine in the USA) was first marketed as an antipsychotic medication in Great Britain in 1954. In 1956, clinical studies confirmed the effectiveness in treating depression of both the monoamine oxidase inhibitor iproniazid, which was first used in 1951 in tuberculosis causing euphoria in some of those so treated, and the tricyclic antidepressant imipramine.

The Percy Commission, The Royal Commission on the Law relating to Mental Illness and Mental Deficiency, was appointed in 1953. Its report in 1957 formed the basis for the new **Mental Health Act 1959** in England and Wales as well as the **Mental Health (Scotland) Act 1960** and the **Mental Health (Northern Ireland) Act 1961.**

The **Mental Health Act 1959** led to voluntary informal admissions being the usual method of psychiatric hospital admission. No longer was a positive statement of such willingness to be admitted on the part of the patient required. All judicial controls on compulsory admission were removed. Applications for admissions were to be made by a mental welfare officer (social worker) or by the patient's nearest relative. Mental disorder was defined as including mental illness, severe subnormality, subnormality and psychopathic disorder. Provisions included a 28-day compulsory order for admission for observation (Section 25), which was non-renewable and required two medical certificates, a 72-hour emergency order (Section 29) on the basis of one medical certificate, which could be converted by the addition of a further medical certificate into an order for observation, and a treatment order (Section 26) for a maximum period of 12 months in the first instance, on the basis of two medical certificates, renewable after 12 months and thereafter for periods of two years. Appeals to a Mental Health Review Tribunal were allowed once in the first period of detention and once in each period for which detention was renewed.

In 1961, Minister of Health, J. Enoch Powell, announced that 'in 15 years' time there would be needed not more than half as many places in hospital for mental illness as there are today', which would represent '75,000' fewer hospital beds.

The antipsychotic oral medication haloperidol was introduced in 1959.

The 1962 White Paper, Hospital Plan for England and Wales, proposed the creation of new and large district general hospitals, but made no specific reference to provision for long-stay psychiatric patients. The Seebohm Report of 1968 noted that community care was, for many parts of the country, a 'sad illusion' and was likely to remain so for many years ahead.

The Royal College of Psychiatrists received its charter in 1971.

In 1975, the Butler Committee report on Mentally Abnormal Offenders recommended the establishment of regional (medium) secure units, pending the development of which temporary interim secure units were to be established in each region.

The **Local Authorities Social Services Act 1970** created social services departments. In the same year, the **Chronically Sick and Disabled Persons Act 1970** was passed, which also applied to mentally disordered persons.

In 1980, the Boynton Report of the Review of Rampton Hospital was published. This followed allegations of abuse at this special hospital that had been made in a Yorkshire Television documentary, The Secret Hospital.

The Mental Health (Amendment) Act of 1982, introduced as a Bill in November 1981, led to The **Mental Health Act 1983** for England and Wales. Under this Act, voluntary admissions were still to be encouraged but the legislation was more legalistic in its approach to mental health. Changes were made to the definition of mental disorder. Mental disorder was defined as including mental illness (which was undefined), severe mental impairment and mental impairment (which replaced subnormality), and psychopathic disorder. (The corresponding **Scottish Mental Health Act 1984** used the term mental handicap rather than mental impairment.) The Mental Health Act 1983 also introduced a separate treatability test for psychopathic disorder and mental impairment. Detention orders were effectively halved in length and opportunities to apply for a Mental Health Review Tribunal hearing effectively doubled. Tribunal hearings were to be made available to 28-day assessment order (Section 2) patients. Also introduced were powers for a Mental Health Review Tribunal to order delayed discharge and to recommend, but not order, leave of absence or transfer. Tribunals, when chaired by a Judge or Queen's Counsel (QC or 'Silk'), could now also discharge from restriction orders (Section 41), which previously only the Home Secretary could do. Provisions for consent to treatment were specified and the Mental Health Act Commission was introduced. There were also changes to guardianship and a requirement for training of social workers before appointment as approved social workers under the Act. Informal inpatients were allowed to retain voting rights and their access to the courts and were also entitled to the provision of after-care services (Section l17). The proposed Mental Health Act Code of Practice was eventually laid before Parliament in December 1989 (pursuant to Section 118(4) of the Mental Health Act 1983) and published in 1990.

The **Police and Criminal Evidence Act 1984 (PACE)** with its code of practice used the term 'mental disorder' as in the 1983 Mental Health Act and the term 'mental handicap', defined as 'a state of arrested or incomplete development of mind which includes significant impairment of intelligence and social functioning'.

In the late 1980s, newer classes of safer antidepressants were marketed, for example, the selective serotonin re-uptake inhibitors (SSRIs), such as fluvoxamine (marketed as Faverin) and fluoxetine (marketed as Prozac).

In 1989, Ashworth Special Hospital was formed when two Liverpool special hospitals in close proximity were amalgamated – Moss Side Hospital, which had opened in 1919, and Park Lane Hospital, which had opened in 1974. In the same year, a new authority, the Special Hospitals Service Authority, took charge of Broadmoor, Ashworth and Rampton special hospitals.

Clozapine, an oral atypical antipsychotic medication for treatment-resistant schizophrenia, was re-introduced from 1990, with strict requirements for blood monitoring after its original failed introduction owing to mortality from induced low white cell counts in the 1970s.

In 1990, the **National Health Service and Community Care Act 1990** was introduced.

The Care Programme Approach Circular was published in 1990, which was to take effect from April 1991. The issue of the adequacy of community care was highlighted by the killing by Christopher Clunes, who suffered from schizophrenia, of Jonathon Zito at Finsbury Park tube station in London in December 1992 and also, on New Year's Day 1993, by Ben Silcock, then aged 27 years and who also suffered from schizophrenia, who climbed into the lions' enclosure at London Zoo and was severely mauled and injured by the lions.

A revised Mental Health Code of Practice came into effect in November 1993 following publication in August of that year. The Secretary of State for Health, Virginia Bottomley, introduced a 10-point plan for the care of mentally disordered people.

In April 1995, the publication of HSG (94)(5) heralded the introduction of supervision registers in October 1994. The Department of Health published *Building Bridges: A Guide to Inter-agency Working* in November 1995.

The **Mental Health (Patients in the Community) Act 1995,** with its provisions for supervised discharge/after-care under supervision, came into effect in April 1996.

In September 1998, Professor Genevra Richardson of Queen Mary and Westfield College, London, was appointed to lead a root-and-branch review of the Mental Health Act 1983. The expert committee, chaired by Professor Richardson, reported to Ministers at the Department of Health in July 1999, having consulted a wide range of organisations and individuals in formulating their proposals. They issued their Draft Outline Proposals to over 350 key stakeholders to consider the practicability of the proposals. In 1999, the Report of the Expert Committee was published.

In 1999, the revised Code of Practice to the Mental Health Act 1983 came into force.

In 2000, the **Human Rights Act 1998** became operational, with a delay allowing judges and others to be trained in how to operate the new legislation. This Act is considered in more detail in the corresponding chapter later in this book.

In 2002, a Draft Mental Health Bill was published by the Department of Health.

In 2004, a Revised Draft Mental Health Bill was published.

The **Mental Capacity Act 2005** received Royal Assent in April 2005. It provides a statutory framework to empower and protect vulnerable people who are unable to make their own decisions. It makes it clear who can take decisions, in which situations, and how they should go about this. It enables people to plan ahead for a time when they may lose capacity. Further details are given in the corresponding chapter later in this book.

The **Mental Health Act 2007** received Royal Assent in July 2007. It amended the Mental Health Act 1983, the Mental Capacity Act 2005 and the Domestic Violence, Crime and Victims Act 2004. The main changes made to the Mental Health Act 1983 by the Mental Health Act 2007 included:

- *Changes to the definition of mental disorder:* it changed the way the 1983 Act defined mental disorder, so that a single definition applies throughout the 2007 Act, abolishing references to categories of disorder.
- *Criteria for detention:* it introduced a new appropriate medical treatment test which applies to all the longer-term powers of detention. It is not now possible for a patient to be compulsorily detained, or for their detention to be continued, unless appropriate medical treatment and all other circumstances of the case are available to him. (These criteria abolished the treatability test.)
- *ECT:* it introduced new safeguards for patients.
- *Independent mental health advocacy:* it placed a duty on the appropriate national authority to make arrangements for help to be provided by independent mental health advocates.
- *Nearest relative:* it gave patients the right to make an application to the county court to displace their nearest relative and it enabled county courts to displace a nearest relative whom it thinks is not suitable to act as nearest relative. Also, the provisions allowing determination of the nearest relative were amended to include civil partners amongst the list of relatives.
- *Professional roles:* it broadened the group of practitioners who can take on

the functions performed under the 1983 Act by approved social workers and responsible medical officers.

- *Services made age-appropriate:* it required hospital managers to ensure that patients aged under 18 years, admitted to hospital for mental disorder, are accommodated in an environment that is suitable for their age (subject to their needs).
- *Supervised Community Treatment (SCT):* it introduced SCT for patients following a period of detention in hospital. SCT allows certain patients with a mental disorder to be discharged from detention, subject to the possibility of recall to hospital if necessary. The intention was to help avoid situations in which some patients leave hospital and do not continue with their treatment, with the result that their health deteriorates and they require detention again (the revolving door).
- *Tribunals:* it reduced the periods after which hospital managers must refer certain patients' cases to the Tribunal if they do not apply themselves. It introduced an order-making power to make further reductions in due course.

Further details of the 2007 Act are given in relevant chapters of this book.

In 2008, a further revised Code of Practice to the Mental Health Act 1983 came into force. Further details are given in the corresponding chapter later in this book.

For greater detail, *See* Chapter 2.

Further reading

Fennell, P (1996). *Treatment without Consent: Law, Psychiatry and Treatment of Mentally Disordered People since 1845*. London: Routledge.

Formigoni, W (1996). *Pithanon a Paulo Epitomatorum libri VIII: Sulla funzione critica del commento del giurista Iulius Paulus*. Milan: Giuffrè.

Scull, A (2005). *The Most Solitary of Afflictions: Madness in Society in Britain 1700–1900*. London: Yale University Press.

Scull, A (2011). *Madness: A Very Short Introduction*. Oxford: Oxford University Press.

2 Definitions used in mental health legislation

Many of the definitions are set out or summarised in Sections 1 and 145 of the Mental Health Act 1983, amended by the Mental Health Act 2007. Definitions regarding patients concerned in criminal proceedings or under sentence are not considered in this chapter but can be found in Chapter 9.

Structure of the Amended 1983 Act

The Parts (Roman numbers) and Sections (Arabic numbers) of the 1983 Act are as follows.

Part I: Application of the Act

1 Application of Act: 'mental disorder'

Part II: Compulsory Admission to Hospital and Guardianship

Procedure for hospital admission

2 Admission for assessment
3 Admission for treatment
4 Admission for assessment in cases of emergency
5 Application in respect of patient already in hospital
6 Effect of application for admission

Guardianship

7 Application for guardianship
8 Effect of guardianship application, etc.
9 Regulations as to guardianship
10 Transfer of guardianship in case of death, incapacity, etc. of guardian

General provisions as to applications and recommendations

11 General provisions as to applications
12 General provisions as to medical recommendations
12A Conflicts of interest
13 Duty of approved mental health professionals to make applications for admission or guardianship
14 Social reports

15 Rectification of applications and recommendations
17 Leave of absence from hospital
17A Community treatment orders
17B Conditions
17C Duration of community treatment order
17D Effect of community treatment order
17E Power to recall to hospital
17F Powers in respect of recalled patients
17G Effect of revoking community treatment order
18 Return and readmission of patients absent without leave
19 Regulations as to transfer of patients
19A Regulations as to assignment of responsibility for community patients
20 Duration of authority
20A Community treatment period
20B Effect of expiry of community treatment order
21 Special provisions as to patients absent without leave
21A Patients who are taken into custody or return within 28 days
21B Patients who are taken into custody or return after more than 28 days
22 Special provisions as to patients sentenced to imprisonment, etc
23 Discharge of patients
24 Visiting and examination of patients
25 Restrictions on discharge by nearest relative

Functions of relatives of patients

26 Definition of 'relative' and 'nearest relative'
27 Children and young persons in care
28 Nearest relative of minor under guardianship, etc
29 Appointment by court of acting nearest relative
30 Discharge and variation of orders under Section 29

Supplemental

31 Procedure on applications to county court
32 Regulations for purposes of Part II
33 Special provisions as to wards of court
34 Interpretation of Part II

Part III: Patients Concerned in Criminal Proceedings or under Sentence

Remands to hospital

35 Remand to hospital for report on accused's mental condition
36 Remand of accused person to hospital for treatment

Hospital and guardianship orders

37 Powers of courts to order hospital admission or guardianship
38 Interim hospital orders
39 Information as to hospitals
39A Information to facilitate guardianship orders
40 Effect of hospital orders, guardianship orders and interim hospital orders

Restriction orders

41 Power of higher courts to restrict discharge from hospital
42 Powers of Secretary of State in respect of patients subject to restriction orders
43 Power of magistrates' courts to commit for restriction order
44 Committal to hospital under Section 43
45 Appeals from magistrates' courts

Hospital and limitation directions

45A Power of higher courts to direct hospital admission
45B Effect of hospital and limitation directions

Transfer to hospital of prisoners, etc.

47 Removal to hospital of persons serving sentences of imprisonment, etc.
48 Removal to hospital of other prisoners
49 Restriction on discharge of prisoners removed to hospital
50 Further provisions as to prisoners under sentence
51 Further provisions as to detained persons
52 Further provisions as to persons remanded by magistrates' courts
53 Further provisions as to civil prisoners and persons detained under the Immigration Acts

Supplemental

54 Requirements as to medical evidence
54A Reduction of period for making hospital orders
55 Interpretation of Part III

Part IV: Consent to Treatment

56 Patients to whom Part 4 applies
57 Treatment requiring consent and a second opinion
58 Treatment requiring consent or a second opinion
58A Electro-convulsive therapy, etc
59 Plans of treatment
60 Withdrawal of consent
61 Review of treatment
62 Urgent treatment
62A Treatment on recall of community patient or revocation of order
63 Treatment not requiring consent
64 Supplementary provisions for Part IV

Part 4A: Treatment of Community Patients Not Recalled to Hospital

64A Meaning of 'relevant treatment'
64B Adult community patients
64C Section 64B: supplemental
64D Adult community patients lacking capacity
64E Child community patients
64F Child community patients lacking competence
64G Emergency treatment for patients lacking capacity or competence
64H Certificates: supplementary provisions

64I Liability for negligence
64J Factors to be considered in determining whether patient objects to treatment
64K Interpretation of Part 4A

Part V: Mental Health Review Tribunals

Constitution etc.

65 Mental Health Review Tribunals for Wales
66 Applications to tribunals
67 References to tribunals by Secretary of State concerning Part II patients
68 Duty of managers of hospitals to refer cases to tribunal
68A Power to reduce periods under Section 68
69 Applications to tribunals concerning patients subject to hospital and guardianship orders
70 Applications to tribunals concerning restricted patients
71 References by Secretary of State concerning restricted patients

Discharge of patients

72 Powers of tribunals
73 Power to discharge restricted patients
74 Restricted patients subject to restriction directions
75 Applications and references concerning conditionally discharged restricted patients

General

76 Visiting and examination of patients
77 General provisions concerning tribunal applications
78 Procedure of Mental Health Review Tribunal for Wales
78A Appeal from the Mental Health Review Tribunal for Wales to the Upper Tribunal
79 Interpretation of Part V

Part VI: Removal and Return of Patients within United Kingdom, etc.

Removal to and from Scotland

80 Removal of patients to Scotland
80ZA Transfer of responsibility for community patients to Scotland
80A Transfer of responsibility for patients to Scotland; 80A Transfer of responsibility for conditionally discharged patients to Scotland
80B Removal of detained patients from Scotland
80C Removal of patients subject to compulsion in the community from Scotland
80D Transfer of conditionally discharged patients from Scotland
81 Removal of patients to Northern Ireland
81ZA Removal of community patients to Northern Ireland
81A Transfer of responsibility for patients to Northern Ireland
82 Removal to England and Wales of patients from Northern Ireland
82A Transfer of responsibility for conditionally discharged patients to England and Wales from Northern Ireland

Removal to and from Channel Islands and Isle of Man

83 Removal of patients to Channel Islands or Isle of Man
83ZA Removal or transfer of community patients to Channel Islands or Isle of Man
83A Transfer of responsibility for conditionally discharged patients to Channel Islands or Isle of Man
84 Removal to England and Wales of offenders found insane in Channel Islands and Isle of Man
85 Patients removed from Channel Islands or Isle of Man
85ZA Responsibility for community patients transferred from Channel Islands or Isle of Man
85A Responsibility for conditionally discharged patients transferred from Channel Islands or Isle of Man

Removal of aliens

86 Removal of alien patients

Return of patients absent without leave

87 Patients absent from hospitals in Northern Ireland
89 Patients absent from hospitals in the Channel Islands or Isle of Man

General

90 Regulations for purposes of Part VI
91 General provisions as to patients removed from England and Wales
92 Interpretation of Part VI

Part VIII: Miscellaneous Functions of Local Authorities and the Secretary of State

Approved mental health professionals

114 Approval by local social services authority
114A Approval of courses etc for approved mental health professionals
115 Powers of entry and inspection

Visiting patients

116 Welfare of certain hospital patients

After-care

117 After-care

Functions of the Secretary of State

118 Code of practice
119 Practitioners approved for Part IV and Section 118
120 General protection of relevant patients
120A Investigation reports
120B Action statements
120C Provision of information
120D Annual reports
122 Provision of pocket money for in-patients in hospital
123 Transfers to and from special hospitals

Part IX: Offences

126 Forgery, false statements, etc.
127 Ill-treatment of patients
128 Assisting patients to absent themselves without leave, etc.
129 Obstruction
130 Prosecutions by local authorities

Part X: Miscellaneous and Supplementary

Miscellaneous provisions

130A Independent mental health advocates: England
130B Arrangements under Section 130A
130C Section 130A: supplemental
130D Duty to give information about independent mental health advocates
130E Independent mental health advocates: Wales
130F Arrangements under Section 130E for Welsh qualifying compulsory patients
130G Arrangements under Section 130E for Welsh qualifying informal patients
130H Independent mental health advocates for Wales: supplementary powers and duties
130I Welsh qualifying compulsory patients
130J Welsh qualifying informal patients
130K Duty to give information about independent mental health advocates to Welsh qualifying compulsory patients
130L Duty to give information about independent mental health advocates to Welsh qualifying informal patients
131 Informal admission of patients
131A Accommodation, etc for children
132 Duty of managers of hospitals to give information to detained patients
132A Duty of managers of hospitals to give information to community patients
133 Duty of managers of hospitals to inform nearest relatives of discharge
134 Correspondence of patients
134A Review of decisions to withhold correspondence
135 Warrant to search for and remove patients
136 Mentally disordered persons found in public places
137 Provisions as to custody, conveyance and detention
138 Retaking of patients escaping from custody
139 Protection for acts done in pursuance of this Act
140 Notification of hospitals having arrangements for special cases
141 Members of Parliament suffering from mental illness
142A Regulations as to approvals in relation to England and Wales
142B Delegation of powers of managers of NHS foundation trusts

Supplemental

143 General provisions as to regulations, orders and rules
144 Power to amend local Acts
145 Interpretation
146 Application to Scotland
147 Application to Northern Ireland
148 Consequential and transitional provisions and repeals
149 Short title, commencement and application to Scilly Isles

Mental disorder

Mental disorder means any disorder or disability of the mind. The term *mentally disordered* is construed accordingly.

Learning disability

Learning disability means a state of arrested or incomplete development of the mind which includes significant impairment of intelligence and social functioning. A person with learning disability is not considered by reason of that disability to be suffering from mental disorder for the purposes of this Act, or to be requiring treatment in hospital for mental disorder, unless that disability is associated with abnormally aggressive or seriously irresponsible conduct. Note that the requirement for association with conduct etc. only applies to certain sections of the Act and not to all parts of it (*see* Section 1(2B))

Dependence on alcohol or drugs

Such dependence is not considered to be a disorder or disability of the mind for the purposes of the Act.

Other definitions

Leave of absence from hospital (Section 17)

The key Subsections of Section 17 are as follows:

(1) The responsible clinician may grant, to any patient, who is for the time being liable to be detained in a hospital under Part II of the Act, leave to be absent from the hospital subject to such conditions (if any) as that clinician considers necessary in the interests of the patient or for the protection of other persons.

(2) Leave of absence may be granted to a patient under Section 17 either indefinitely or on specified occasions or for any specified period; and where leave is so granted for a specified period, that period may be extended by further leave granted in the absence of the patient.

(2A) But longer-term leave may not be granted to a patient unless the responsible clinician first considers whether the patient should be dealt with under Section 17A (Community treatment orders) instead.

(2B) For these purposes, longer-term leave is granted to a patient if:

- (a) leave of absence is granted to him under this section either indefinitely or for a specified period of more than seven consecutive days; or
- (b) a specified period is extended under this section such that the total period for which leave of absence will have been granted to him under this section exceeds seven consecutive days.

(3) Where it appears to the responsible clinician that it is necessary so to do in the interests of the patient or for the protection of other persons, he may, upon granting leave of absence under this section, direct that the patient remain in custody during his absence; and where leave of absence is so granted, the patient may be kept in the custody of any officer on the staff of the hospital, or of any other person authorised in writing by the managers of the hospital or, if the patient is required in accordance with conditions

imposed on the grant of leave of absence to reside in another hospital, of any officer on the staff of that other hospital.

(4) In any case where a patient is absent from a hospital in pursuance of leave of absence granted under this section, and it appears to the responsible clinician that it is necessary so to do in the interests of the patient's health or safety or for the protection of other persons, that clinician may, subject to Subsection (5) below, by notice in writing given to the patient or to the person for the time being in charge of the patient, revoke the leave of absence and recall the patient to the hospital.

(5) A patient to whom leave of absence is granted under this Section shall not be recalled under Subsection (4) above after he has ceased to be liable to be detained under this Part of this Act.

(7) For the purpose of giving effect to a direction or condition imposed by virtue of a provision corresponding to Subsection (3) above, the person may be conveyed to a place in, or kept in custody or detained at a place of safety in, England and Wales by a person authorised in that behalf by the direction or condition.

Absent without leave

This refers to a patient being absent without permission from any hospital or other place and being liable to be taken into custody and returned under Section 18 (Return and readmission of patients absent without leave) of the Mental Health Act. Specifically, Section 18 states that a patient who at the time is liable to be detained under Part I of the Act in a hospital is considered to be absent without leave if any of the following apply:

- He absents himself without leave granted under Section 17 of the Act (often referred to as 'Section 17 leave').
- He fails to return to the hospital at the end of 'Section 17 leave'.
- He fails to return to the hospital upon being recalled under Section 17.
- He absents himself without permission from any place where he is required to reside in accordance with conditions imposed on the grant of leave under Section 17.

Such a patient who is absent without leave may, subject to the provisions of Section 18, be taken into custody and returned to the hospital or place by any approved mental health professional, by any officer on the staff of the hospital, by any constable, or by any person authorised in writing by the managers of the hospital.

Under Subsection (4) of Section 18, a patient shall not be taken into custody under this Section after the later of:

(a) the end of the period of six months beginning with the first day of his absence without leave; and

(b) the end of the period for which (apart from Section 21) he is liable to be detained or subject to guardianship or, in the case of a community patient, the community treatment order is in force.

Under Subsection (4) of Section 18, a patient shall not be taken into custody under this Section if the period for which he is liable to be detained is that specified in Section 2(4), 4(4) or 5(2) or (4) and that period has expired.

Appropriate medical treatment

In the Act, references to appropriate medical treatment, in relation to a person suffering from mental disorder, are references to medical treatment which is appropriate in his case, taking into account the nature and degree of the mental disorder and all other circumstances of his case.

Approved clinician

This refers to a person approved by the Secretary of State (in relation to England) or by the Welsh Ministers (in relation to Wales) to act as an approved clinician for the purposes of the Act.

Approved mental health professional

Under Section 114 of the Act, an *approved mental health professional* means a person approved under the Act (Section 114(1)) by any local social services authority in England or Wales in relation to acting on behalf of a local social services authority whose area is in England or Wales, respectively. A local social services authority may not approve a registered medical practitioner to act as an approved mental health professional.

Community patient

Under Section 17A(7), a *community patient* means a patient in respect of whom a community treatment order is in force.

Hospital

This means:

- any health service hospital within the meaning of the National Health Service Act 2006 or the National Health Service (Wales) Act 2006;
- any accommodation provided by a local authority and used as a hospital by or on behalf of the Secretary of State under the National Health Service Act 1977;
- any hospital as defined by Section 206 of the National Health Service (Wales) Act 2006 which is vested in a Local Health Board.

Local social services authority

A *local social services authority* means a council which is a local authority for the purpose of the Local Authority Social Services Act 1970.

Managers

Hospital

In relation to a hospital as defined above, *the managers* refer to the Primary Care Trust, Strategic Health Authority, Local Health Board or Special Health Authority responsible for the administration of the hospital. In relation to a hospital vested in a Primary Care Trust, a National Health Service Trust, or an NHS Foundation Trust, *the managers* refer to the Trust. In relation to a hospital vested in a Local Health Board, *the managers* refer to the Board.

In relation to a special hospital (*see* below), *the managers* refer to the Secretary of State.

Registered establishment

If the establishment is in England, *the managers* refer to the person or persons registered as a service provider under Chapter 2 of Part 1 of the Health and Social Care Act 2008 in respect of the regulated activity (within the meaning of that Part) relating to the assessment or medical treatment of mental disorder that is carried out in the establishment. If the establishment is in Wales, *the managers* refer to the person or persons registered in respect of the establishment under Part 2 of the Care Standards Act 2000.

Medical treatment

Under the Act *medical treatment* includes:

- nursing
- psychological intervention
- specialist mental health habilitation
- specialist mental health rehabilitation
- specialist mental health care.

Any reference in this Act to medical treatment, in relation to mental disorder, shall be construed as a reference to medical treatment the purpose of which is to alleviate, or prevent a worsening of, the disorder or one or more of its symptoms or manifestations.

Nearest relative

In Part I of the Act, a relative is defined by Section 26(1) to mean any of the following persons:

- husband or wife or civil partner
- son or daughter
- father or mother
- brother or sister
- grandparent
- grandchild
- uncle or aunt
- nephew or niece.

For the purposes of the definition of *nearest relative*:

- half-blood relationships are treated in the same way as whole-blood relationships;
- an illegitimate person is treated as the legitimate child of his mother and, if his father has parental responsibility for him under Section 3 of the Children Act 1989, his father.

With the exceptions given below, the *nearest relative* is defined as being the surviving person first described in the above list (Section 26(1)), with preference being given to:

- whole-blood relations over half-blood relations;
- the elder or eldest of two or more relatives at a given position in the list, regardless of sex.

Preference is also given to a relative with whom the patient ordinarily resides or by whom he is ordinarily cared for.

Exceptions

Where the person who would be the nearest relative under the above definition —

- in the case of a patient ordinarily resident in the United Kingdom, the Channel Islands or the Isle of Man, is not so resident; or
- is the husband or wife or civil partner of the patient, but is permanently separated from the patient, either by agreement or under a court order, or has deserted or been deserted by the patient for a period which has not come to an end; or
- is a person other than the husband, wife, civil partner, father or mother of the patient, and is for the time being under 18 years old; the nearest relative is determined as if that person were dead.

Spouse

- The terms *husband*, *wife* and *civil partner* include a person who is living with the patient as the patient's husband or wife or as if they were civil partners, as the case may be (or, if the patient is for the time being an in-patient in a hospital, was so living until the patient was admitted), and has been or had been so living for a period of at least six months. However, this does not apply to a person living as the patient's spouse or civil partner if the patient is married, unless the legal spouse or civil partner is permanently separated from the patient, either by agreement or under a court order, or has deserted or been deserted by the patient for a period which has not come to an end.

Other non-relatives

- A person, other than a relative, with whom the patient has ordinarily been residing for at least five years is treated as a relative who comes last in the above list of relatives. In the case of a married patient or a patient in a civil partnership, this non-relative cannot count as the nearest relative unless the patient's spouse or civil partner can be disregarded by virtue of permanent separation or desertion (as outlined above).

Children and young persons in care

Under Section 27 of the Act, where:

(a) a patient who is a child or young person is in the care of a local authority by virtue of a care order within the meaning of the Children Act 1989; or
(b) rights and powers of a parent of a patient who is a child or young person are vested in a local authority by virtue of Section 16 of the Social Work (Scotland) Act 1968, the authority shall be deemed to be the nearest relative of the patient in preference to any person except the patient's husband or wife or civil partner (if any).

Patient

A *patient* is a person suffering from or appearing to be suffering from mental disorder.

Responsible clinician

Detention under Section 2 or 3

In relation to a patient liable to be detained by virtue of an application for admission for assessment (Section 2) or an application for admission for treatment (Section

3), the *responsible clinician* is the approved clinician with overall responsibility for the patient's case. He is usually a consultant psychiatrist.

Community patient

In relation to a community patient, the *responsible clinician* is the approved clinician with overall responsibility for the patient's case.

Guardianship

In relation to a patient subject to guardianship, the *responsible clinician* is the approved clinician authorised by the local social services authority to act (either generally or in any particular case or for any particular purpose) as the responsible clinician.

Special hospital

Under Section 4 of the National Health Service Act 1977 a *special hospital* is defined as being an establishment for:

> 'persons subject to detention under the Mental Health Act 1983 who in the Secretary of State's opinion, require treatment under conditions of special security on account of their dangerous, violent or criminal propensities.'

At the time of writing there are three special hospitals:

- Broadmoor
- Ashworth
- Rampton.

3 Professional roles

As mentioned in the first chapter of this book, an important change made by the Mental Health Act 2007 **to the** Mental Health Act 1983 **is allowing a broader range of professionals to carry out functions under the Act. This chapter considers aspects of professional roles within the context of the** Mental Health Act 2007.

Approved mental health professional

The new role of the approved mental health professional (replacing approved social workers under the Mental Health Act 1983) has been opened up, by the Mental Health Act 2007, to include nurses, occupational therapists and psychologists. In addition to helping with potential recruitment problems, this change can allow for better continuity of care for patients. Local social services authorities are responsible for the approval of approved mental health professionals, and for ensuring that sufficient numbers of approved mental health professionals are available in their respective geographic areas.

The Mental Health Act 2007 makes a distinction between:

- having approval as an approved mental health professional;
- having permission to carry out the functions of an approved mental health professional on behalf of a local social services authority.

While an approved mental health professional may be approved by only one local social services authority, he (or she) may have agreed permission to act on behalf of one or more additional local social services authorities. The approved mental health professional does not need to be employed by the local social services authority from which he has approval or for which he has permission to act; an approved mental health professional does not need to be employed by any local social services authority (in contradistinction to the situation that prevailed in respect of approval social workers under the previous Mental Health Act 1983).

Eligible and non-eligible professionals

Local social services authorities may approve members of the following professional categories to become approved mental health professionals:

- Registered social workers
- First-level nurses practising in mental health or learning disabilities
- Registered occupational therapists
- Chartered psychologists.

Registered medical practitioners are not eligible to become approved mental health professionals. This applies even to a medical practitioner who may also fulfil the criteria to fit into one of the above eligible professional categories.

Main functions

Approved mental health professionals have overall responsibility for co-ordinating the process of assessment.

Gathering information/liaison with others

Approved mental health professionals should consider consulting relatives, carers or friends and should take their views into account. Where those being assessed are under the age of 18 years, approved mental health professionals should, in particular, consider consulting with the parents or with those who have parental responsibility.

Approved mental health professionals should, whenever possible, consult with other people who have been involved with the care of the patient. They may include people working for statutory, voluntary or independent mental health services and other service providers.

Organising an assessing team

The assessment team should include the following three people: the approved mental health professional; a doctor approved under Section 12 (who may have previous acquaintance with the person to be assessed); and a second doctor who has previous acquaintance with the patient. A patient being assessed should, where possible, be seen jointly by the approved mental health professional and at least one of the two doctors.

In the case of the assessment of a person who is under the age of 18 years, at least one of the three professionals conducting the assessment (that is, either the approved mental health professional or one of the two doctors) should be a clinician specialising in child and adolescent mental health.

Risk assessment

The approved mental health professional should be conversant with the provisions of Section 135 (Warrant to search for and remove patients) of the Act.

The Code of Practice recommends that 'everyone involved in an assessment should be alert to the need to provide support for colleagues, especially where there is a risk of the patient causing physical harm. People carrying out assessments should be aware of circumstances in which the police should be asked to provide assistance.'

The approved mental health professional should also be able to carry out an appropriate risk assessment for the conveyance of a patient.

Interviewing/assessment

The approved mental health professional should identify himself to the person being assessed, members of the person's family, carers or friends and other professionals present. The approved mental health professional should ensure that the purpose of the visit and the roles of the professionals present are explained. Patients should usually be given the opportunity of speaking alone to the approved mental health professional. Furthermore, if the patient expresses a wish that someone else be present, then under normal circumstances, the approved mental health professional should assist in securing that person's attendance.

The approved mental health professional should ensure that: the interview is conducted in a suitably professional manner; if applicable, the statutory criteria for detention are met; in all the circumstances of the case, detention in hospital is the most appropriate way of providing the care and medical treatment the patient needs; if applicable, relevant provisions of the Mental Capacity Act are implemented; the patient's wishes and view of his own needs, age and physical health, cultural background, social and family circumstances are taken into account; the impact of deterioration on children, relatives, carers and others is considered; and that due consideration is paid to the effect of a decision to admit or not to admit the patient under the Act on the patient, and those close to the patient.

Decision making

The role of the approved mental health professional is crucial. As Lord Bingham stated, referring to the previous corresponding role of the approved social worker (ASW), 'I would ... resist the lumping together of the ASW and the recommending doctor or doctors as "the mental health professionals". It is the ASW who makes the application, not the doctors.' Moreover, Von Brandenburg stated that the approved mental health professional 'will be a "public authority" for the purpose of the Human Rights Act 1998'.

The approved mental health professional must take into account, and professionally balance, many factors when making the application, including: implementation of the Human Rights Act 1998; the possibility of exercising discretion not to apply even where the statutory criteria are met; and the relative advantages and disadvantages of an informal admission and of detention itself. There is no lower age for the use of detention under the Act, and for those aged less than 16 years, both competence and the child's views must be taken into account, while capacity must be considered in the case of 16- and 17-year-olds.

Disagreements between members of the assessment team must be handled with tact and the utmost professionalism by the approved mental health professional.

Conveyance

Approved mental health professionals should make the decision regarding the most appropriate method of transportation to use. They should consider: local policies; police and ambulance assistance; risk assessment; and delegation to others.

Alternative support

The approved mental health professional should consider alternatives to hospital admission, and the nearest relative should be advised of his right to be an applicant. In order to be able to give due consideration to alternative support, the approved mental health professional must ensure that he is aware of the appropriate available local resources.

Recording and informing

Having decided whether or not to make an application for detention, the approved mental health professional should inform the following people:

- the patient
- the patient's nearest relative
- the doctors involved in the assessment
- the care co-ordinator
- the patient's GP.

Consideration should, naturally, be given to patient confidentiality.

An outline report is written by the approved mental health professional at the hospital, while a full report is written by him for the appropriate local social services authority.

Approved clinician and responsible clinician

The Mental Health Act 2007 has introduced the new roles of the approved clinician and the responsible clinician. The former is a person approved by the appropriate national authority to act as an approved clinician for the purposes of the Mental Health Act, while a responsible clinician is an approved clinician who has been allocated overall responsibility for a patient. This new role of the approved clinician has been opened up, by the Mental Health Act 2007, to include nurses, occupational therapists, psychologists and social workers. In like manner to the new role of the approved mental health professional, the opening up of the role of the approved clinician can, in addition to helping with potential recruitment problems, allow for better continuity of care for patients.

Eligible professionals

Strategic Health Authorities may approve members of the following professional categories to act as an approved clinician:

- Registered medical practitioners
- Chartered psychologists
- First-level nurses practising in mental health or learning disabilities
- Registered occupational therapists
- Registered social workers.

Main functions of the approved clinician

It is generally only an approved clinician who may be in charge of the treatment administered under the Mental Health Act to a patient who has not consented to such treatment; this lack of consent may be because consent is refused by the patient or because the patient is unable to give consent. For the following functions, the approved clinician does not also need to be the responsible clinician for the patient concerned; a responsible clinician may exercise the following functions only if he is also the clinician in charge of the relevant treatment. (As an example, if the patient's responsible clinician is not qualified to prescribe medication, then he could not direct that his patient be administered medication without consent; another approved clinician in charge of the medication would be required.)

Treatment without consent

Only the approved clinician in charge of the patient's treatment may give, or supervise the provision of, treatment without consent, and without a second opinion doctor certificate, under Section 63 (Treatment not requiring consent) of the Act. This also applies to treatment provided under Section 63 because it is defined under Section 62 (Urgent treatment) as being 'immediately necessary'.

An approved clinician must be in charge of medication given to a detained patient who has not consented to it but where such treatment has been approved by a second opinion doctor under Section 58 (Treatment requiring consent or a second opinion).

ECT

An approved clinician must be in charge of ECT given to a detained patient who cannot consent to it but where such treatment has been approved by a second opinion doctor under Section 58A (Electro-convulsive therapy, etc.).

Continuation of treatment

It is only the approved clinician who is in charge of the patient's treatment who may decide that treatment should be continued to avoid serious suffering by the patient, under Section 62 (Urgent treatment) or Section 62A (Treatment on recall of community patient or revocation of order), while the process of obtaining a new certificate under Section 58 (Treatment requiring consent or a second opinion) or Section 58A (Electro-convulsive therapy, etc.) is pursued.

Supervised community treatment

In the case of a supervised community treatment patient who has not been recalled to hospital and who is unable to consent to treatment owing to lack of competence or capacity, when no one else with authority has consented on his behalf, then treatment may only be administered to that patient if there is an approved clinician in charge of the treatment and it is given by, or under the supervision of, that approved clinician. Further details are given in Part 4A (Treatment of Community Patients Not Recalled to Hospital) of the Mental Health Act 2007.

Reports

The approved clinician in charge of a patient's treatment must submit periodic reports to the Mental Health Act Commission, under Section 61 (Review of treatment), in respect of medication given to that patient (supported by a second opinion doctor certificate under Section 58) and/or ECT given to the patient (supported by a second opinion doctor certificate under Section 58A). Similarly, the approved clinician in charge of a supervised community treatment patient's treatment must submit reports as required to the Mental Health Act Commission in respect of treatment given to the patient on the basis of a second opinion doctor's Part 4A certificate.

Certifying consent

The approved clinician in charge of a patient's treatment is the professional who can sign a certificate under Section 58, certifying that the patient has consented to receiving medication, or under Section 58A, certifying that the patient has consented to being treated with ECT.

Allocation of the responsible clinician

Hospital managers should use local protocols for the process of allocation of the responsible clinician, paying particular attention to the need to provide a seamless continuity of responsibility when patients move between hospitals and services. In principle, a patient's responsible clinician should be the available approved clinician with the most appropriate expertise to meet the patient's main therapeutic needs. In practice, a temporary responsible clinician may initially have to be allocated to a patient when he is first detained in hospital in order to provide him with a responsible clinician at that stage, but as soon as is practicable and the patient's main treatment needs are known, the available approved clinician with the most appropriate expertise for that patient should be allocated as his responsible clinician.

Even while a patient remains in the same treatment centre, as his therapeutic needs change, his responsible clinician may also need to change. Hospital managers should keep the appropriateness of each patient's responsible clinician under review.

Main functions of the responsible clinician

Detained patients

All patients detained under Part II (Compulsory Admission to Hospital and Guardianship) and Part III (Patients Concerned in Criminal Proceedings or Under Sentence), with the exception of those remanded for a report under Section 35 (Remand to hospital for report on accused's mental condition) of Part III, require a responsible clinician, whose functions include having:

- overall responsibility for the patient's care within the context of a multi-disciplinary team;
- responsibility for reviewing the patient's progress, including regular assessment of whether the patient still meets the criteria for detention;
- the power to grant leave of absence or discharge;
- the power to block discharge of the patient by his nearest relative;
- the power to renew detention, with the agreement of another professional from a profession different from that of the responsible clinician and who is also involved in the patient's treatment.

Supervised community treatment

A supervised community treatment patient's responsible clinician may:

- make a community treatment order, if an approved mental health professional also agrees that the necessary criteria are met and that this is appropriate;
- include conditions in the community treatment order, if an approved mental health professional agrees, and thereafter, vary these conditions or suspend any of them temporarily without the agreement of an approved mental health professional;
- recall the patient to hospital for medical treatment for his mental disorder, if the responsible clinician believes that not to do so would lead to risk of harm to the patient's health or safety or to that of others;
- recall the patient to attend for examination if he is not complying with any of the mandatory conditions;
- discharge the patient;
- block discharge of the patient by his nearest relative;
- extend the supervised community treatment period with the agreement of an approved mental health professional.

Guardianship

The responsible clinician is not formally in overall charge of the patient's case. He can discharge a patient from guardianship.

Confidentiality and liability

Contractual liability for service provision

The law of contract

A contract is an agreement that can be enforced by law. Note that while all contracts are agreements, an agreement is not necessarily a contract. The characteristic components of a contract are as follows:

- Offer
- Acceptance
- Consideration
- Intention
- Capacity.

Liability

A doctor cannot be expected, under law, to guarantee success; a proposed course of treatment might fail in spite of the best efforts of the medical profession, for example. Thus, liability may not normally be imposed on a doctor purely on the basis of failing to achieve an intended clinical goal. In order for this to be the case, the doctor (or clinical team) must exercise reasonable care and skill; under Section 13 of the **Supply of Goods and Services Act 1982**:

> *'In a contract for the supply of a service where the supplier is acting in the course of a business, there is an implied term that the supplier will carry out the service with reasonable care and skill.'*

This rule on liability also requires that the doctor does not give a prior guarantee that the service to be offered will definitely succeed. (It is also possible that the giving of such a guarantee might not be covered by the doctor's medical professional indemnity.)

Breach of duty of confidentiality

Except under the specific circumstances described below, a doctor has a duty of confidentiality toward his patients. Not only is information about a patient confidential during the time that the doctor is treating the patient, but it should also remain so after the end of such treatment.

Justified disclosure of patient information

The General Medical Council (Confidentiality, 2009) have issued guidance in relation to circumstances in which it is appropriate to disclose confidential patient information. This is available from their website (www.gmc-uk.org/guidance/ethical_guidance/confidentiality.asp).

If you decide to disclose confidential information you must be prepared to explain and justify your decision.

Close and direct proximity

A duty of care is owed by a medical professional to his patient and to those in 'close proximity' to the patient, that may include the immediate family of the patient.

Breach of duty of care

Bolam test

In the case of *Bolam* v. *Friern Hospital Management Committee* (1957), a psychiatric patient was given ECT without the use of a muscle relaxant. Apart from his lower jaw, which was controlled manually, there was no use of restraints either. During this treatment, the patient sustained orthopaedic injuries (pelvic fractures and dislocation of the hip joints). The patient sued. At the time the patient had sustained these injuries, the issues of muscle relaxation, sedation and restraint during ECT were the subjects of debate within the medical profession, and no definitive protocol had been laid down in respect of these. The patient lost his case. Having established that there exists the 'man on the Clapham omnibus', who is not a highly trained medical specialist, the case held that:

> *'...where you get a situation which involves the use of some special skill or competence, then the test of whether there has been negligence or not is not the test of the man on the Clapham omnibus, because he has not got this special skill. The test is the standard of the ordinary skilled man exercising and professing to exercise that special skill. A man need not possess the highest skill at the risk of being found negligent. It is well-established law that is sufficient if he exercises the ordinary skill of an ordinary man exercising that particular act...A doctor is not guilty of negligence if he has acted in accordance with a practice accepted as proper by a responsible body of medical opinion of medical men skilled in that particular act.'*

This is the *Bolam* test, and is central in cases of alleged professional negligence. Note that the 'practice accepted as proper by a responsible body of medical opinion of medical men skilled in that particular act' refers to the accepted practice at the material time, and not to accepted practice at the later time of a trial, by when it may have changed owing to advances in medicine, for example. Also, in the case of medical specialties, the medical doctors 'skilled in that particular act' should be taken as referring to a doctor exercising the ordinary skills of their speciality (*see Maynard* v. *West Midlands Regional Health Authority* (1984)).

Professional liability

So far as the medical profession is concerned, medical professional liability may be attached to a person correctly designated a 'registered medical practitioner' or to a person who makes a false declaration that they are qualified as a 'registered medical practitioner'; in the latter case, criminal liability also attaches.

Tort

Central to medical profession liability is tort. This is a civil wrong, other than a breach of contract, which gives the right to bring an action in a civil court. (Such actions might include nuisance, negligence, defamation, trespass.)

Duty of care

Line of duty of care

The legal duty of medical care to a patient may be considered to have a linear form, beginning with the presentation, in some manner, of a person requiring some form of care, and ending with completion of the relevant treatment(s).

Emergencies

Although a 'Good Samaritan' law does not formally exist within English law, the General Medical Council advises medical practitioners that:

> *'In an emergency, wherever it may arise, you must offer anyone at risk the assistance you could reasonably be expected to provide.'*

It could be argued that English case law would tend to agree. For example, the judge in *Barnes* v. *Crabtree* (1955) stated:

> *'In a case of real acute emergency a doctor under the NHS scheme was under an obligation to treat any patient who was acutely ill; for example, if there was a motor accident and someone was lying seriously injured.'*

Duty of confidence

The duty of confidentiality has been detailed earlier in this chapter.

In respect of the issue of disclosure in the public interest, the case of *W* v. *Egdell* (1990) is instructive. Patient W suffered from schizophrenia and was detained in a secure unit under a restriction order made under Section 60 and Section 65 of the Mental Health Act 1959; he had been convicted of the manslaughter of five people and had also wounded two others. He subsequently exercised his right, under Section 41 of the Mental Health Act 1983, to apply for review by a mental health review tribunal for discharge (or transfer with a view to discharge). The responsible medical officer for W was of the opinion that the patient's schizophrenic symptomatology could be adequately controlled by pharmacotherapy, and supported his application. W's solicitors instructed Dr Egdell, another psychiatrist, to review W and prepare a report on him. This report was unfavourable to W and recommended against the patient being transferred from the secure unit. In his report, Dr Egdell suggested that W had an abnormal, possibly psychopathic, personality. Dr Egdell expressed concern about the fact that the patient had an interest in what he (the patient) referred to as 'fireworks', by which he meant explosive devices (pipes filled with explosives). On reading Dr Egdell's report, W's solicitors withdrew the application to the mental health review tribunal. Dr Egdell asked that a copy of his report be included in W's hospital records, but this was refused by W's solicitors. Dr Egdell then disclosed a copy of his report to the medical director of the hospital in which W was a patient, and in due course the Home Office also received a copy.

The case came up for review again, this time under Section 67 of the Mental Health Act 1983. Although W's solicitors obtained an injunction barring Dr Egdell from disclosing his report at the hearing, The Home Secretary was able to put forward information gathered by Dr Egdell. As a result, W brought actions in equity and contract against Dr Egdell, alleging a breach of duty of confidence.

At trial, the issue of concern was not whether or not Dr Egdell was under a duty of confidence; it was clear that he was. Rather,

> *'The question is as to the breadth of that duty. Did the duty extend so far as to bar disclosure to the medical director of the hospital? Did it bar disclosure to the Home Office?'*

The Court of Appeal ruled that in this case the public interest of the protection and safety to the public was greater than the public interest in maintaining confidence.

Conflicts of interest

The circumstances in which a potential conflict of interest would prevent an approved mental health professional from making an application for detention or guardianship and would prevent a medical practitioner from making a recommendation in support of such an application are given in the *Mental Health*

(Conflict of Interest) (England) Regulations 2008 and in the 2008 revision of the *Code of Practice Mental Health Act 1983*. It is convenient to refer to both approved mental health professionals and medical practitioners as 'assessors' in this section.

Financial conflict

If a patient is to be admitted to an independent hospital, then there will be a potential conflict of interest if both medical practitioners giving medical recommendations are on the staff of that same independent hospital. If one of these two doctors is on the staff of the independent hospital, then the other doctor must be a medical practitioner who is not on the staff of that hospital.

There is a conflict of interest if the assessor stands to make a financial gain (or loss) from his decision; this does not apply in respect of a fee for making an application or giving a medical recommendation when that fee is received irrespective of the assessment outcome.

Business conflict

An assessor has a potential conflict of interest if both he and one of the other assessors, the patient or the nearest relative (if the nearest relative is the applicant) are closely involved in the same business venture when this is a commercial enterprise from which an assessor stands to profit, for example, through a business partnership or a partnership in a GP practice.

Professional conflict

There is a conflict of interest if the assessor is in a line management or employment relationship with one of the other assessors, the patient or the nearest relative (if the nearest relative is the applicant).

There is a conflict of interest if the assessor is in the same team as the patient, where a team is defined to be a group of professionals who work together for clinical purposes on a routine basis, for instance, a community mental health team, a crisis resolution or home treatment team, or staff working in the same in-patient unit.

There is a conflict of interest if, where there are three assessors, all three are members of the same team, with a team being defined as above.

Urgent necessity

According to the Code of Practice:

> *'If there is a case of urgent necessity, all three assessors may be from the same team. However, this should happen only in a genuine emergency, where the patient's need for urgent assessment outweighs the desirability of waiting for another assessor who has no potential conflict of interest. Any decisions made to proceed despite a potential conflict of interest should be recorded, with reasons, in case notes.'*

Other potential conflicts

There may be other circumstances, not formally covered by current regulations, which may amount to a potential conflict of interest. The Code of Practice advises that 'Assessors should work on the principle that, in any situation where they believe that the objectivity or independence of their decision is (or could be seen to be) undermined, they should not become involved or should withdraw.'

In respect of supervised community treatment, the responsible clinician and the approved mental health professional responsible for deciding whether or not to place a patient on supervised community treatment, or for deciding to revoke a community treatment order, should not have any financial interest in the outcome of the decision. Neither the responsible clinician nor the approved mental health professional should be a relative of the patient or of each other.

An approved mental health professional's decision regarding whether or not to make an application under the Mental Health Act must be an independent decision.

Further reading

Department of Health (2008). *Mental Health Act 1983: Code of Practice.* London: Department of Health.

General Medical Council (2009). *Confidentiality.* London: General Medical Council.

National Institute for Mental Health in England (2008). *Mental Health Act 2007 New Roles.* London: National Institute for Mental Health in England.

4 Safeguards for patients under the Mental Health Act

The use of compulsion under the Mental Health Act is balanced by a number of safeguards for the patient. These are summarised briefly in this chapter and some of them are visited in more detail in subsequent chapters. The training for the professionals who have powers under the Act is a form of safeguard in itself, and this training was referred to in the preceding chapter. When the Bournewood case reached Strasbourg, the European Court noted that the following 'substantive and procedural safeguards' were available to those detained under the Mental Health Act 1983:

(a) statutory criteria need to be met and applied by 2 doctors and an applicant;
(b) Part IV consent to treatment procedures;
(c) Applications and automatic referrals to MH Review Tribunals;
(d) Nearest relative powers (including powers of discharge);
(e) Section 117 after-care services;
(f) The Code of Practice and the Mental Health Act Commission;
(g) Section 132 rights to information.

(Para 54 of *HL* v. *UK*, 2004)

The main concerns for the current chapter are to summarise those safeguarding functions that are not covered in detail elsewhere. In addition to those identified by the European Court the following safeguards will also be considered:

- hospital managers' discharge powers
- Independent Mental Health Advocates
- criminal offences protecting people with mental disorders
- The European Convention on Human Rights (ECHR).

Nearest Relatives

There are several areas where the nearest relative provides a potential safeguard for a patient. The Act places a duty upon Approved Mental Health Professionals (AMHPs) to inform or consult the nearest relative where 'practicable' or 'reasonably practicable' when considering use of Section 2 (admission for assessment), Section 3 (admission for treatment), or Section 7 (application for guardianship). Where an application for either Sections 3 or 7 is being considered, an AMHP is prevented from proceeding with the application if the patient's nearest relative objects. In these circumstances, the AMHP would need to apply to the County Court for displacement of the nearest relative if they wished to proceed. The nearest relative is not necessarily the patient's next of kin and is identified by following a somewhat complex procedure set out in Section 26. One new safeguard in this area is that if the nearest relative is seen as an unsuitable person to carry out the function, an application can be made to the County Court to displace them. Such an application could be made by the patient themselves but is more likely to be made by an AMHP.

As mentioned below, it is also possible for the responsible clinician (RC) to exercise a barring power.

There are also certain circumstances where the nearest relative can discharge the patient from compulsory powers. This places a check on professional powers. Unless the patient is likely to behave in a manner dangerous to themselves or others (a higher risk threshold than that used for admission, i.e. that detention is needed for the patient's 'health, safety or protection of others') a nearest relative can order the discharge of a patient who is detained on Sections 2 or 3.

Hospital Managers

Hospital managers have the power under Section 23 to discharge some patients from compulsion. Patients may apply for a managers' hearing in addition to a tribunal, but the managers do not have to proceed with a hearing if a tribunal hearing is due shortly. The managers should also consider holding a hearing if the RC bars a nearest relative's discharge. If an RC renews detention or extends a community treatment order (CTO) they do not have a choice, and must hold a hearing. The Act does not identify criteria to be considered regarding the decision-making process. The Code of Practice gives some guidance stating that managers should focus on whether the initial criteria for detention or a CTO continue to be met. Where the legal criteria are not met, the patient must be discharged.

The Tribunal

The Mental Health Review Tribunal still exists in Wales but in England its functions are now performed by the First Tier Tribunal. Here, we will just refer to 'the Tribunal'. Section 66 of the Act allows patients to apply to a Tribunal in specified circumstances. The tribunal gives most detained patients a legal right to challenge their detention. This meets the requirements of Article 5(4) of the ECHR. Tribunals have the power to discharge patients from detention immediately or at a future specified date. They can also make the following recommendations for patients on treatment orders: that the patient should be granted Section 17 leave, transferred to another hospital, transferred into guardianship, or made subject to a CTO. If the recommendation is not followed they can reconvene. In many cases, they uphold detention. Tribunals consist of three members: a legal chair (a judge); a medical member; and a third member. The tribunal must consider the evidence before them and comply with the requirements of law when making decisions. Patients are entitled to non-means tested public funding, and can have a solicitor or someone else to represent them at the Tribunal.

Consent to Treatment Provisions and Second Opinion Appointed Doctors

Chapter 6 sets out these provisions in some detail. Before the 1983 Act, there were no specific safeguards. It was just assumed that if a patient was detained for treatment you could treat without their consent if necessary. The rules set out in Part IV were an attempt to clarify that treatment could be given in some circumstances without the patent's valid consent but, to balance this, there would be safeguards. One of the main safeguards is that to continue treating with medication beyond three months without consent there is a requirement that the patient is seen by a second opinion appointed doctor (SOAD). SOADs are doctors appointed by the Care Quality Commission (CQC) to provide independent medical views. They are required to assess patients' capacity to consent to treatment, and to give a view regarding the continuation of medical treatment for mental disorder. To assist them in this role they are required to visit and interview patients, as well as relevant professionals concerned with the patient's treatment. SOADs have access to any relevant records.

Mental Health Act Commissioners

The Mental Health Act Commission has now been subsumed within the Care Quality Commission in England and within the Healthcare Inspectorate in Wales. These bodies have responsibility for keeping under review the exercise of the powers and duties conferred by the Mental Health Act in relation to the detention of patients, including those liable to be detained and patients subject to CTOs. In England, the visiting function is still performed by Mental Health Act Commissioners; in Wales, the equivalent role is that of Inspector. These individuals visit wards, interview patients, investigate complaints, and review decisions regarding the withholding of patients' post. They produce annual statements on Trusts and private providers. They do not have the ability to discharge patients from detention, but the CQC has powers to impose sanctions where services do not conform to national standards. The CQC (or Health Inspectorate Wales) appoint second opinion doctors. Chapter 14 takes a more detailed look at these bodies.

Independent Mental Health Advocates

The amending Mental Health Act 2007 introduced Independent Mental Health Advocates (IMHAs), who are available to certain patients subject to compulsion. Qualifying patients are those subject to detention, those liable to be detained (e.g. those on leave of absence) and patients subject to conditional discharge, guardianship or a CTO. In very rare circumstances, some informal patients will also be entitled to an IMHA if, for example, they are being considered for treatment under Section 57 of the Act, or if ECT is being considered as a means of treatment for a young person or child under the age of 18. Those patients who are subject to short-term detention (Sections 4, 5(2), 5(4), 135 and 136) are not entitled to an IMHA. The intention is that advocates should be independent of those professionals who are concerned with the care and treatment of the patient. The role of the IMHA is to ensure that the patient understands their rights, the rights of others (such as the nearest relative and the RC), any conditions placed upon them and what treatments can be given. IMHAs are able to visit and interview patients and, in some circumstances, have access to relevant medical and social care records. IMHAs are also able to visit and interview any professionals who are concerned with the patient's treatment. Those who can request the involvement of an IMHA include the patient, the patient's nearest relative, an AMHP or the patient's RC. IMHAs have to comply with such a request but the patient is not required to accept the support of an IMHA.

Criminal offences protecting people with mental disorders

Under Section 126, it is an offence for anyone to forge or make false statements in applications, recommendations or other Mental Health Act forms. Section 127 makes it an offence for staff or managers to ill-treat or wilfully neglect a patient at a hospital. The same applies to patients in guardianship. This provides protection additional to that given by the common law duty of care. If someone assists a patient to go absent without leave (AWOL) that is an offence under Section 128. The last of the relevant Mental Health Act Sections is 129 which makes it an offence if someone without reasonable cause:

'(a) refuses to allow the inspection of any premises; or
(b) refuses to allow the visiting, interviewing or examination of any person by a person authorised in that behalf by or under this Act or to give access to any person to a person so authorised; or
(c) refuses to produce for the inspection of any person so authorised any document or record the production of which is duly required by him; or
(d) otherwise obstructs any such person in the exercise of his functions...'

Proceedings can be instituted by a local social services authority.

There are a number of other safeguards which are enshrined in the Sexual Offences Act 2003 such as the offence of 'sexual activity with a person with mental disorder impeding choice' or 'inducement, threat or deception to procure sexual activity with a person with a mental disorder'. The recent amendments in this area of law extend to care workers, which now makes it an offence for any care worker to: have sexual activity with a person with mental disorder; cause or incite sexual activity with a person with mental disorder; or, engage in sexual activity in the presence of a person with mental disorder. There are additional safeguards for people who are covered by the Mental Capacity Act 2005 (*see* details in Chapter 19).

The Code of Practice

Chapter 13 is devoted to the Code of Practice so this chapter has just a brief section emphasising the Code's safeguarding aspects. The Mental Health Act Code of Practice provides guidance to doctors, approved clinicians, the managers and staff of hospitals, and AMHPs. It is also relevant for others, but those listed here must have regard to the Code and may only depart from it if they have cogent reasons; usually these will rely on human rights arguments. There is specific guidance in the Code on assessment and treatment under the Act and it contains the details of the principles that are referred to in the Act itself.

The European Convention on Human Rights

The Human Rights Act (HRA) is discussed in Chapter 21. In effect, this enshrined most of the European Convention on Human Rights within English statute law. This strengthened the effect of the ECHR in practice in England and Wales and there are several areas where this has assisted in the safeguarding of patients. One key area is that issues concerning Article 5 (which were key in the *HL* v. *UK* case) now drive English courts. Courts are required to interpret legislation if possible in a way which is compatible with Convention rights. The HRA also provides that it is unlawful for a public authority to act in a way which is incompatible with a Convention right. This includes anyone 'certain of whose functions are functions of a public nature'. This means that health and social care professionals carrying out their obligations under the Mental Health Act are covered by the provisions of the HRA. An example of this protecting a patient's rights could be seen in the case of *R(E)* v. *Bristol City Council* where Article 8 was critical in determining the judge's decision that AMHPs do not always have to consult with the nearest relative (e.g. where this may be detrimental to the patient).

In conclusion, a range of safeguards are now enshrined in the Mental Health Act and in related legislation. They are not all as robust or effective as everyone would like but they are, nonetheless, very significant from a patient's point of view.

References

Council of Europe (1950) *The European Convention on Human Rights.*

Department of Health (2008) *Mental Health Act 1983: Code of Practice.* London: TSO.

1983 Mental Health Act.

1998 Human Rights Act.

2005 Mental Capacity Act.

2007 Mental Health Act.

Cases

HL v. *UK* (2004) 40EHHR761.

R (E) v. *Bristol City Council* (2005) EWHC 74 (Admin).

Welsh Assembly (2008) *Mental Health Act 1983, Code of Practice.* Welsh Assembly Government.

5 Compulsory Admission to Hospital: (Sections 2, 3 and 4 of the Mental Health Act)

Compulsory admission to hospital is covered in Part II of the Mental Health Act under Sections 2, 3 and 4.

Section 2

Purpose

The aim of Section 2 is an admission to hospital for assessment.

Grounds for admission

Under Subsection (2), an application for admission for assessment may be made in respect of a patient on the grounds that:

'(a) he is suffering from mental disorder of a nature or degree which warrants the detention of the patient in a hospital for assessment (or for assessment followed by medical treatment) for at least a limited period; and
(b) he ought to be so detained in the interests of his own health or safety or with a view to the protection of other persons.'

An application for admission for assessment shall be founded on the written recommendations in the prescribed form of two registered medical practitioners, including, in each case, a statement that in the opinion of the practitioner the conditions set out in Subsection (2) above are complied with. At least one of these two doctors should be approved under Section 12 of the Act. If the Section 12 approved doctor does not have previous acquaintance with the patient then, if practicable, the second doctor should be one who does have such previous acquaintance. The two doctors may examine the patient jointly or separately. However, no more than five clear days must elapse between the days of the two examinations.

Duration

Under this section, a patient admitted to hospital for admission for assessment may be detained for up to 28 days, beginning with the day of admission. The patient must not be detained after the expiration of this period unless, before it has expired, he has become liable to be detained under some other provision of the Mental Health Act.

Discharge

The patient may be discharged by any of the following:

- his responsible clinician
- the hospital managers
- his nearest relative.

Before giving a discharge order, the nearest relative must give the hospital managers at least 72 hours' notice in writing of his intention to discharge the patient, during which time, the patient's responsible clinician can block the discharge by issuing a 'barring report' stating that, if discharged, the patient is likely to act in a manner dangerous to himself or others. According to the Code of Practice, this question focuses on the probability of dangerous acts, such as causing serious physical injury or lasting psychological harm, not merely on the patient's general need for safety and others' general need for protection.

Section 3

Purpose

The aim of Section 3 is an admission to hospital for treatment.

Grounds for admission

Under Subsection (2), an application for admission for treatment may be made in respect of a patient on the grounds that:

'(a) he is suffering from mental disorder of a nature or degree which makes it appropriate for him to receive medical treatment in a hospital; and
(b) it is necessary for the health or safety of the patient or for the protection of other persons that he should receive such treatment and it cannot be provided unless he is detained under this section; and
(c) appropriate medical treatment is available for him.'

An application for admission for assessment shall be founded on the written recommendations in the prescribed form of two registered medical practitioners, including, in each case, a statement that in the opinion of the practitioner the conditions set out in Subsection (2) above are complied with. These statements must specify whether other methods of dealing with the patient are available and, if so, why they are not appropriate. At least one of these two doctors should be approved under Section 12 of the Act. If the Section 12 approved doctor does not have previous acquaintance with the patient then, if practicable, the second doctor should be one who does have such previous acquaintance. The two doctors may examine the patient jointly or separately. However, no more than five clear days must elapse between the days of the two examinations.

Duration

Under this section, a patient admitted to hospital for admission for treatment may be detained for up to six months initially and the section may be renewed.

Discharge

The patient may be discharged by any of the following:

- his responsible clinician
- the hospital managers
- his nearest relative.

Before giving a discharge order, the nearest relative must give the hospital managers at least 72 hours' notice in writing of his intention to discharge the patient, during which time, the patient's responsible clinician can block the discharge by issuing a 'barring report' stating that, if discharged, the patient is likely to act in a manner dangerous to himself or others. According to the Code of Practice, this question focuses on the probability of dangerous acts, such as causing serious physical injury or lasting psychological harm, not merely on the patient's general need for safety and others' general need for protection.

Assessment for Sections 2 and 3

Factors to consider

According to the Code of Practice (4.6), factors to be considered in deciding whether a patient should be detained for his own health or safety include:

- evidence suggesting that he is at risk of suicide, self-harm, self-neglect or being unable to look after his own health or safety;
- evidence suggesting that he is jeopardising his own health or safety accidentally, recklessly or unintentionally;
- evidence that his mental disorder is otherwise putting his health or safety at risk;
- any evidence suggesting that his mental health will deteriorate if he does not receive treatment;
- the reliability of such evidence, including what is known of the history of his mental disorder;
- his views and the views of any carers, relatives or close friends, especially those living with him, about the likely course of the disorder and the possibility of it improving;
- his skills and experience in managing his own condition;
- the potential benefits of treatment, which should be weighed against any adverse effects that being detained might have on his well-being;
- whether other methods of managing the risk are available.

According to the Code of Practice (4.7), factors to be considered in deciding whether a patient should be detained for the protection of others include:

- the nature of the risk to other people arising from his mental disorder;
- the likelihood that harm will result;
- the severity of any potential harm.

Taking into account:

- that it is not always possible to differentiate risk of harm to the patient from the risk of harm to others;
- the reliability of the available evidence, including any relevant details of the clinical history and past behaviour, such as contact with other agencies and any criminal convictions and cautions;
- the willingness and ability of those who live with the patient and those who provide care and support to him to cope with and manage the risk;
- whether other methods of managing the risk are available.

The Code of Practice (4.8) points out that harm to other people includes psychological as well as physical harm.

Mental Capacity Act 2005

According to the Code of Practice (4.14–4.16), if a patient cannot consent to the treatment needed, or to being admitted to hospital, this does not automatically mean that the Mental Health Act must be used. It may be possible to rely instead on the provisions of the Mental Capacity Act 2005 to provide treatment in the best interests of patients who are aged 16 years or over, and who lack capacity to consent to treatment, and this may be possible even if the provision of treatment unavoidably involves depriving the patient of his liberty. Deprivation of liberty for the purposes of care or treatment in a hospital or care home can be authorised to be in a patient's best interests under the deprivation of liberty safeguards in the Mental Capacity Act if the patient is aged 18 years or over. If admission to hospital for assessment or treatment for mental disorder is necessary, for a patient who lacks capacity to consent to it, an application under the Mental Health Act should be made if:

- providing appropriate care or treatment will unavoidably involve depriving the patient of his liberty and the Mental Capacity Act deprivation of liberty safeguards cannot be used; or
- the assessment or treatment needed cannot be safely or effectively delivered by relying on the Mental Capacity Act alone.

According to the Code of Practice (4.18), the key points when considering whether an application for detention should be made under the Mental Health Act instead of relying on the Mental Capacity Act Deprivation of Liberty Safeguards are that those safeguards cannot be used if any of the following apply:

- The patient is aged less than 18 years.
- The patient has made a valid and applicable advance decision refusing a necessary element of the treatment for which he is to be admitted to hospital.
- The use of the safeguards would conflict with a decision of the person's attorney or deputy or of the Court of Protection.
- The patient meets the criteria in Sections 2 or 3 of the Mental Health Act and is objecting to being admitted to (or remaining in) hospital for mental health treatment unless an attorney or deputy consents on his behalf.

Choosing between Sections 2 and 3

It can sometimes be difficult to decide whether to use Section 2 or 3 of the Mental Health Act.

The Code of Practice (4.26) advises using Section 2 if any of the following apply:

- The full extent of the nature and degree of a patient's condition is unclear.
- There is a need to carry out an initial in-patient assessment in order to formulate a treatment plan, or to reach a judgement about whether the patient will accept treatment on a voluntary basis following admission.
- There is a need to carry out a new in-patient assessment in order to re-formulate a treatment plan, or to reach a judgement about whether the patient will accept treatment on a voluntary basis.

Conversely, the Code of Practice (4.27) advises using Section 3 if any of the following apply:

- The patient is already detained under Section 2 (since detention under Section 2 cannot be renewed by a new Section 2 application).
- The nature and current degree of the patient's mental disorder, the essential elements of the treatment plan to be followed and the likelihood of the patient accepting treatment on a voluntary basis are already established.

Assessment process

An application for detention may be made by an approved mental health professional or the nearest relative; the former is usually the more appropriate applicant. The application should be supported by two medical practitioners in accordance with the Mental Health Act, as mentioned above. Note that a doctor should never advise a nearest relative to make the application in order to avoid the involvement of an approved mental health professional in the assessment process.

The Code of Practice (4.37–4.47) gives advice on setting up the assessment:

- Local arrangements should, as far as possible, ensure that assessments are carried out by the most appropriate approved mental health professional and doctors in the particular circumstances.
- Where a patient is known to belong to a group for which particular expertise is desirable (e.g. he is aged less than 18 years or has a learning disability), at least one of the professionals involved in the assessment should have expertise in working with people from that group, wherever possible; and if this is not possible, then at least one of the professionals involved in the assessment should, if at all possible, consult with one or more professionals who do have relevant expertise and involve him (them) as closely as the circumstances of the case allow.
- Unless different arrangements have been agreed locally between the relevant authorities, approved mental health professionals who assess patients for possible detention under the Act have overall responsibility for co-ordinating the process of assessment. In doing so, the approved mental health professional should be sensitive to the patient's age, gender (and gender identity), social, cultural, racial and religious background and sexual orientation, and should consider how any disability the patient has may affect the way the assessment needs to be carried out.

- The professionals involved in the assessment should be able to communicate with the patient effectively and reliably to prevent potential misunderstandings. The approved mental health professional should establish, as far as possible, whether the patient has any particular communication needs or difficulties and take steps to meet them, for example, by arranging for the services of a signer or a professional interpreter. The approved mental health professional should also be in a position, where appropriate, to supply suitable equipment to make communication easier with a patient who has impaired hearing, but who does not have his own hearing aid.
- Unless there is good reason for undertaking separate assessments, the patient should, where possible, be seen jointly by the approved mental health professional and at least one of the two doctors involved in the assessment.
- If the patient is not examined by both doctors at the same time, both doctors should discuss the case with the person considering making an application for his detention.
- Those involved in an assessment should be alert to the need to provide support for colleagues, especially where there is a risk of the patient causing physical harm. They should be aware of circumstances in which the police should be asked to provide assistance, in accordance with arrangements agreed locally with the police, and of how to use that assistance to maximise the safety of everyone involved in the assessment.
- Locally agreed arrangements on the involvement of the police should include a joint risk assessment tool to help determine the level of risk, what (if any) police assistance may be required and how quickly it is needed. In cases where no warrant for the police to enter premises under Section 135 of the Mental Health Act is being applied for, the risk assessment should indicate the reasons for this and explain why police assistance is still necessary.

Once the decision as to whether or not to make an application under Section 2 or Section 3 of the Mental Health Act has been made, the approved mental health professional should inform the patient, together with the relevant reasons. Subject to considerations of patient confidentiality, this decision should also be communicated to all of the following individuals:

- the nearest relative
- the doctors involved in the assessment
- the patient's care co-ordinator (if any)
- the patient's GP, if he was not one of the two doctors involved in the assessment.

'Difficult' patients

Although a variety of problems may arise, most can be pre-empted by taking a few precautions. For instance, it is worth checking whether a bed is booked at the admission unit. Similarly, if the patient is known to be aggressive, then the police may be approached for assistance.

A patient with a previous history of psychiatric admission or with partial insight, who wishes to avoid compulsory admission, may attempt to do so in a number of ways. The patient may take flight; if this is assessed as being likely to occur, perhaps because of such an incident in the past, the doctor can try to prevent it happening by carefully explaining the benefits of admission to the patient. Often such a patient may recognise, albeit at an unconscious level, the need for admission. Again, as with certain prisoners in forensic psychiatric assessments, a patient in the community may attempt to give a misleading picture of his mental state; however, whereas the former may try to feign mental illness, the latter may endeavour to suppress evidence of mental illness, for example, by being very guarded in replies to questions, or indeed electively mute. Such a manoeuvre is very likely to fail, however, if the assessment is thorough and includes interviews with relatives and informants, a consideration of the past history and discussion with others involved in the care of the patient either previously or at the time of the assessment. It should be noted that muteness may in itself be a function of a mental illness, for example, severe depression or catatonic schizophrenia. In such cases, other features of the underlying mental illness will be present and can be elicited.

If a person living alone refuses access to his home and there is reasonable reason to believe that he has been, or is being, ill-treated or neglected, or that he is unable to care for himself, for example, as the result of auditory hallucinations or persecutory delusions, then an application may be made to a justice of the peace for a warrant to be issued to allow the police to enter, by force if need be, search for and remove a patient, under Section 135(1) of the Mental Health Act. Note that the requirement for association with conduct etc. only applies to certain sections of the Act and not to all parts of it (*see* Section 1(2B)).

Disagreement between the assessors

There may infrequently be a disagreement between the assessors as to whether compulsory admission is indicated. In such cases, it is important that each assessor sets out his reasoning clearly during a joint discussion. If there is still no resolution, the approved mental health professional and the doctor(s) may offer to reassess the patient at a later date. However, it is vital in the event of a decision against compulsory admission, that an alternative package of care be implemented to ensure continued support for both the patient and his family. The patient should also be encouraged to attend a psychiatric outpatient appointment made for the earliest date possible. The Code of Practice (4.101) advises:

Where there is an unresolved dispute about an application for detention, it is essential that the professionals do not abandon the patient. Instead, they should explore and agree an alternative plan – if necessary on a temporary basis. Such a plan should include a risk assessment and identification of the arrangements for managing the risks. The alternative plan should be recorded in writing, as should the arrangements for reviewing it. Copies should be made available to all those who need them (subject to the normal considerations of patient confidentiality).

Section 4

Purpose

The aim of Section 4 is an admission to hospital for assessment in cases of emergency. This section should only be used in exceptional circumstances. An application made under this section is referred to as 'an emergency application'.

Grounds

The emergency application must state that it is of urgent necessity that the patient should be admitted and detained for assessment, and that compliance with the normal procedures would involve undesirable delay. This must be confirmed by the doctor making the medical recommendation. In particular, all the following criteria must be fulfilled:

- The criteria for detention for assessment under Section 2 are met.
- The patient's detention is required as a matter of urgent necessity.
- Obtaining a second medical recommendation would cause undesirable delay.

Procedure for admission

The procedure for admission under Section 4 is as follows.

- The application should preferably be made by an approved mental health professional (but, in special circumstances, the nearest relative can make the application).
- The applicant must have seen the patient within the previous 24 hours.
- One registered medical practitioner who, if possible (but not necessarily if this is not practicable), has previous acquaintance with the patient (and who need not necessarily be approved under Section 12 of the Mental Health Act if this is not practicable) must examine the patient; the doctor must give his signed written recommendation on the appropriate form.
- The patient must be admitted to hospital within 24 hours of either the medical examination or the application, whichever is earlier.

Duration

A patient may be detained under Section 4 for a maximum of 72 hours from the time of admission, unless a second medical recommendation is provided to the hospital managers in accordance with the Mental Health Act (*see* below) to allow detention under Section 2.

Discharge

By the end of the 72 hours one of the following options is implemented:

- The patient is discharged.
- The patient remains informally.
- A second medical recommendation is received which, together with the first medical recommendation, thereby allows compliance with the requirements for detention under Section 2 of the Act.
- Application for compulsory admission under Section 3 is initiated; if such an application is made while the patient is being detained under Section 4, then two fresh medical recommendations are required.

Good practice

The Mental Health Commissioners recommend that, whenever possible, two doctors should be involved in the decision to admit a patient to hospital under the Mental Health Act. That is, Sections 2 and 3 should always be used in preference to Section 4 (for which only one doctor is required). They further recommend that the use of Section 4 should be confined to emergencies when it is only possible to secure the attendance of one doctor. Section 4 is for genuine emergencies and should never be used for administrative convenience.

Note that patients detained on the basis of emergency applications may not be treated without their consent under Part IV of the Act unless, or until, the second medical recommendation is received.

References

Department of Health (2008) *Mental Health Act 1983: Code of Practice*. London: TSO.

Department of Health (2008) *Reference Guide to the Mental Health Act 1983*. London: TSO.

1983 Mental Health Act.

2007 Mental Health Act.

6 Consent to Treatment Provisions under the Mental Health Act

Part IV of the Mental Health Act 1983

Part IV of the Mental Health Act 1983 is concerned with the issue of consent to treatment and applies to any patient liable to be detained under this Act *except*:

- a patient detained (for up to 72 hours) in an emergency, under Section 4;
- an informal patient detained (for up to 72 hours) under Section 5(2) to prevent him from leaving hospital;
- an informal patient detained (for up to six hours) under Section 5(4) to prevent him from leaving hospital;
- an accused person remanded to hospital by a court for a report on their mental condition, under Section 35;
- a patient believed to be suffering from mental disorder who is detained (for up to 72 hours) in a place of safety under Section 135;
- a person found in a public place who appears to be suffering from mental disorder who is removed by the police and detained (for up to 72 hours) in a place of safety under Section 136;
- a convicted patient detained (for up to 28 days) in a place of safety awaiting transfer to hospital under Section 37;
- a patient who has been conditionally discharged under Sections 42, 73 or 74 and who has not been recalled to hospital.

Treatment requiring consent and a second opinion (Section 57)

The treatments which come under the umbrella of Section 57 of the Mental Health Act 1983 are psychosurgery and implantation of sex hormones. They cannot be carried out without the patient's capable consent and a second opinion.

Treatment requiring consent or second opinion (Sections 58 and 58A)

This section covers physical treatments of mental disorder including medication (Section 58) and electroconvulsive therapy (Section 58A).

Relevant patients can be treated for three months on medication for their mental disorder without their consent. This does not apply to medical treatment for physical illness which must be covered under the **Common Law for valid consent and Mental Capacity Act 2005** if the patient does not consent to it.

There is no medication certification required for the first 28 days of a community treatment order (or the first three months since the commencement of detention, if this is later). After the first 28 days, all medication for mental disorder must be authorised by a second opinion appointed doctor (SOAD), whether the patient has capacity and voluntarily consents or lacks capacity.

Electroconvulsive therapy (ECT) cannot be administered, except in an emergency, if a patient has capacity and refuses this treatment. Note that the requirement for association with conduct etc. only applies to certain sections of the Act and not to all parts of it (*see* Section 1(2B)). No ECT may be administered, unless in an emergency, if a patient lacks capacity but has a valid advanced decision refusing ECT or has an attorney who refuses ECT for his client under the powers of the lasting power of attorney of the Mental Capacity Act 2005.

Physical investigations necessary for the administration of medication or ECT can be undertaken against the patient's wishes, if the medication or ECT is being imposed on the patient under the Mental Health Act consent to treatment provisions. In the case of ECT, treatment entails taking blood samples. Similarly, in the situation where lithium treatment is used, thyroid function and creatinine clearance monitoring and serum lithium levels in guidance with the British National Formulary can be carried out. With regard to clozapine administration, this will also include regular venepuncture. Note that the requirement for association with conduct etc. only applies to certain sections of the Act and not to all parts of it (*see* Section 1(2B)).

Urgent treatment (Section 62)

In respect of urgent treatment, under Section 62 of the Mental Health Act 1983 it is the case that Sections 57 and 58 do not apply to *any* of the following cases:

- The treatment is immediately necessary to save a patient's life.
- The treatment, not being irreversible, is immediately necessary to prevent a serious deterioration of a patient's condition.
- The treatment, not being irreversible or hazardous, is immediately necessary to alleviate serious suffering by a patient.
- The treatment, not being irreversible or hazardous, is immediately necessary and represents the minimum interference necessary to prevent a patient from behaving violently or being a danger or himself/herself or to others.

Irreversible treatment

For the purposes of Section 62, a treatment is considered irreversible if it has unfavourable irreversible physical or psychological consequences.

Hazardous treatment

For the purposes of Section 62, a treatment is considered hazardous if it entails significant physical hazard.

Part IVA of the Mental Health Act

This is concerned with the treatment of patients who are subject to Community Treatment Orders (CTOs). Apart from where a CTO patient has been recalled to hospital, they cannot be given treatment for mental disorder unless the requirements of Part 4A are met. This means that the person giving the treatment must have the authority to do so and, in most cases, there will be a certification requirement. Form CTO11 is needed for those treatments which would require a certificate under Sections 58 or 58A for detained patients i.e. medication after the initial three-month period as well as ECT and any related medication. A certificate is not required during the first month following a patient's discharge from detention on to a CTO.

When giving Part 4A certificates, SOADs are stating whether the treatment is appropriate. They do not have to certify whether or not a patient has capacity to consent to the treatments in question, nor whether a patient with capacity is consenting or refusing. The certificate, by itself, is not enough for treatment to be given. There is also an authorisation requirement such as valid consent.

Under Part IVA the SOAD consults with two other people who have been professionally concerned with the patient's medical treatment. Only one of these may be a doctor and neither of them can be the patient's responsible clinician or the approved clinician in charge of any of the treatments that are to be specified on the certificate.

With regard to authorisation where a patient has capacity to consent to treatment then this provides the authority to treat. In some cases, there may be a donee of an LPA, or a deputy appointed by the Court of Protection, who is able to consent on the patient's behalf.

If a community patient lacks capacity to consent to the treatment, the person wishing to have authority to treat must take reasonable steps to establish that the patient lacks capacity to consent to the treatment. When giving the treatment, he must then reasonably believe that the patient lacks capacity to consent to it. He must have no reason to believe that the patient objects to being given the treatment; or, if he does have reason to believe that the patient objects, it must not be necessary to use force against the patient in order to give the treatment. The treatment giver must be the person in charge of the treatment and an approved clinician or the treatment must be given under the direction of that clinician. He must ensure that giving the treatment will not conflict with an advance decision which he is satisfied is valid and applicable, or with a decision made by a donee or deputy or the Court of Protection.

If treatment is to be given in an emergency without a certificate, the treatment must fall into one of the following categories set out in Section 64G(5):

'(a) *it is immediately necessary to save the patient's life; or*

(b) *it is immediately necessary to prevent a serious deterioration of the patient's condition and is not irreversible; or*

(c) *it is immediately necessary to alleviate serious suffering by the patient and is not irreversible or hazardous; or*

(d) *it is immediately necessary, represents the minimum interference necessary to prevent the patient from behaving violently or being a danger to himself or others and is not irreversible or hazardous.*'

In these circumstances, if it is necessary to use force against the patient in order to give the treatment, this can only be to prevent harm to the patient. The use of such force must be a proportionate response to the likelihood of the patient's suffering harm, as well as to the seriousness of that harm.

Recalled Community Patients are covered by Part IVA.

7 Community Treatment Orders, Leave of Absence and After-care

Community Treatment Orders (CTOs)

Sections 17A–G cover Community Treatment Orders. These orders were introduced as part of the Mental Health Act 2007 reforms and provide a framework for ensuring that certain patients receive compulsory care and treatment within the community. The Code of Practice refers to the treatment regime as Supervised Community Treatment. However, it should be noted that this term does not exist anywhere in the 1983 Act as revised, and many try to avoid its use.

CTOs replaced Supervised Aftercare which was regarded by some as not being sufficiently robust in terms of requiring patients to take medication in the community. CTOs have proved both popular and controversial with professionals and their use has outstripped that of guardianship. There were 3 525 patients who were subject to CTOs in England on 31 March 2010 compared with only 836 on guardianship. As with guardianship, the use of CTOs varies considerably by area.

The effect of Section 17(2A) is that the responsible clinician (RC) must consider the use of a CTO in any case where he is granting Section 17 leave that will exceed seven consecutive days. This does not prevent the use of longer term leave; it just requires the RC to justify it. In practice, many RCs seem to prefer the use of the CTO rather than leave. A number of factors have been suggested to explain this: pressure from managers because CTOs look better on the statistics than Section 17 leave, which makes it look as though bed-occupancy is high (when in fact there is no requirement for a bed); responsibility for the patient may transfer to another professional with the CTO, while remaining with the original RC with Section 17 (this varies across the country); there are more safeguards with the CTO (e.g. involvement of an improved mental health professional (AMHP) and Part IVA Consent to Treatment rules); the CTO is less restrictive than Section 17 leave, which leaves the patient still liable to be detained.

Grounds for a CTO

Patients who are liable to be detained under Sections 3, 37, 45A, 47 and 48 can be made subject to a CTO by their RC, if they obtain the agreement of an AMHP, and if the criteria set out in Section 17A(5) are met. These are:

(a) the patient is suffering from mental disorder of a nature or degree which makes it appropriate for him to receive medical treatment;
(b) it is necessary for his health or safety or for the protection of other persons that he should receive such treatment;
(c) subject to his being liable to be recalled as mentioned in paragraph (d) below, such treatment can be provided without his continuing to be detained in a hospital;
(d) it is necessary that the responsible clinician should be able to exercise the power under Section 17E(1) below to recall the patient to hospital;
(e) appropriate medical treatment is available for him.

The application form (CTO1 in England, CP1 in Wales) requires both the RC and the AMHP to state that these criteria are met. The AMHP also needs to state that it is appropriate to make the CTO. If discretionary conditions are set, the AMHP must agree that they are necessary or appropriate or the CTO cannot go ahead. The form is not ideal from the AMHP's point of view, as there is no space for them to explain their decision and some agencies have produced their own supplementary form (much like the social circumstances form required by the Code when the AMHP applies for detention).

Conditions

All CTOs will have two conditions attached to the order and these are set out on the form itself. Section 17B(3) states that the order will specify:

(a) a condition that the patient make himself available for examination under Section 20A below; and
(b) a condition that, if it is proposed to give a certificate under Part 4A of this Act in his case, he make himself available for examination so as to enable the certificate to be given.

The RC may also specify discretionary conditions if he obtains the agreement of the AMHP. Such discretionary conditions must be considered necessary or appropriate for one or more of the following purposes:

(a) ensuring the patient receives medical treatment;
(b) preventing risk of harm to the patient's health or safety;
(c) protecting other persons.

One slightly contentious fact is that although the RC needs the agreement of the AMHP before making these conditions, they can subsequently vary or suspend them at any time without the agreement of an AMHP. The Code provides a limited safeguard at Paragraph 25.31 where it states:

> *'The responsible clinician does not need to agree any variation or suspension with the AMHP. However, it would not be good practice to vary conditions which had recently been agreed with an AMHP without discussion with that AMHP.'*

Conditions might cover where the patient should live, what treatment they should receive and a range of other matters that would address risk as above. The cumulative effect of the conditions imposed on a patient should not amount to a deprivation of liberty. If they are living in a relevant place, an incapacitated patient whose care and treatment amounts to a deprivation of liberty could be made subject to the Deprivation of Liberty Safeguards (DOLS) whilst remaining on the CTO.

If a patient does not comply with a mandatory condition, this provides grounds for the RC to recall a patient. Breaching a discretionary condition is not enough by itself to justify recall. The RC would additionally need to believe that the patient required treatment in hospital and that there would be a risk of harm to the health or safety of the patient or to others if they were not recalled to hospital for treatment of their mental disorder.

Time periods for a CTO

A CTO lasts for six months in the first instance, but can be extended for a further six months, and then yearly. Section 20A sets out the provisions and criteria for the extension of CTOs. Essentially, the RC and an AMHP both need to be satisfied that the criteria for a CTO are still met. This is recorded on the appropriate form (CTO7 in England, CP3 in Wales). A CTO can only be revoked if the patient is currently subject to recall in hospital. This means that time can be very tight if, for example, the patient has already been in hospital for a day or two before the RC reaches the conclusion that revocation may be necessary.

Recall

A patient who is subject to a CTO may be recalled to hospital by the RC. Notice of recall should be in writing and, as we have seen, can only take place if either the patient has failed to comply with a mandatory condition or they require medical treatment in hospital for their mental disorder, and there would be a risk of harm to the health or safety of the patient or to others if they were not recalled to hospital. In deciding whether to recall a patient to hospital, the RC may take into account any failure to comply with a discretionary condition. The Code (at Paragraph 25.51) states:

> *The responsible clinician should consider, in each case, whether recalling the patient to hospital is justified in all of the circumstances. For example, it might be sufficient to monitor a patient who has failed to comply with a condition to attend for treatment, before deciding whether the lack of treatment means that recall is necessary.*

Where a patient is served with a notice of recall but does not comply they can be returned under Section 18 of the Act. If the patient refuses access, this may require obtaining a warrant under Section 135(2).

Where a patient has been recalled, they can be detained in hospital for up to 72 hours, during which time the RC may decide to treat the patient and allow them to return home within 72 hours, or revoke the CTO which would have the effect of making the patient subject to Section 3 again (this requires the agreement of an AMHP), or discharge the CTO completely so the patient is not subject to any compulsion.

The use of recall went up in England after the first five months of CTOs. Of 2 109 CTOs up to March 2009 in NHS facilities there were 206 recalls, but of the 4 020 in the following year 1 197 were recalled. There was a similar increase in the use of revocation.

Revocation

Revocation has the effect of placing the patient back under detention on their original treatment section. The RC, with the support of an AMHP, may revoke a

CTO in writing using the appropriate form (CTO5 in England, CP7 in Wales) if the criteria for detention under Section 3 are met, i.e.:

- the patient is suffering from a mental disorder of a nature or degree which makes it appropriate for him to receive medical treatment in a hospital; and
- it is necessary for the health or safety of the patient or for the protection of other persons that he should receive such treatment and it cannot be provided unless he is detained under this section; and
- appropriate medical treatment is available for him.

The effect of revocation is that the patient remains in hospital under their original detention section. The patient starts a new detention period of six months from the time of revocation. The fact that it is regarded as the original detention order preserves the patient's rights for consent to treatment purposes. In other words, the patient does not have to restart a period of 3 months medication before being eligible for a Second Opinion Appointed Doctor (SOAD).

Revocation will lead to an automatic Mental Health Tribunal hearing.

Discharging a CTO

The RC can discharge a CTO at any time and the numbers of discharges appear to be increasing, which may suggest that the honeymoon period for CTOs is over. The patient can apply for a Mental Health Tribunal hearing once in each period. Although the tribunal can discharge the CTO, it does not have any powers to vary the conditions which may prove a frustration. Hospital Managers have the power of discharge and the patient may request a hearing. Unless the patient had formerly been on a Part III Section (e.g. Section 37) rather than subject to Section 3, the nearest relative (NR) can discharge the patient (giving 72 hours written notice). The RC can block the NR discharge if they believe the patient is likely to behave in a manner dangerous to themselves or others. A discharge from a CTO has the effect of discharging the initial liability for detention.

Section 17 leave

A Responsible Clinician may grant leave of absence to any patient who is liable to be detained under Part II of the Act. Section 37 Hospital order patients may also be granted leave by the RC but restricted patients may only be granted leave with the permission of the Secretary of State for Justice. Patients subject to Sections 35, 36 or 38 may not be granted leave.

The Code of Practice states:

> '*21.6 Only the patient's responsible clinician can grant leave of absence to a patient detained under the Act. Responsible clinicians cannot delegate the decision to grant leave of absence to anyone else. In the absence of the usual responsible clinician (e.g, if they are on leave), permission can be granted only by the approved clinician who is for the time being acting as the patient's responsible clinician.*'

Leave of absence may be subject to any conditions the RC thinks are necessary in the interests of the patient or for the protection of others. Leave may be granted indefinitely, on specified occasions, or for a specified period. However, it may not go beyond the renewal date for the section. The RC may also direct that the patient should remain in custody when on leave. A patient on leave is still liable to be detained and, therefore, is still subject to the consent to treatment provisions of Part IV of the Act (unlike a CTO patient who is covered by Part 4A). A Community Treatment Order could be made while a patient is on Section 17 leave.

If the RC considers it necessary in the interest of the patient's health or safety or for the protection of others, they may revoke leave in writing and recall the patient to hospital.

There is no statutory form for granting leave but the code states that hospitals should establish a system by which responsible clinicians can record the leave they authorise and specify the conditions attached to it. A copy should then be given to the patient.

A virtual Community Treatment Order

A patient who is liable to be detained under Section 3 may have the section renewed, even if they are on leave, as long as the RC considers that there is a hospital element to the treatment plan (*B* v. *Barking, Havering and Brentwood Community Healthcare NHS Trust* (1999), 1FLR 106 and *R. (on the application of DR) v. Mersey Care NHS Trust*, (2002)).

In a further case, a patient who had been on Section 17 leave for three months challenged a tribunal's failure to discharge from detention. Attendance at a hospital was limited to a ward round every four weeks, and sessions with a ward psychologist weekly. The judge, in upholding the tribunal's decision, stated that the RMO was encouraging progress to discharge. Her purpose was to break a revolving-door pattern and the judge considered that the use of long-term leave in these circumstances was justified (*R (CS)* v. *MHRT* (2004).

Given that hospitals could include places without beds that are used for out-patient clinics, Section 17 leave in some areas has become a virtual community treatment order. Some examination of its use compared with Section 17A or guardianship would be interesting.

Choice of compulsion in the community

There is guidance in the Code as to which might be the most appropriate community provision in situations where any one of the three options would be possible (i.e. where the patient is currently detained in hospital for treatment). Paragraph 28.4 states that Section 17 leave:

> *'is primarily intended to allow a patient detained under the Act to be temporarily absent from hospital where further in-patient treatment as a detained patient is still thought to be necessary. It is clearly suitable for short-term absences, to allow visits to family and so on. It may also be useful in the longer term, where the clinical team wish to see how the patient manages outside hospital before making the decision to discharge.'*

As we have seen, case law requires that there is some hospital element which forms a significant part of the care plan if Section 17 leave is to be used longer term. This could, however, include attendance at a day hospital or for out-patient appointments.

At Paragraph 28.5 the Code looks at the CTO as a way of preventing the 'revolving door' problem. It states that the CTO is:

> *'a more structured system than leave of absence and has more safeguards for patients. A key feature of SCT is that it is suitable only where there is no reason to think that the patient will require further treatment as a detained in-patient for the time being, but the responsible clinician needs to be able to recall the patient to hospital.'*

A key feature of the after-care plan is to require the patient to live at a particular address, however, there may be a problem with the CTO in that there is no way of enforcing such a requirement. Guardianship allows the patient to be returned to a place of residence if they abscond. The CTO looks as though it may be at its most effective where medical treatment is a key issue, but where the patient would not voluntarily accept it.

Finally, with regard to guardianship, the Code states at Paragraph 28.3 that it is:

> *'social care-led and is primarily focused on patients with welfare needs. Its purpose is to enable patients to receive care in the community where it cannot be provided without the use of compulsory powers.'*

Section 117 after-care

This places a duty on health and social services authorities (in co-operation with relevant voluntary agencies) to provide after-care to a patient who has been detained under Sections 3, 37, 45A, 47 or 48 and who is discharged and leaves hospital. This still applies if there is a gap between the section being lifted and the patient leaving hospital.

A problem has arisen in terms of financial responsibility of the authorities in that the services under Section 117 should continue to be provided, until both health and social services authorities are satisfied that the person concerned no longer needs the services, and there is no way of charging the patient for these services. Services provided under Section 117 are community care services for the purposes of the NHS and Community Care Act 1990. If a need is then identified, it must be provided, but there is some discretion as regards the level and precise nature of the service. (*R* v. *Gloucestershire CC ex p. Barry* (1997))

Charging for services remains a contentious area. As we have seen Section 117 services should be free to the patient. The Bournewood case highlighted the fact that there are some benefits derived from being detained on Section 3. Subsequent residential and other services can be very expensive but will be free if covered by Section 117. In *R.* v. *Manchester City Council, ex p. Stennett* (2002) the House of Lords ruled that Section 117 imposes a freestanding duty to provide aftercare services rather than being a passport to services provided under other legislation. This would include any medication which was part of the patients' psychiatric treatment. A number of authorities have had to reimburse people as a result of the Stennett judgment.

As yet, there are no moves to introduce a way of charging for Section 117 services.

8 Guardianship (Sections 7 or 37 of the Mental Health Act)

Guardianship, compared with detention, is a little used part of the Mental Health Act 1983. However, it is both important and contentious, especially as community based powers have changed with the introduction of Community Treatment Orders under the amended Mental Health Act and the new Deprivation of Liberty Safeguards (DOLS) under the amended Mental Capacity Act. Under the 1959 Mental Health Act, guardianship was seen as a community version of compulsory treatment in hospital but it was very little used. The guardian had all the powers of a parent over a child under the age of 14. With the reforms that led to the Mental Health Act 1983, the powers were limited to three essential areas: where the person should live; where they should go during the day; and who should be allowed access to them.

The use of guardianship varies considerably in different parts of England and Wales but the overall number of people subject to guardianship remains low, in stark contrast to the number who are subject to Community Treatment Orders.

From a low base of 60 new guardianships in England in the period from April 1983 to March 1984, there were 139 new cases in 1988–9 and 667 by 1999–2000. The number of new cases then dipped. There were 561 new cases in 2001–02 and by 2009–10 the number was only 420.

In terms of continuing cases on a given date, the numbers have also declined in recent years. On March 31st 2010, there were 836 people in guardianship compared with 984 in March 2002. However, this figure is still significantly higher than the 161 who were in guardianship in 1984.

Table 8.1 and Figure 8.1 illustrate the overall use as well as significant variations around England.

Figure 8.1 ends in 2008 because the changes in law that year resulted in no classifications of mental disorder following that date.

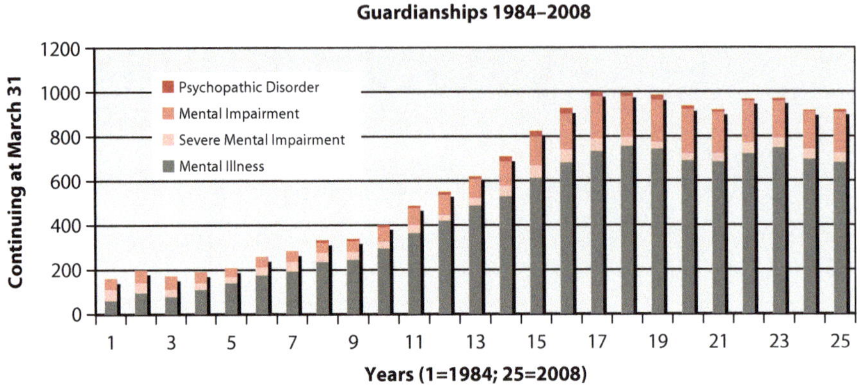

Figure 8.1 Guardianships by classification of mental disorder.

Table 8.1 Continuing Guardianships at 31.03.10 for some English local authorities

Local authority	Total	Population	Per 100 000
Middlesbrough	13	134 855	9.64
Bath	13	169 040	7.69
Halton (Widnes)	9	118 208	7.61
Liverpool	33	439 473	7.51
Southampton	11	217 455	5.06
Poole	7	138 288	5.06
Bolton	13	260 000	5.00
Bristol	19	380 615	4.99
Isle of Wight	6	132 731	4.52
Lancashire	49	1 134 974	4.32
Newcastle	10	259 536	3.85
Bracknell	5	129 706	3.85
Gloucestershire	19	564 559	3.37
Kent	44	1 329 718	3.31
Torbay	4	122 900	3.25
Devon	21	704 493	2.98
Swindon	4	180 051	2.22
Cornwall	11	501 267	2.19
Hertfordshire	19	1 033 977	1.84
Bournemouth	3	163 400	1.84
Plymouth	4	240 720	1.66
Portsmouth	3	186 701	1.61
Somerset	6	498 093	1.20
Wiltshire	5	432 973	1.15
Westminster	2	181 286	1.10
Lewisham	2	248 922	0.80
Hampshire	8	1 240 103	0.65
South Gloucestershire	1	245 641	0.41
Surrey	4	1 059 015	0.38
Lambeth	0	261,150	0.00
Total in sample	**348**	**12 709 850**	**2.74**
Total England	**836**	**49 138,831**	**1.70**

Sources: Government Statistical Service.

Purpose of guardianship

Paragraph 26.2 of the English Code states:

> *'The purpose of guardianship is to enable patients to receive care outside hospital when it cannot be provided without the use of compulsory powers. Such care may or may not include specialist medical treatment for mental disorder.'*

The Code continues at Paragraph 26.4:

> *'Guardianship therefore provides an authoritative framework for working with a patient, with a minimum of constraint, to achieve as independent a life as possible within the community. Where it is used, it should be part of the patient's overall care plan.'*

Two examples are then given at Paragraph 26.8 of the Code of positive examples of situations where guardianship might be suitable:

> *'Guardianship is most likely to be appropriate where:*
>
> - *the patient is thought to be likely to respond well to the authority and attention of a guardian and so be more willing to comply with necessary treatment and care for their mental disorder; or*
> - *there is a particular need for someone to have the authority to decide where the patient should live or to insist that doctors, AMHPs or other people be given access to the patient.'*

Where the patient lacks the capacity to make decisions such as where to live, guardianship can be very helpful in that it will provide a decision-maker while providing certain safeguards for the patient (the right to appeal to the Tribunal) and for the nearest relative (the right to object to the guardianship, or to discharge it).

Routes into guardianship

Guardianship is possible through a civil route (Section 7) or via the courts (Section 37). The guardian may be either the local authority or a private individual who has been approved by the local authority. On 31 March 2010, there were 831 cases where the local authority was the guardian and only 5 where the guardian was a private individual. The Law Commission wanted to abolish the private individual as guardian but it remains an option.

For the civil route, the application is usually made by an Approved Mental Health Professional (AMHP) (although it could be made by the nearest relative (NR)) and this application is based on two medical recommendations (much like a Section 3 application). As with Section 3 one doctor should, where possible, have previous acquaintance of the patient and one must be approved under Section 12 of the Mental Health Act. The AMHP must consult with the nearest relative, where practicable and, if the nearest relative objects the guardianship cannot go ahead unless the nearest relative is displaced by the County Court on the basis that they have acted unreasonably in making their objection. This involvement of the nearest relative is an important limitation on the state's interference with family matters. Once a patient is received into guardianship, a nearest relative has the right to order their discharge (and there is no blocking power for the RC on dangerousness grounds, in contrast with the position with Section 3).

The decision whether to accept the guardianship is made by the local authority. This can sometimes be a fairly drawn-out process which may make guardianship a less than attractive proposition for mental health practitioners.

Under Section 37, courts can make guardianship orders if the local authority agrees.

Social Services Departments vary in their procedures for making decisions on guardianship applications (or requests from the courts) and some are explicit in their attitude to this piece of legislation, either being against its use or encouraging it. The relevant local authority is the one in which the patient lives unless the guardian is a private individual when their address determines the relevant authority.

In either case, the guardian has certain essential powers to enable them to provide for the patient's care. They involve requirements to reside in a particular place, to attend places for treatment etc., and to allow greater access to the patient by relevant professionals. This limitation on powers is in stark contrast to the Mental Health Act 1959 where we have already noted that the guardian had the equivalent powers to the parent of a child under the age of 14. It was believed (probably erroneously) that the powers were seen as too great and that to reduce them would encourage the use of guardianship.

Apart from the reduction from general to specific powers, there was one other major change in 1983 compared with the earlier 1959 Act, and with hindsight, it seems like a mistake. The change from 'subnormality' to 'mental impairment' drastically reduced the use of guardianship for people with learning difficulties. Although guardianship is often seen as having a strong protective function, many people who might benefit from its provisions were excluded from guardianship as a result of the new definition of 'mental impairment', i.e. the requirement for abnormal aggression or seriously irresponsible conduct. By way of contrast, the inclusion of dementia within the classification of 'mental illness' led to a significant increase in the use of guardianship with this group. The changes brought about by the 2007 amending Act removed the term 'mental impairment' but kept exactly the same limitations in the use of guardianship for people with learning disabilities.

The grounds for using guardianship

Firstly, no-one under the age of 16 can be received or placed in guardianship. For a mentally disordered child under 16 who requires some supervision in the community, Child Care Law (including the rights of parents and the local authority) is available.

The grounds for guardianship under Sections 7 or 37 are slightly different. Here we will concentrate on the more common civil route as Section 37 is rarely used. Section 7(2) states:

> *'A guardianship application may be made in respect of a patient on the grounds that:*
>
> (*a*) *he is suffering from mental disorder of a nature or degree which warrants his reception into guardianship under this section; and*

> (b) *it is necessary in the interests of the welfare of the patient or for the protection of other persons that the patient should be so received.'*

As we have seen, if the patient is suffering from a learning disability this must be associated with abnormally aggressive or seriously irresponsible conduct on the part of the patient.

The guardian's powers are set out in Section 8(1) and give the guardian:

> '(a) *the power to require the patient to reside at a place specified by the authority or person named as guardian;*
>
> (b) *the power to require the patient to attend at places and times so specified for the purpose of medical treatment, occupation, education or training;*
>
> (c) *the power to require access to the patient to be given, at any place where the patient is residing, to any medical practitioner, approved social worker or other person so specified.'*

The Reference Guide gives examples for the use of each of these powers:

> *'19.5 The* residence power *allows a guardian to require that a patient lives at a specified place. This may be used, for example, to discourage a patient from sleeping rough or living with people who may exploit or mistreat them, or to ensure that they reside in a particular hostel or other facility.*
>
> *19.6 The* attendance power *lets a guardian require a patient to attend specified places at specified times for medical treatment, occupation, education or training. Such places might include a day centre, or a hospital, surgery or clinic, for example.*
>
> *19.7 The* access power *entitles a guardian to require that access to the patient be given at the place where the patient is living, to any doctor, approved mental health professional (AMHP), or other specified person. This power could be used for example, to ensure that patients do not neglect themselves.'*

The changes which were implemented in November 2008 gave the power to convey to the place of residence in addition to the existing power to return the person when they had absconded from the place of residence.

Note that Part IV of the Act on consent to treatment does **not** apply to guardianship. Thus, there is no statutory route to make a patient accept treatment, such as medication, against their will. Because guardianship does not give any powers in relation to property and affairs it sometimes goes hand in hand with the use of the Court of Protection.

Time limits

Guardianship lasts for up to 6 months, is renewable for a further 6 months, and then on a yearly basis. The renewal process involves the Responsible Clinician (or Nominated Medical Attendant where there is a private guardian) examining the patient in the last two months of the order and confirming in writing that the grounds for guardianship are still met. The local authority then has a duty to inform the patient of the renewal. There is no automatic reference to the Tribunal for a guardianship patient but he may make an application for a hearing once in each period of guardianship.

Discharge from guardianship

The local authority may discharge a patient from guardianship whether they were received under Section 7 or 37(courts). This decision may be taken on behalf of the authority by any three or more members of the authority or of a committee or subcommittee that is authorised for the purpose. If the decision is taken by three people, they must be unanimous in their decision to discharge. If the decision is taken by more than three people, as well as needing a majority in favour, that majority must consist of at least three people who are in favour of discharge before a decision to discharge can be made.

The RC can discharge a patient from guardianship at any time. The NR can discharge a patient who has been received into guardianship under Section 7 but not where they are subject to a Section 37 guardianship order (where they would need to make application to the Tribunal). Unlike the similar power for Section 3 there is no need for the NR to give 72 hours notice of this and the RC has no power to bar this on the grounds of dangerousness.

The First–tier Tribunal may discharge a patient from guardianship and, as we have seen, the patient may apply for a hearing once in each period of guardianship.

Mental Capacity Act or Guardianship?

It will be difficult for practitioners to decide when to seek to use guardianship and when to rely on the Mental Capacity Act if the person lacks capacity to make certain key decisions. The Code of Practice notes that there may be many occasions, including moving into residential care, when it will be seen as appropriate to rely on the Mental Capacity Act but at Paragraph 26.12 it points out that:

> *'guardianship may still be appropriate in such cases if:*
>
> - *there are other reasons – unconnected to the move to residential care – to think that the patient might benefit from the attention and authority of a guardian;*
> - *there is a particular need to have explicit statutory authority for the patient to be returned to the place where the patient is to live should they go absent; or*
> - *it is thought to be important that decisions about where the patient is to live are placed in the hands of a single person or authority – for example, where there have been long-running or particularly difficult disputes about where the person should live.'*

In unusual or finely balanced cases, the Code recommends that consideration is also given to seeking a decision from the Court of Protection.

Local Authority responsibilities

There is a list at Paragraph 26.15 where the Code of Practice states that Local Social Services Authorities (LSSAs) should have policies for:

'• *receiving, scrutinising and accepting or refusing applications for guardianship. Such arrangements should ensure that applications are properly but quickly dealt with;*
- *monitoring the progress of each patient's guardianship, including steps to be taken to fulfil the authority's statutory obligations in relation to private guardians and to arrange visits to the patient;*
- *ensuring the suitability of any proposed private guardian, and that they are able to understand and carry out their duties under the Act;*
- *ensuring that patients under guardianship receive, both orally and in writing, information in accordance with regulations under the Act;*
- *ensuring that patients are aware of their right to apply to the Tribunal and that they are given the name of someone who will give them the necessary assistance, on behalf of the LSSA, in making such an application;*
- *authorising an approved clinician to be the patient's responsible clinician;*
- *maintaining detailed records relating to guardianship patients;*
- *ensuring that the need to continue guardianship is reviewed in the last two months of each period of guardianship in accordance with the Act; and*
- *discharging patients from guardianship as soon as it is no longer required.*'

The local authority may discharge the patient following the procedures noted above.

Information to patients and nearest relatives

When a patient is received into guardianship, the responsible LSSA must take whatever steps are reasonably practicable to ensure that the patient is informed of their rights to apply to the First-tier Tribunal for their discharge and (where applicable) of the right of their nearest relative to discharge them from guardianship. This information needs to be given both orally and in writing. Whatever steps are reasonably practicable must also be taken to ensure that the person the LSSA thinks is the patient's nearest relative is given the same information in writing, unless the patient has requested otherwise. Information given to a nearest relative or private guardian must be in writing, but may be communicated by electronic means (e.g. by email) if the nearest relative or private guardian agrees.

Under the new Section 130D, the LSSA must also take steps to ensure that a patient subject to guardianship is told about the independent mental health advocacy service. The LSSA must also take steps to give the same information to the person they think is the patient's nearest relative, unless the patient has requested otherwise. This needs to be done as soon as practicable after the patient becomes subject to guardianship.

Restriction of movement or deprivation of liberty?

Requiring someone to live in a particular place, without their agreement, is clearly a significant restriction of their movement, but the Government has been at pains to state that this, of itself, will not amount to a deprivation of liberty. For example, the point is made in Paragraph 26.29 of the Code of Practice when considering the power to take and convey:

'The power to take or return patients to the place they are required to live may be used, for example, to discourage them from:

- *living somewhere the guardian considers unsuitable;*
- *breaking off contact with services;*
- *leaving the area before proper arrangements can be made; or*
- *sleeping rough.*

But it may not be used to restrict their freedom to come and go so much that they are effectively being detained.

26.30 *The power to require patients to reside in a particular place may not be used to require them to live in a situation in which they are deprived of liberty, unless that is authorised separately under the MCA. That authorisation will only be possible if the patient lacks capacity to decide where to live.'*

Such authorisation may be obtained from the Court of Protection or, depending on where the patient was required to live, via the Deprivation of Liberty Safeguards (DOLS) procedures in the revised Mental Capacity Act.

Comment

The introduction of the DOLS procedures as a result of the *HL* v. *UK* judgment has led to a labyrinthine system which seeks to provide a procedure prescribed by law for those cases of deprivation of liberty that fall outside the scope of Sections 2 and 3 of the Mental health Act. In effect, a new industry has grown up to meet the requirements of Article 5 of the European Convention of Human Rights. A simple change to guardianship to allow it to include cases of deprivation of liberty in the community would have avoided this expensive new structure. It would also not have limited the provision to residential and nursing homes and some would argue it would have provided more safeguards than the new system. Perhaps there will be a move to take this approach in the future when the full impact of DOLS has been felt.

Comparison of Community Treatment Orders (17A) with Guardianship (Section 7)

	Community Treatment Order	Guardianship
Existing status	No age limit but liable to detention on ss3, 37, 45A, 47 or 48	Aged at least 16
Mental disorder	Any mental disorder as defined in S1 except that for learning disability this needs to be associated with abnormally aggressive or seriously irresponsible conduct	Any mental disorder as defined in S1 except that for learning disability this needs to be associated with abnormally aggressive or seriously irresponsible conduct
Risk level	It is necessary for the patient's health or safety or for the protection of other persons that he should receive medical treatment	Guardianship is necessary in the interests of the welfare of the patient or for the protection of others
Application	RC	AMHP or Nearest Relative
Supported by?	AMHP	2 doctors
Who accepts?	Health authority	Local authority
Duration	6 m, 6 m, yearly	6 m, 6 m, yearly
Mental Health Tribunal	Patient or NR (for Part III CTOs) can apply	Patient can apply
Who can discharge?	RC, Tribunal or Hospital Managers & Nearest Relative for Part II CTOs	RC, Tribunal, Nearest Relative or the Local Authority
When does it end automatically?	If detained on Section 3 or placed in guardianship	If detained on Section 3
Requirements	Patient must see RC when extension of period is considered Must see SOAD if certificate under Part 4A is considered Other conditions may be specified	Reside where specified Attend for treatment etc. Grant access as authorised by the guardian
Power to convey?	Only if recalled to hospital	Yes. And power to return to required place of residence
Consent to Treatment rules?	Covered by Part 4A (and by Part IV if recalled)	Not covered by Part IV
Will S117 after-care apply?	Yes	Only if patient previously on S3, 37, 45A, 47 or 48
Covered by CPA	Yes	Yes

Comment

9 Patients concerned in criminal proceedings or under sentence

In this chapter, the following topics will be considered:

- detention at a police station
- court procedure
- disposal/sentencing.

Ultimately, nowadays, the aim of the criminal justice system is to try to divert away from the court system as many mentally disordered people as possible.

Criminal Responsibility

Criminal responsibility is a legal concept related to justice and determined adversarily. It begins at the age of 10 years in England and Wales (*doli incapax*) and technically 10 years in Scotland, although, confusingly, a child may not come before the Criminal Courts there until age 12 years (Criminal Justice and Licensing (Scotland) Act 2010). In the Republic of Ireland, it begins at 10 years of age. For the most serious offences, e.g. murder, but is 12 years for other offences (Children Act 2001 as amended by The Criminal Justice Act 2006). It is questionable how good psychiatrists are in judging responsibility, as opposed to clinically diagnosing mental disorder, which is key to their role.

Most offences require some form of intent (*mens rea*) as well as an unlawful act (*actus reus*). These offences are divided into those that require specific intent, such as murder, rape and arson, and those that require only basic intent. Some minor offences, such as motoring offences, do not require *mens rea*. Certain mental states interfere with the defendant's (patient's) intent and may give rise to defences in law to the offences.

Insanity has always been regarded as a defence in English law. For example, as mentioned in Chapter 1, a judge in King Alfred's time was hanged for having ordered the hanging of an insane man. By the early eighteenth century, for insanity to be a defence in law, it had to be such as to cause the subject to be like a 'wild beast', devoid of all reason and memory. However, in 1780, a soldier was acquitted of murder because he was found to be suffering from a delusion about the victim, as a result of insanity.

Mentally disordered offenders involved with the police courts

Police custody

Following an arrest, an individual may be:

- admitted informally to a psychiatric hospital; *or*
- detained compulsorily under civil sections of the Mental Health Act (*e.g.*, Sections 2, 3, 4 or 136); *and/or*
- cautioned by the police, so long as the individual accepts his guilt; *or*
- charged and taken to court (where the individual may be remanded on bail or into custody).

In any event, the police will check to determine whether the person is an absconding patient; if so, the police will return him to hospital under Section 18 (Return and readmission of patients absent without leave) or Section 138 (Retaking of patients escaping from custody).

Under the **Police and Criminal Evidence Act 1984** (PACE), there is a Code of Practice, Code C, which covers the detention, treatment and questioning of suspects not related to terrorism in police custody by police officers. This Code of Practice must be readily available at all police stations for consultation by:

- police officers
- police staff
- detained persons
- members of the public.

If an officer has any suspicion, or is told in good faith, that a person of any age may be mentally disordered or otherwise mentally vulnerable, in the absence of clear evidence to dispel that suspicion, the person shall be treated as such for the purposes of Code C.

If the custody officer authorises the detention of a person who is mentally vulnerable or appears to be suffering from a mental disorder, the custody officer must, as soon as practicable, inform 'the appropriate adult' of the grounds for detention and the person's whereabouts, and ask the appropriate adult to come to the police station to see him. The appropriate adult should be present while the individual is told his rights and can advise the person being interviewed, observe the fairness of the interview, and facilitate communication with the interviewee. In this context, 'the appropriate adult' means:

(a) a relative, guardian or other person responsible for the detainee's care or custody;
(b) someone experienced in dealing with mentally disordered or mentally vulnerable people but who is not a police officer or employed by the police;
(c) failing these, some other responsible adult aged 18 years or over who is not a police officer or employed by the police.

The detainee may also require the presence of a lawyer. If the appropriate adult, having been informed of the right to legal advice, considers legal advice should be taken, the appropriate provisions apply as if the mentally disordered or otherwise mentally vulnerable person had requested access to legal advice.

The custody officer must make sure a person receives appropriate clinical attention as soon as reasonably practicable if the person appears to be suffering from a mental disorder or, in urgent cases, immediately call the nearest healthcare professional or an ambulance.

Under Paragraph 3.16 of the revised Code C, it is imperative that a mentally disordered or otherwise mentally vulnerable person, detained under Section 136 of the Mental Health Act, be assessed as soon as possible. If that assessment takes place at a police station, then an approved mental health professional and a registered medical practitioner should be called to the police station as soon as possible in order to interview and examine the detainee. Once he has been interviewed and examined,.and suitable arrangements have been made for his treatment or care, he can no longer be detained under Section 136. A detainee must be immediately discharged from detention under Section 136 if a registered medical practitioner, having examined him, concludes that he is not mentally disordered within the meaning of the Act.

For summary only offences (i.e. those that can only be tried by a magistrate's court), a decision can be taken by the police to prosecute. Other more serious cases are passed to the Crown Prosecution Service (CPS), which will also consider the public interest and the likely adverse effects of prosecution of a mentally disordered individual. The principle applied is that people with mental health problems should be diverted from the courts in cases where the public interest does not require their prosecution. Box A summarises liaison by psychiatrists with the police and courts.

Box A: Police and court liaison

Terminology

- *Diversion or early diversion:* transfer to the healthcare system of a mentally disordered individual in police custody or at first court hearing.
- *Diversion or police or court diversion schemes:* specific psychiatric services provided to the police or courts, usually to a magistrate's court, where 98 per cent of offenders are tried. Such services reduce the time on remand in custody for mentally ill individuals but may not affect the long-term risk of offending. However, it is unlikely that serious offenders, such as those charged with murder, will be suitable for such diversion.

Psychiatric issues relevant to police and court liaison

- Evidence of mental disorder.
- Need for out- or in-patient psychiatric treatment.
- Urgency if in-patient psychiatric treatment required.
- Nature of alleged offence and risk to others.
- Fitness to remain in police custody.
- Fitness to be interviewed by police.
- Fitness to plead if individual is to appear in court.

Remember that the technical legal offence may not reflect the actual risk. For example, arson may be of a wastepaper bin in front of others on a busy hospital ward or committed with intent to endanger the lives of others in a tower block. Similarly, possession of an offensive weapon may have been with a view to seriously harming others.

Fitness to remain in police custody

- There is no legal definition.
- An individual may be unfit to remain in police custody due to physical illness or psychiatric disorder.
- Serious and immediate risk to an individual's health will usually make the individual unfit to remain in police custody. Detention under a civil section of the Mental Health Act may then be indicated.

Fitness to be interviewed by police

- There is no legal definition.
- The individual should be able to understand the police caution after it has been explained.
- Full orientation to time, place and person is required.
- Fitness may be questioned if the individual is likely to give answers due to their mental disorder that may be wrongly interpreted by the court.
- If the individual is fit to be interviewed but has a history of mental disorder, then an appropriate adult should be present. Such individuals can be provided by appropriate adult schemes.

False confessions (after Gudjonsson, 2003)

Three types of false confession have been described:

- *Voluntary*: e.g. due to depression or morbid guilt.
- *Coerced-compliant*: due to being pressurised during interrogation. Individuals often retract such false confessions after interrogation.
- *Coerced-internalised*: the individual becomes confused by interrogation and comes to believe the false story. This is seen particularly in people with learning disability.

In cases of possible suggestibility and false confessions:

- assess the individual's intellectual level;
- use the Gudjonsson Suggestibility Scale.

Court procedure

The presumption is normally in favour of remanding an individual on bail rather than in custody. Bail could include a condition of residence in a psychiatric hospital, although the individual would be an informal patient there unless otherwise detained under the Mental Health Act.

Where a person might otherwise be remanded to prison, the Mental Health Act allows for the following three possibilities:

- Remand to hospital for a report on the accused's mental condition, under Section 35.
- Remand of the accused person to hospital for treatment, under Section 36.
- Removal to hospital of other prisoners (including those on remand in custody), under Section 48.

At many magistrates' courts there are diversion teams in attendance on certain days. These teams are made up of a psychiatrist plus a community psychiatric nurse (CPN) and social worker (approved mental health professional) and are there to assess mentally disordered defendants. The benefit of these teams is that they allow defendants in custody to be assessed quickly and diverted into the mental health system if appropriate. The scheme also allows for the courts, the defence and prosecution to be appraised of a defendant's condition more quickly than may be the case otherwise.

Section 35: Remand to hospital for a report on the accused's mental condition

The court shall not remand an accused person to a hospital under Section 35 unless satisfied, on the written or oral evidence of the approved clinician who would be responsible for making the report, or of some other person representing the managers of the hospital, that arrangements have been made for his admission to that hospital and for his admission to it within the period of seven days beginning with the date of the order; and if the court is so satisfied it may, pending his admission, give directions for his conveyance to and detention in a place of safety. Subject to this proviso, this order can be made under Subsection (3) if:

(a) the court is satisfied, on the written or oral evidence of a registered medical practitioner, that there is reason to suspect the accused person is suffering from mental disorder; and
(b) the court is of the opinion that it would be impractical for a report on his mental condition to be made, if he were remanded on bail;

but those powers are not to be exercised by the Crown Court in respect of a person who has been convicted before the court, if the sentence for the offence of which he has been convicted is fixed by law, e.g. murder.

Thus, a hospital bed must be available within seven days. If awaiting a bed, the accused must be kept in a 'place of safety', e.g., 'police station, prison or remand centre or any hospital, the managers of which, are willing temporarily to receive him' (Section 55(1)).

The remand is for a maximum period of 28 days, although it is renewable for further periods of 28 days, without the need for the patient to attend court, up to a maximum of 12 weeks. Part IV provisions on Consent to Treatment do not apply, so an individual cannot be treated without their consent except in an emergency under common law. Some psychiatrists, therefore, additionally detain such individuals under Sections 2 or 3 when they wish to treat them without their consent and the Code of Practice states that this may be considered if there is a delay in getting to court. The use of Section 36, however, may then be more appropriate.

Section 36: Remand of the accused person to hospital for treatment

This may only be used by the Crown Court and is an alternative to remanding an accused person in custody. It can apply to those awaiting trial or sentence. It requires the written or oral evidence of two medical practitioners, that:

(a) the accused is suffering from mental disorder of a nature or degree which makes it appropriate for him to be detained in a hospital for medical treatment; and
(b) appropriate medical treatment is available for him.

It cannot be used for those charged with murder.

The remand is for a maximum of 28 days, although this may be renewed for further periods of 28 days, without the need for the patient to attend court, up to a maximum of 12 weeks. Part IV provisions of Consent to Treatment apply.

A hospital bed must be available within seven days and the individual must meanwhile be kept in a 'place of safety' (Section 55(1)).

Problems arise if an individual has to wait for more than the maximum 12 weeks of the order to appear in the Crown Court. In these circumstances, detention under a civil section or the use of Section 48 may be required.

Section 48: Removal to hospital of other prisoners

This section gives the Justice Secretary (Secretary of State, Ministry of Justice) powers to direct the removal to hospital of the following types of prisoner:

(a) persons detained in a prison or remand centre, not being persons serving a sentence of imprisonment;
(b) persons remanded in custody by a magistrates' court;
(c) civil prisoners, that is, persons committed by a court to prison for a limited term (who are not covered by Section 47);
(d) persons detained under the Immigration Act 1971 or under Section 62 of the Nationality, Immigration and Asylum Act 2002 (detention by Secretary of State).

The Justice Secretary requires two medical reports, which do not need to specify the availability of a bed at a particular hospital, stating that:

(a) that person is suffering from mental disorder of a nature or degree which makes it appropriate for him to be detained in a hospital for medical treatment; and
(b) he is in urgent need of such treatment; and
(c) appropriate medical treatment is available for him.

The period of detention is variable and can continue to the time of sentence. This order has been increasingly used to divert severely mentally disordered (psychotic) offenders from custody to hospital, even when the need may not be 'urgent'. It has the advantage that it does not require a court hearing to impose the order. On occasions, for instance when an acutely mentally ill offender has appeared in court, such an individual may only nominally be remanded to a named custodial facility and, by arrangement with the Ministry of Justice, is transferred directly to hospital without being actually placed in custody.

Mental Abnormality as a defence in court

In some cases, a person charged with an offence offers evidence of his mental disturbance either:

(a) to excuse his being tried (not fit to plead); or
(b) to agree to having done the act but not to have been fully responsible at the time (insane or diminished responsibility or automatism or infanticide).

Thus, in these cases, the psychiatric evidence is presented as part of the arguments to the court and is heard before conviction.

Unfit to Plead – Criminal Procedure (Insanity and Unfitness to Plead) Act 1991

A mentally disordered defendant may assert that he is unfit to plead (under 'disability' in relation to trial). This refers to the time of trial. The defendant would have to prove, using medical evidence, in a Crown Court hearing that he was not fit to do at least one of the following (based on the original test used in *R* v. *Pritchard* (1836)):

- instruct counsel ('so as to make a proper defence')
- appreciate the significance of pleading
- challenge a juror
- examine a witness
- understand and follow the evidence of court procedure.

Note that the defendant does *not* specifically have to be fit to give evidence himself, (although the ability to do so is often assessed), as it is the right of those in court not to have to give evidence.

If it appears that a defendant is unfit to plead but may, in time and with treatment, become fit, then the case is often adjourned to allow for improvement in the defendant's mental state. If, however, the defendant does not become fit, then the unfitness to plead procedure will have to be followed. If raised by the judge or the prosecution, this must be proved beyond reasonable doubt, but if raised by the defence, this only has to be proved on the balance of probabilities. This is a very rare plea and is only likely to be successful in cases such as severe mental impairment or for patients who are extremely paranoid, e.g. about the court or their legal representatives. Physical illness, e.g. pneumonia, may also result in unfitness to plead and stand trial.

If the individual is found unfit to plead, a decision for a Crown Court judge since the Domestic, Violence, Crime and Victims Act 2004 (see Box B), then there is a provision for a trial of facts. The Court will have to have evidence (written or oral) from at least two Section 12 Mental Health Act approved doctors before reaching their decision. If the defendant is fit to plead, then he will stand trial as normal in front of a jury. If a defendant is found unfit to plead, then there is a trial of the facts (Section 4A hearing), but only to determine whether or not the defendant committed the act alleged (*actus reus*) and not to consider the defendant's mental state (*mens rea*).

If found unfit to plead, and to have committed the act, then a defendant can be sentenced only to a hospital order, guardianship order, supervision and treatment order or absolute discharge.

Box B: Domestic Violence, Crime and Victims Act 2004

Provisions for unfitness to plead and insanity:

1. Judge rather than jury will determine fitness to plead.
2. Justice Secretary loses role in deciding whether defendant is admitted to hospital. Now a matter for Court.
3. Court can no longer order psychiatric hospital admission without medical evidence that justifies detention on grounds of mental disorder.
4. New range of disposals.

a. Section 37 Mental Health Act 1983 with or without a Restriction Order under Section 41. (Also Section 38 Interim Hospital Order.) N.B. Court can now require a hospital to admit.
b. Supervision Order for physical and/or mental disorder, but not as inpatient without consent.
c. Absolute Discharge.

Extension of Victim Contact Scheme to victims of mentally disordered offenders. Includes offenders:

- Transferred from prison to hospital
- Subject to Hospital Orders with Restriction Orders

Historically, the concept originates from dealing with deaf mutes. In medieval times, defendants were pressed under weights to give a plea, without which they could not be convicted or executed or their property given to the Exchequer; hence the phrase 'press for an answer'.

On rare occasions, one may be asked to help the court decide whether an offender who appears to be mute (i.e. there is no speech at all) is being **mute *'by malice or by visitation of God'***. If **mute *'by malice'***, the case proceeds with a not guilty plea entered on the defendant's behalf. If **mute *'by visitation of God'***, i.e. if deaf and dumb, the question of fitness to plead will arise with a view to disposal under the Criminal Procedure (Insanity and Unfitness to Plead) Act 1991.

In Scotland, individuals are found unfit to plead more commonly, including in cases where in England they would be convicted and detained under a Section 37 hospital order. Fitness to plead is also often a major issue in the USA where the term 'competency' is used.

Note that the unfit to plead procedure relates only to Crown Court cases; there is no such procedure in a magistrates' court. In less serious summary cases, which can only be tried by a magistrates' court, where there is evidence that the defendant is mentally disordered, then cases can be dealt with in the magistrates' court under Section 37(3) of the Mental Health Act. This procedure allows for the facts of an alleged offence (*actus reus*) to be proved so that the court is satisfied that the defendant did the act or made the omission charged, again without regard to the defendant's mental state at the time of the offence. If the defendant is proved to have committed the act, then he will be made the subject of a hospital order.

Criticism of the law based on the Pritchard Criteria includes it not adequately reflecting modern psychiatric thinking, its disproportionate emphasis on low-intellectual ability and a lack of emphasis on the accused's decision-making capacity. These criticisms have led to proposals for reform by the Law Commission which, at the time of writing, appear likely to be incorporated into law. It is proposed that the Pritchard Test be replaced by a test of decision-making capacity for meaningful participation in the trial. A new procedure for the Section 4A hearing to determine the facts of the case is also proposed, which would result in one of three possible outcomes:

1. A finding that the accused has done the act or made the omission for which charged and that there are no grounds for acquittal.
2. An outright acquittal.
3. An acquittal qualified by reason of mental disorder.

Not Guilty by Reason of Insanity ('Special Verdict'; Insanity Defence; McNaughton Rules) – Criminal Procedure (Insanity and Unfitness to Plead) Act 1991

Historically, this defence arose from the case of Daniel McNaughton in 1843. McNaughton, believing himself to be poisoned by Whigs, attempted to shoot the then Prime Minister Robert Peel, missed (or alternatively misidentified) and shot and killed Peel's secretary. Because McNaughton was deluded and insane, he was acquitted, but this caused a great deal of argument, including from Queen Victoria ('Insane he may be, but not guilty he is not'), and the law lords were asked to issue guidance for the courts in response to five questions. Their guidance is known as the McNaughton Rules.

In this defence, the offender is arguing that he is not guilty (not deserving of punishment) by reason of his insanity. It has to be proved to a court, on the balance of probabilities, that *at the time of the offence*, the offender laboured under such defect of reason that he met the McNaughton Rules, i.e.:

1. That by reason of such defect from disease of the mind, he did not know the nature or quality of his act (this means the physical nature of the act), *or*
2. He did not know that what he was doing was wrong (forbidden by law).
3. If an individual was suffering from a delusion, then his actions would be judged by their relationship to the delusion, i.e. if he believed his life to be immediately threatened, then he would be justified in striking out, but not otherwise.

Technically, this plea may be put forward for any offence but, in practice, it is put forward usually only for murder or other serious offences. In fact, such a plea is rare.

Evidence from two or more medical practitioners, one of whom is approved under Section 12 of the Mental Health Act, is required before the return of the verdict not guilty by reason of insanity. Such a verdict implies lack of intent. However, a psychiatrist can only give evidence regarding an individual's capacity to form intent (a legal concept), not the fact of intent at the time of the offence.

Under the Criminal Procedure Act 1991, if the defendant is found not guilty by reason of insanity, the judge has freedom to decide on the sentencing and disposal of the defendant, i.e. discretionary sentencing, including detention in hospital under forensic treatment orders of the Mental Health Act.

Diminished Responsibility

As a reaction against the fact that mentally disordered people who had killed were still being hanged despite the McNaughton rules, a movement was created to bring in a defence of diminished responsibility, i.e. the responsibility of the offender is not totally absent because of mental abnormality but is only partially impaired; therefore, the offender would be found guilty but the sentence modified. This was made law in the **Homicide Act 1957** and applies only to a charge of murder. The murder charge is reduced to manslaughter on the grounds of diminished responsibility.

Under the 1957 Homicide Act (Section 2), as a defence against the charge (only) of murder, the offender could plead that at the time of the offence he had diminished responsibility. Section 2(1) states that:

'where a person kills or is party to a killing of another, he shall not be convicted of murder if he was suffering from such abnormality of mind (whether arising from a condition of arrested or retarded development of mind or any inherent causes or induced by disease or injury) as substantially impaired his mental responsibility for his acts and omissions in doing or being a party to the killing.'

Section 2(1) of the Homicide Act 1957 has been amended by the Coroners and Justice Act 2009, Section 52 (Persons suffering from diminished responsibility (England and Wales)), Subsection 1, which states (bold added):

In Section 2 of the Homicide Act 1957 (c. 11) (persons suffering from diminished responsibility), for Subsection (1) substitute:

'(1) *A person ("D") who kills or is a party to the killing of another is not to be convicted of murder if D was suffering from an* ***abnormality of mental functioning*** *which:*
- (a) *arose from a* **recognised medical condition,**
- (b) ***substantially impaired*** *D's ability to do one or more of the things mentioned in Subsection (1A), and*
- (c) ***provides an explanation*** *for D's acts and omissions in doing or being a party to the killing.*

(1A) *Those things are:*
- (a) *to understand the nature of D's conduct;*
- (b) *to form a rational judgment;*
- (c) *to exercise self-control.*

(1B) *For the purposes of Subsection (1)(c), an abnormality of mental functioning provides an explanation for D's conduct if it causes, or is a significant contributory factor in causing, D to carry out that conduct.'*

Note that the reference to a *recognised medical condition* is more medically based than the previous reasonable man test of what is abnormal and there must now be a direct causal relationship between it and the offence. It is now a capacity test. The government refused to accept the Law Commission's proposal that developmental immaturity alone could be a cause of abnormality of mental functioning.

Section 5 of the Criminal Justice Act (Northern Ireland) 1966 (c. 20) (effect, in cases of homicide, of impaired mental responsibility) has been amended in a similar way by the Coroners and Justice Act 2009, Section 53 (Persons suffering from diminished responsibility (Northern Ireland)), Subsection 2.

Abnormality of mental functioning

'Abnormality of mental functioning' is left to the defendant (or his medical advisers) to define, and is not synonymous with mental disorder as defined in the Mental Health Act. It does not itself have to be severe. Indeed it can be mild, e.g. an adjustment reaction, and can include personality disorder. It is a more dynamic concept than the previous *abnormality of mind*. It has been ruled in the Court of Appeal that the previous 'abnormality of mind' would have affected at the time of the offence the individual's perception, judgement (between right and wrong, between good and bad) and/or the voluntary control of (capacity to control, a legal concept) his actions. Thus, abnormality of mind was:

> *'A state of mind so different from that of the ordinary human beings that the reasonable man, earlier defined as 'a man with a normal mind,' would term it abnormal. It appears to us to be wide enough to cover the mind's activities in all its aspects, not only the perception of physical acts and matters, and the ability to form a rational judgement as to whether the act was right or wrong, but also the ability to exercise will power to control physical acts in accordance with that rational judgement.'*
>
> (R. v. *Byrne* (1960))

The authoritative interpretation of the term 'abnormality of mind' was given by Lord Parker (R. v. *Byrne* (1960)) as follows:

> *'Whether the accused was at the time of killing suffering from "any abnormality of mind" in the broad sense in which we have indicated above is a question for the jury. On this question medical evidence is, no doubt, important, but the jury are entitled to take into consideration all the evidence including the acts or statements of the accused and his demeanour. They are not bound to accept the medical evidence, if there is other material before them which, in their good judgement, conflicts with it and outweighs it. The aetiology of the abnormality of mind (namely, whether it arose from a condition of arrested or retarded development of mind or any inherent causes or was induced by disease or injury) does, however, seem to be a matter to be determined on expert evidence...'*

Substantially

'Substantially' is also undefined and is theoretically left to the jury to decide, though the Court of Appeal has ruled that doctors may give their opinion. This is the key issue in the defence as any abnormality of mental functioning can be mild.

> *'Substantial does not mean total...At the other end [it] does not mean minimal or trivial. It is something in between.'*
>
> (R. v. *Lloyd* (1966))

Successful plea

The effect of a successful plea is to reduce the charge from murder to manslaughter. Murder carries a statutory sentence of life imprisonment, but the court is free to make any sentence at all with regard to manslaughter, including a hospital or a community rehabilitation (old probation) order or, indeed, a life prison sentence, in which case such individuals may spend longer in custody than those convicted of murder (Dell 1984). The verdict 'unties the judge's hands'. In addition to a report supporting the plea of diminished responsibility, the psychiatrist may also, if appropriate, wish to arrange for the appropriate hospital treatment and offer the appropriate section recommendations to the court to help them with their sentencing.

Use

The diminished responsibility defence has been used where a defence of insanity would have no hope of success. Examples include:

- mercy killing;
- when the subject kills his spouse in a state of reactive depression;

- individuals who kill in jealous frenzies;
- individuals who are subject to an 'irresistible impulse' to kill;
- those who kill who are 'deranged' by psychopathic disorder.

The diminished responsibility defence has largely replaced the insanity defence in England and Wales for individuals charged with murder. However, the number of successful diminished responsibility pleas has reduced in recent years to a range of 13–35 per year, reflecting a less sympathetic view by the courts (and probably society) to this group of mentally abnormal offenders. Those who commit multiple homicides now rarely succeed in making this plea.

Retrospective mental state assessment for the time of the offence

The psychiatrist carries out a retrospective mental state examination for the time of the offence when assessing if the defendant is not guilty by reason of insanity (McNaughton Rules) or if diminished responsibility applies. In the McNaughton Rules, the legal concept used is *disease of mind*. In Diminished Responsibility, the legal concept used is *abnormality of mental functioning*. From case law:

- mental functioning = reason, memory, understanding
- disease = organic/functional, permanent/temporary, treatable/not treatable, is 'internal' (*R* v. *Quick* (1973)) and/or 'manifests in violence and is prone to recur' (*Bratty* v. *A.G.* in Northern Ireland (1961)). It can also include epilepsy (*R.* v. *Sullivan* (1983)).

Criticism of McNaughton Rules and Diminished Responsibility

McNaughton Rules

These rules are now almost obsolete. Points against them include the following:

- Hardly anybody is mad enough to fit the rules (Lord Bramwell). Even McNaughton would not have been.
- The rules assume a doctrine that mind is made up of separate independent compartments, of which cognition is most important (a Victorian view).
- The rules are too unfair, as abnormal mental states do not fit into rigid categories.
- The rules ignore the importance of emotional disturbance and failure of will when cognition is normal.

Diminished responsibility

The most important points in favour of this are:

- It allows for an overall assessment of the person.
- It leads to more flexible sentencing.

Against diminished responsibility are the following points:

- There is a problem of balancing the concept of responsibility with 'determinism', e.g. does a greater propensity to lose one's temper imply less responsibility?
- It assumes that a distinction can be made between psychopathy and wickedness in terms of moral or criminal responsibility.

- Does diminished responsibility mean less power to resist temptation? If so, should the irresponsible be punished less than the responsible?
- Does an irresponsible act in a normally responsible person indicate a greater aberration of mind than irresponsible behaviour in the irresponsible?
- If a person is found to have diminished responsibility, then it may mean that the court will return such a person to society faster than the responsible offender.

In fact, those who are given a custodial sentence following a successful plea of diminished responsibility (Dell 1984) spend longer in custody than those convicted of murder, who serve a mean of 11.5 years before being released on life licence. This may reflect concern that while abnormality of mental functioning was identified in these cases of diminished responsibility, no ameliorating treatment of it was undertaken, for example, in hospital, if the individual received a life prison sentence.

Automatism

This is a rare plea generally restricted (though not entirely) to cases of homicide. The defendant pleads that at the time of the offence his behaviour was automatic (no *mens rea*, a total absence of mind). The law uses this term to mean a state almost near unconsciousness. It refers to unconscious, involuntary, non-purposeful acts where the mind is not conscious of what the body is doing. There is a separation between the will and the act, or the mind and the act ('Mind does not go with what is being done.' *Bratty* v. *A.G.* in Northern Ireland (1961)). Of note, in Canada automatism is considered to be a total absence of control.

- Automatism has been pleaded successfully, particularly in cases of homicide, for offences occurring during hypoglycaemic attacks, sleepwalking and sleep, e.g. fighting tigers and snakes in dreams (theoretically, this should be during night terrors in slow-wave sleep, since during dreams involving complex visual images one should be paralysed in rapid-eye movement sleep, but it has been argued that such offences may occur as an individual wakes from a dream). Such must be the degree of automatism that there is no capacity to form any intent to kill or any capacity to control actions.

In certain cases, e.g. offending while sleepwalking, the accused has walked free from the court on the understanding that he will always lock his bedroom door when sleeping.

Where a defence of *non-insane automatism* is put forward, the subject is hoping to receive a total acquittal. However, the law has become aware that some automatism states are really the result, in the legal sense, of a disease of the mind, e.g. epilepsy, which may recur. Therefore, in such cases, the jury may be invited to consider that the defence of automatism should be regarded as evidence of insanity (*insane automatism*) and to return a special verdict of 'not guilty by reason of insanity', which would allow for discretionary sentencing, including detention in hospital.

While, historically, sleepwalking and night terrors have been accepted as automatisms and have led to acquittal, case law (Lord Justice Lawton) now differentiates *non-insane automatism due to external causes*, e.g. hypoglycaemia caused by insulin, from *insane automatism due to disease of the mind caused by mental illness or brain disease (intrinsic factors)*, e.g. diabetes, epilepsy and even hysterical dissociative fugue states, in which a special verdict of 'not guilty by reason of insanity' should be returned.

Homicide

Definition

Homicide is the killing of another human being. It is not necessarily unlawful.

Epidemiology

There have been around 600–700 homicides each year in England and Wales during the first decade of the twenty-first century. These have included certain exceptional events: the year 2000–01 included 58 Chinese nationals who suffocated in a lorry en route in the UK; the year 2003–04 included 20 cockle pickers who drowned in Morecambe Bay; the year 2005–06 included 52 victims of the 7th July London bombings. A peak during 2002–03 included 172 of the victims of the convicted English serial killer Harold Shipman, a general practitioner who is believed to have murdered over 200 mainly elderly patients; these murders took place before the first decade of the twenty-first century, with Shipman's trial beginning in October 1999.

For the year 2009–10 there were 619 deaths recorded as homicide in England and Wales; the risk of being a victim of homicide in England and Wales was 11 per million of the population; children under the age of one year were the most at-risk age group (33 offences per million population); 68 per cent of victims were male; the most common method of killing was by sharp instrument (34 per cent for 2009–10); female victims were more likely to be killed by someone they knew, with 76 per cent of female victims having known the main suspect, compared with a figure of 50 per cent of male victims; 75 per cent of victims aged under 16 years knew the main suspect (Smith et al., 2011).

Legal classification

Homicide may be lawful or unlawful.

Lawful homicide

Lawful homicide may be:

- justifiable, e.g. on behalf of state – such as actions by the army and police;
- excusable, e.g. a pure accident, an honest or reasonable mistake.

Unlawful homicide

Unlawful homicide is the unlawful killing of any reasonable creature in being and under the Queen's (or King's) Peace. Types of unlawful homicide include:

- murder
- manslaughter
- child destruction
- genocide
- causing death by dangerous driving
- suicide pacts
- infanticide.

Some of these are considered further here.

Murder

Murder is an offence at common law. It is defined as an unlawful killing with *malice aforethought*. Malice aforethought requires either an intention to kill or cause grievous bodily harm. Murder, like any other crime requiring proof of intent, involves proof of a subjective state of mind on the part of the accused. The *actus reus* of murder consists of both of the following:

- an unlawful act
- the act causes the death of another human being.

Murder results in a mandatory life sentence of imprisonment. In England and Wales, an average of 11.5 years is served in prison, and then the prisoner is released on life licence. A few murderers do serve life.

Manslaughter

Manslaughter may be categorised into three groups, namely:

- voluntary manslaughter
- involuntary manslaughter
- corporate liability.

The third of these is on the increase in terms of prosecutions but will not be considered further here.

Voluntary manslaughter

These are cases of homicide in which the defendant would be guilty of murder if it were not for the availability of one of the following partial defences:

- Diminished responsibility (Section 2 Homicide Act 1957 amended by Section 52 of the Coroners and Justice Act 2009).
- Provocation (originally Section 3 Homicide Act 1957) is the sudden or temporary loss of control under provocation that might make a normal person kill. Whether this occurred is for the jury to decide, although a psychiatrist's opinion may be requested. More recently, psychiatric evidence about the propensity of individuals with certain vulnerable personalities or conditions, such as learning disability, to be provoked has been accepted as admissible. Following criticism that this defence was used inappropriately by those who kill after losing their temper and that it is not sufficiently tailored to those who kill out of fear of serious violence, e.g. those subject to prolonged domestic violence, this defence has been replaced in the Coroners and Justice Act (2009) with a new partial defence for those who kill in response to:

    (a) fear of serious violence; and/or
    (b) having a justified sense of being seriously wronged.

- Killing in pursuance of a suicide pact (which the offender has to prove) (Section 4 Homicide Act 1957). A suicide pact is defined as being a common agreement between two or more persons having for its object the death of all of them, whether or not each is to take his or her own life.

Involuntary manslaughter

Involuntary manslaughter refers to cases of homicide without malice aforethought. It can take several forms, including:

- an unlawful and dangerous act – '*constructive manslaughter*': the *actus reus* consists of an unlawful act which is dangerous and causes death;
- gross negligence: the *actus reus* consists of a breach of a duty of care that the accused owes to the victim, with the result that this breach leads to the victim's death.

Infanticide

Under the **Infanticide Acts 1922 and 1938** (Section 1), infanticide is defined as having occurred when a woman by any wilful act caused the death of her child under the age of 12 months, but at the time of the act or omission, the balance of her mind was 'disturbed by reason of her not being fully recovered completely from the effect of giving birth to the child or the effect of lactation consequent upon the birth of the child'. This is technically an offence rather than a defence.

The grounds for this plea, as an alternative to murder, are less stringent than those for diminished responsibility (i.e. there is no need to prove abnormality of mental functioning), nor do they require proof of a mental disorder, e.g. mental illness. It is the policy of the Director of Public Prosecutions (DPP) and the Crown Prosecution Service (CPS) to use this plea for such mothers. It does not apply to adopted children or to any child other than the youngest (otherwise a manslaughter plea has to be used), as it is possible to have two children born within one year.

When originally introduced, many such mothers had acute organic confusional puerperal psychoses. Now few do and infanticide is rather an historical anachronism. Now about one in six have functional puerperal psychoses. The rest are not dissimilar from those who batter their children. It usually results in a sentence of a community rehabilitation order (previously probation), often with a condition of psychiatric treatment (out-patient or in-patient).

Amnesia

Amnesia is not in itself a defence – the underlying condition may be, for example, a post-traumatic state, epileptic fits, or acute psychosis. In the 1959 Podola Appeal case (Podola's amnesia was, in fact, not genuine), it was ruled that even if amnesia is genuine, it is no bar to trial.

Amnesia may be feigned by lying or caused by:

- hysterical amnesia (denial)
- failure of registration owing to over-arousal
- alcohol
- other psychoactive drugs
- head injury.

Between 40 and 50 per cent of those charged with homicide claim amnesia for the actual act.

Drugs and alcohol

It has always been considered that a person is fully responsible for their actions if they knowingly took such substances (voluntary intoxication). It is assumed that everyone knows that drunkenness is associated with aggressive and irresponsible behaviour and therefore one is responsible for not becoming drunk. The same argument applies to drug abuse. This would not apply if an individual were 'slipped' drugs or alcohol, or if their doctor did not inform them of side-effects and interactions (e.g. with alcohol) of medication, e.g. of benzodiazepines which, in particular, have been cited by shoplifters as a defence, although almost never are the cause alone of shoplifting. Such issues may also arise following the consumption of over-the-counter medications such as cold cures and nose drops, which may, for instance, contain ephedrine.

Successful defences have been based on:

- being so drunk as to be incapable of forming intent in offences requiring specific intent;
- developing a mental illness, e.g. psychosis, as the result of the ingestion of a drug or alcohol (as in delirium tremens), and acting under the influence of such a mental illness, which may allow the defence of not guilty by reason of insanity or diminished responsibility;
- where the use of a drug, which might be quite legitimate, produces a mental state abnormality which could not have been anticipated by the subject, e.g. hypoglycaemia after the use of insulin. For such an abnormal mental state to be used as a defence successfully, it must be shown that the accused took reasonable precautions (for instance, in the case of insulin, not to become hypoglycaemic), and yet these precautions failed. In one case, a man, who had drunk 12 pints of beer before an offence, successfully cited the effect of consuming a large amount of fluid as the precipitating cause of his mental state, rather than the alcohol. It was demonstrated that his electroencephalographic recording became disturbed when he drank 12 pints of water and it was argued that the fluid itself, and not the alcohol, had been the cause of his abnormality.

Thus, overall, successful defences following consumption of alcohol or drugs are based on either (i) involuntary intoxication, or (ii) if voluntarily intoxicated, lack of specific intent where offences require this.

Note that the term pathological intoxication (used in ICD-10) refers to a sudden onset of aggression and often violent behaviour, not typical of an individual when sober, very soon after drinking amounts of alcohol (only) that would not produce intoxication in most people.

Sentencing

Courts are bound in Section 157 of the Criminal Justice Act 2003, when sentencing mentally disordered offenders, to obtain a medical report before passing a sentence other than one fixed by law. Disposals (disposal being the legal term for a sentence in such circumstances) available under the Mental Health Act are detailed in Table 9.1 and include:

- hospital order – Section 37
- interim hospital order – Section 38
- restriction order – Section 41
- guardianship order – Section 37
- hospital and limitation directions – Section 45a.

Note a person cannot receive such hospital disposals unless the offence is punishable by imprisonment. The mental disorder requiring in-patient medical treatment does not need to be directly connected to the offence.

Table 9.1 Forensic Treatment Orders for Mentally Abnormal Offenders

	Grounds	Made by	Medical recommendation	Maximum duration	Eligibility for appeal to First Tier Tribunal (Mental Health)
Section 35: Remand to hospital for report	Mental Disorder	Magistrates' or Crown Court	Any doctor	28 days. Renewable at 28-day intervals. Maximum 12 weeks	None
Section 36: Remand to hospital for treatment	Mental Disorder. **(Not if charged with murder)**	Crown Court	Two doctors: one approved under Section 12	28 Days. Renewable at 28-day intervals. Maximum 12 weeks	None
Section 37: (Hospital and Guardianship Orders) (Section 37(3): without conviction)	Mental Disorder. Accused or convicted of an imprisonable offence	Magistrates' or Crown Court	Two doctors: one approved under Section 12	6 months. Renewable for further six months and then annually	During second six months. Then every year. Mandatory every 3 years
Section 41: Restriction Order	Added to Section 37. To protect public from serious harm	Crown Court	Oral evidence from one doctor	Usually without limit of time. Effect: leave, transfer or discharge only with consent from Justice Secretary	As Section 37
Section 38: Interim Hospital Order	Mental Disorder. To establish if Section 37 order is appropriate	Magistrates' or Crown Court	Two doctors: one approved under Section 12	12 weeks. Renewable at 28-day intervals. Maximum 12 months	None
Section: 47 Transfer of sentenced prisoner to hospital	Mental Disorder	Justice Secretary (Secretary of State, Ministry of Justice)	Two doctors: one approved under Section 12	Until earliest date of release (EDR) from sentence	Once in the first six months. Then once in the next six months. Thereafter, once a year
Section: 48 Urgent transfer to hospital of remand prisoner	Mental Disorder	Justice Secretary (Secretary of State, Ministry of Justice)	Two doctors: one approved under Section 12	Until date of trial or sentence	Once in the first six months. Then once in the next six months. Thereafter, once a year
Section 49 Restriction Direction	Added to Section 47 or Section 48	Justice Secretary (Secretary of State, Ministry of Justice)	—	Until end of Section 47 or 48. Effect: leave, transfer or discharge only with consent of Justice Secretary	As for Sections 47 and 48 to which applied

In addition, a community rehabilitation order (previously probation) with a condition of psychiatric treatment, if accepted by the offender, is available.

Each of these is now considered in turn.

Section 37: Hospital order

This may be made by the Crown Court or a magistrates' court, the latter being able to make such an order without conviction in the case of summary offences (i.e. those that can only be tried in a magistrates' court) under Section 37(3) so long as the court is satisfied that the offender committed the act or omission in question. The individual has to be charged with an imprisonable offence, not just any offence.

For this sentence to be made, a hospital bed must be available within 28 days, beginning from the date of the order. The patient, meanwhile, must be kept in a 'place of safety' (Section 55(1)). The availability of a bed within 28 days and the evidence of two registered medical practitioners, at least one of whom is approved under Section 12 of the Mental Health Act, are essential before the court can impose such an order.

Section 38: Interim Hospital Order

If the court is uncertain that a full Section 37 hospital order is appropriate, this can be tested out by making an interim hospital order. It can be made for up to 12 weeks in the first instance and then renewed by the court for periods of up to 28 days at a time to a maximum of one year. The patient does not have to attend court in person when the order is renewed.

This order is also useful for psychiatrists who are uncertain as to whether the individual's mental disorder is going to be amenable to psychiatric treatment, as may, for example, occur in cases of personality disorder.

If, in the end, a Section 37 hospital order is not considered appropriate, the court can use its discretion to otherwise sentence the individual, including to prison.

Section 41: Restriction order

Section 41(1) states:

> *'Where a hospital order is made in respect of an offender by the Crown Court, and it appears to the court, having regard to the nature of the offence, the antecedents of the offender and the risk of him committing further offences if set at large, that it is necessary for the protection of the public from serious harm so to do, the court may, subject to the provisions of this section, further order the offender shall be subject to special restrictions set out in this section; and an order under this section shall be known as "a restriction order"'.*

Note that magistrates' courts can commit a case to the Crown Court for imposition of a restriction order and under Section 44 direct the offender be detained in hospital meanwhile.

Since the amending Mental Health Act 2007, a restriction order can no longer be made for a fixed period of time as opposed to 'without limit of time'. This reflects the reality of the therapeutic uncertainty of how quickly an individual will progress. One of the two doctors recommending Section 37 must attend court to give evidence, but it is for the Court to decide if a Section 41 restriction order should be imposed. The main restrictions are that the patient can only be absolutely or conditionally discharged, given leave of absence or transferred to another hospital with the approval of the Justice Secretary. A restriction order, therefore, is an added safeguard, so that the decision to discharge, etc., is not left to the responsible clinician alone. A First Tier Tribunal (Mental Health) hearing can order an absolute or conditional discharge, or a deferred conditional discharge pending the conditions being in place. It can only recommend leave or hospital transfer.

If conditionally discharged, the usual conditions relate to supervision, residence, and medical treatment. The main advantage of this order for professionals is that it facilitates the long-term management of mentally abnormal serious offenders by specifying the conditions of their discharge (such as place of residence, e.g. a supervised hostel, and compliance with psychiatric treatment, including medication) upon threat of recall to hospital.

If recalled to hospital, the individual is subject to a mandatory First Tier Tribunal (Mental Health) hearing within the first six months.

Section 37: Guardianship order

The grounds are as for a Section 37 hospital order. It is used rarely. A proposed guardian (the local authority social services or a named individual) must agree to it. If the patient absconds from a place where they are required to live, they may be recaptured and returned there. There are, however, no effective sanctions for a patient refusing to co-operate with psychiatric treatment (such as medication), although attendance to see a psychiatrist can be enforced. Consent provisions for those detained in hospital under the Mental Health Act do not apply.

It was hoped in the Butler Report (Home Office and Department of Health and Social Security 1975) that this order might be increasingly used, but many social services departments are reluctant to use this order for mentally abnormal offenders, although, again, it can facilitate the management of a mentally abnormal offender in the community.

Section 45A: Hospital and limitation directions

This was brought in by the **Crime (Sentences) Act 1997** (*see* Table 9.2) on 1st October 1997. It is referred to as the 'hybrid order', as it is a prison sentence accompanied by hospital and limitation (equivalent to a restriction order) directions. It is only available to the Crown Court and, currently, for persons over age 21 years suffering from mental disorder (previously, prior to the amending of the Mental Health Act 2007, it was for psychopathic disorders only).

Table 9.2 Mentally disordered offenders and the Crime (Sentences) Act 1997

1	Mandatory life sentence for second 'serious offence' (attempted murder, manslaughter, rape, attempted rape) unless exceptional circumstances (which do not include mental disorder alone)
2	Hospital direction and limitation directions (equivalent to restriction order) for mental disorder
3	Transfers to hospital Court and Home Secretary specify unit Justice Secretary's consent required for transfer of restricted patients between hospitals, even if in the same Trust
4	Interim hospital order Maximum duration extended from 6 months to 1 year Can use before a hospital direction

Written or oral evidence from two doctors are required and appropriate treatment must be available.

Community rehabilitation orders with a condition of psychiatric treatment

Under Section 41 of the Powers of the Courts (Sentencing) Act 2000, community rehabilitation orders can be made in any court for any offence, other than one with a fixed penalty (such as murder, which carries a mandatory life prison sentence), but they do require conviction. Supervision by a probation officer is for a specified period between six months and three years.

In cases where there is a condition of psychiatric treatment, the court will require evidence from a doctor approved under Section 12 of the Mental Health Act. Conditions may include that the subject receive treatment as an in-patient or in a nursing home and/or as an out-patient at a specified hospital or place from or under the direction of a named doctor.

The court must explain the requirements of the order to the offender and obtain the offender's consent. If the individual subsequently refuses to co-operate with psychiatric treatment, the doctor can only report this to the supervising probation officer, who may take proceedings on these grounds for breach of the community rehabilitation order. Detention in hospital under the civil provisions of the Mental Health Act may be an alternative disposal, if appropriate, in such circumstances, but it would not constitute a formal court sentence.

After sentencing

Transfer direction from prison: Section 47 of the Mental Health Act

This allows the Secretary of State to order the transfer of a sentenced prisoner following conviction if he is suffering from a mental disorder. The patient is subject to consent to treatment provisions. This order can continue until the earliest date of release, whereupon a notional Section 37 hospital order automatically follows without the need for further completion of legally required medical recommendation reports. Almost inevitably, a restriction direction is also made under Section 49, which has the same effect as a restriction order under Section 41. Such individuals can be returned to prison to complete a sentence before their earliest date of release, for example, if they recover from their mental illness or they no longer require in-patient treatment. Individuals most frequently transferred from prison on this order are those who either develop mental illness during a prison sentence or where the mental illness was missed at the time of sentence.

Forensic psychiatric assessment

See Table 9.3.

Table 9.3 Forensic psychiatric assessment

1	Full history and mental state examination of patient, including exploration of fantasies and impulses to offend
2	Objective account of offence, e.g. from arresting police officer or from statements (despositions) in Crown Court cases
3	Objective accounts of past offences, if any, e.g. obtain list of previous convictions
4	Additional information gathering, such as interviews with informants, e.g. relatives, reading a pre-sentence report from a probation officer, if prepared
5	Review of previous psychiatric records, e.g. to ascertain relationship of mental disorder to previous behaviour and response to psychiatric treatment and need for security

Psychiatric expert evidence

See Table 9.4.

Table 9.4 Psychiatric expert evidence

Fitness to plead
Mental responsibility, e.g. not guilty by reason of insanity, diminished responsibility
Mental disorder, e.g. mental illness, learning disability, personality disorder
Is the client treatable?
Have arrangements been made for such treatment, e.g. community rehabilitation (previously probation) order, personality disorder with condition of out-patient treatment, or in-patient treatment under Section 37 of the Mental Health Act 1983?
Is the client dangerous? e.g. Section 41 Mental Health Act 1983, placement in a special hospital
Suggestions about non-psychiatric management, e.g. probation order, supervised hostel

Psychiatric court reporting

See Table 9.5

Table 9.5 Psychiatric court reporting

A report may be requested:

- By a court (magistrates', Crown or higher), usually through the probation service. Written authorisation by the court must be given
- By the defence solicitors, in which case the patient's written permission is required before giving a report to the solicitor, which remains their property to use or not in court

Information required for a report includes:

- A social enquiry report from a probation officer
- A list of previous convictions
- Previous medical hospital records
- Previous reports (social and medical)
- Depositions where available, e.g. for crown court, but not magistrates' cases

The history will be taken from the patient and, if possible, a relative or friend.
The client should ideally be examined fully physically.
Questions that the court or solicitor will be particularly interested in include the following:

- Does he or she have a mental disorder?
- Is it susceptible to or requiring specific treatment?
- Can arrangements be made for such treatment, e.g. hospital, out-patient?
- Is the client dangerous?
- Have you any suggestions as to the client's management, apart from the psychiatric aspects?

After interview and examination of other reports, etc., one can valuably discuss the case again with the probation officer or others, such as other psychiatrists involved in the case:

- Discuss particularly your findings and compare them with other professionals' observations, which may reveal gross discrepancies
- Discussion may reveal unexpected channels for disposal or unforeseen difficulties

The general principles of the written report are as follows:

- It should be in clear English, and technical terms should be avoided if possible. If such terms are used, an explanation of them should be given, e.g. paranoid (persecutory) delusions (false beliefs), auditory and visual hallucinations (voices and visions)
- Use the report to help the court reach the most appropriate disposal for the patient
- The report is a recommendation to the court. The court may have other psychiatric opinions that oppose yours and may itself be unconvinced by your opinion. Thus, the onus is on you to provide the evidence in the report for your opinion
- The onus is also on the reporting doctor to make all the necessary medical arrangements for the disposal and management of the patient
- Be accurate, complete and brief. The court is extremely busy and will resent a turgid, overwritten report. For magistrates' courts, which may deal with dozens of cases a day, around two pages may suffice; even then, only the opinion may be read

People use different forms for their report, but the following is suggested. Paragraph numbers and headings can be used for clarity:

Para 1 – Introduction: inform the court of when and where the patient was seen, and at whose request, what information was available, who the informants were, and sometimes what information was not available. State the current offence(s) for which the patient is charged and its date(s), and the plea if known, i.e. guilty or not guilty

Para 2 – Past medical history: inform the court of this and of the result of any medical examination, e.g. 'Physical examination revealed no abnormality'

Para 3 – Family history: report the important, relevant points, including family history, or not, of psychiatric disorder and criminality

Para 4 – Personal history: report the important points of the patient's physical development (e.g. birth, milestones), early development (e.g. bedwetting (enuresis)), schooling (e.g. truancy) and occupational history (e.g. difficulties with a job, sackings, sustaining employment, difficulties with colleagues or supervisors at work)

Para 5 – Sexual history: be reasonably discreet. The report may be read in open court

Para 6 – Previous personality: report details of personality in terms of social interaction, emotions and habits, e.g. drinking, gambling, drugs

Para 7 – Past forensic history: technically, past convictions should not be admissible before conviction, but they are admissible when the report is to assist sentencing. In practice, usually only one psychiatric report is prepared for both trial and sentencing

Para 8 – Past psychiatric history: report dates, diagnosis, relevant details and relationship of mental disorder and treatment to offending

Para 9 – Circumstances surrounding index offence(s): report the circumstances leading to current offence(s) and the defendant's state of mind at the time of the offence(s), sticking to the phenomena reported, e.g. 'for the time of the offence, the patient gives a history of tearfulness, loss of hope, poor sleeping… These are symptoms of a depressive mental illness'

Para 10 – Interview: report the result of the interview, e.g. 'the patient showed/did not show evidence of mental illness'. Then give a brief outline of the evidence, e.g. 'the patient muttered and looked around the room as though hearing voices (auditory hallucinations)', or list the symptoms and say, for example, 'these are symptoms of the severe mental illness of schizophrenia'.

Information in Paragraphs 1–10 should be factual, verifiable and ideally agreed by all, even if others' opinions differ from your own.

Para 11 – Opinion: the final paragraph should express your opinion. The court will be interested particularly in your opinion regarding the following:

- Is the individual fit to plead and stand trial?
- Does the individual have a mental disorder as defined in the Mental Health Act 1983?
- Where appropriate, comment on issues of responsibility, e.g. not guilty by reason of insanity, diminished responsibility, in cases of homicide.
- If so, can arrangements be made for the patient's treatment (sort this out if you can)? Make suggestions to the court about which disposal would be appropriate, e.g. Section 37 hospital order with or without a Section 41 restriction order, or out-patient psychiatric treatment as a condition of a Community Rehabilitation (old probation) order.

For example:

This man is fit to plead and stand trial.

In my opinion he suffers from a mental disorder as defined in the Mental Health Act 1983, the severe mental illness of schizophrenia, characterised by delusions (false beliefs) of passivity (being externally controlled) and auditory hallucinations (voices) talking about him in a derogatory way in the third person.

In my opinion, at the time of the alleged offence of murder, Mr X was suffering from an abnormality of mental functioning, due to the severe mental illness of paranoid schizophrenia, affecting his perception, judgment and voluntary control of his actions, as substantially impaired his responsibility for his acts.

I consider he would benefit from treatment in a psychiatric hospital. I have made arrangements for a bed to be reserved for him at X Hospital under Section 37 of the Mental Health Act 1983 if the court considers that this would be appropriate.

I recommend, if the court so agrees, that he additionally be made subject to restrictions under Section 41 of the Mental Health Act 1983 to protect the public from serious harm and to facilitate his long-term psychiatric management, including by specifying the conditions of his discharge from hospital, e.g. of residence and compliance with out-patient treatment, and by providing the ability to recall him to hospital should his mental state or behaviour deteriorate or he otherwise gives rise to concern.

As an alternative:

In my opinion this man does not suffer from mental disorder and is not detainable in hospital under the Mental Health Act 1983. He has an immature personality and requires considerable support and would benefit from group psychotherapy as an out-patient. If the court is prepared to consider an alternative to a custodial sentence in this case, I would recommend that, subject to the probation service's agreement, he be made subject to the direction of a Community Rehabilitation (old probation) order with a condition that he attend an outpatient group under my direction at X Mental Health Unit.

Other Issues:

Comment on any mitigating circumstances, e.g. marital or work stress, and on the prognosis.

Express any doubts you may have as to the likelihood of benefit from or risks associated with treatment in this person's case.

If you have no psychiatric recommendation, say so: for example, 'I have no psychiatric recommendation to make in this case'.

Finally, if essential information is lacking, or if time is not sufficient to make the necessary arrangements for a hospital bed, then do not hesitate to state your findings to date, state what you would like to do, and ask for a further period of remand.

References

Dell, S (1984) *Murder into Manslaughter: The Diminished Responsibility Defence in Practice* (Maudsley Monographs). Oxford: Oxford University Press.

Gudjonsson, GH (2003) *The Psychology of Interrogations and Confessions: a handbook*. Chichester: John Wiley & Sons.

Home Office and Department of Health (1975) *Report of Committee of Mentally Abnormal Offenders (Butler Committee)*. CMMD6244. London: HMSO.

Smith, K (ed.), Coleman, K., Eder, S., Hall, P (2011) *Homicides, Firearm Offences and Intimate Violence 2009/10*. Supplementary Volume 2 to Crime in England and Wales 2009/10. London: Home Office.

10 Mental Health Tribunals

Mental Health Tribunals are covered in Part V (Sections 65–79) of the Mental Health Act 1983. In Wales, they are still Mental Health Review Tribunals. In England, they are First-tier Tribunals (Health, Education and Social Care Chamber) often referred to as 'Mental Health Tribunals'. There is a new Upper Tribunal to deal with appeals on points of law against first-tier decisions.

Constitution and related aspects

Tribunals meet the requirement of Article 5(4) of the European Convention on Human Rights to have a mechanism whereby a person can appeal so that 'the lawfulness of his detention shall be decided speedily by a court and his release ordered if the detention is not lawful'. Although their establishment is provided for by Section 65 of the Mental Health Act 1983, Mental Health Tribunals are independent. Their membership is appointed by the Lord Chancellor having been chosen by the Judicial Appointments Commission, which was set up by the Constitutional Reform Act of 2005.

There exists one Mental Health Tribunal for England, and one Mental Health Review Tribunal for Wales. On the advice of the Judicial Appointments Commission the Lord Chancellor appoints the following three types of members of Tribunals:

- *Legal members*: having such legal experience as the Lord Chancellor considers suitable.
- *Medical members*: registered medical practitioners appointed by the Lord Chancellor after consultation with the Secretary of State. They are expected to be Members or Fellows of the Royal College of Psychiatrists and to have been Consultants for at least three years.
- *Other members*: appointed by the Lord Chancellor after consultation with the Secretary of State and having experience in administration, knowledge of social services or other qualifications or experience considered suitable by the Lord Chancellor.

Members are expected to retire at 70. There are about one thousand tribunal members in England and 90 in Wales.

The chair of each Mental Health Tribunal is a legal member who is known as a tribunal judge. There are usually three tribunal members at a hearing, one legal member, one medical member, and one other member, as defined above. Any three or more such members, constituted in this manner, may exercise the jurisdiction of a Mental Health Tribunal.

Applications and references concerning Part II patients

Table 10.1 summarises the Sections of Part II of the Mental Health Act 1983 under which an application may be made to a Mental Health Tribunal, the period during which such application may be made (known as the relevant period), and by whom such application may be made.

Table 10.1 Access to Mental Health Tribunal – Part II patients

Section	Purpose of Section	Relevant period	Who can apply
2	Admission for assessment	Within 14 days of admission	The patient
3	Admission for treatment	Within 6 months of admission	The patient
7	Reception into guardianship	Within 6 months of the application being accepted	The patient
17A	Community Treatment Order	Within 6 months of the order	The patient
19	Transfer from guardianship to hospital	Within 6 months of the patient being transferred	The patient
20	Renewal of authority	The period for which authority for the patient's compulsion is renewed	The patient
29	Appointment of acting nearest relative by court	Within 12 months of the date of the order, and in any subsequent 12 months	The nearest relative

References to Tribunals by Secretary of State

The Secretary of State may, at any time, refer to a Mental Health Tribunal the case of a patient who is liable to be detained or subject to guardianship under Part 2 of the Mental Health Act 1983. In order to furnish information for this purpose, any registered medical practitioner authorised by or on behalf of the patient may, at any reasonable time, visit the patient, examine the patient in private, and require the production of and inspect any records relating to the detention or treatment of the patient in any hospital.

Duty of Managers of Hospitals to refer cases to Tribunal

Provision is made for the automatic referral to a Mental Health Tribunal by hospital managers of the cases of patients detained under certain sections of Part II of the Mental Health Act 1983 when such patients have not exercised their right of such referral. This provides a safeguard against such patients being detained compulsorily for unduly long periods. This was strengthened in the reforms brought about by the 2007 Act. If a patient is admitted on Section 2 and this is followed by Section 3 the managers must refer for a hearing six months from the first date of admission on the Section 2 (unless the patient applied for a hearing while on Section 3). The new law also affects patients who were admitted on Section 2 which was then frozen because of an application to county court to displace the nearest relative. They cannot now go for more than six months without a tribunal hearing.

If the duration of authority for the detention of a patient in a hospital is renewed under Section 20 of the Mental Health Act 1983, and a period of 3 years (or, in the case of a patient who has not reached 16 years of age, 1 year) has elapsed since his or her case was last considered by a Mental Health Tribunal, then the hospital managers must refer the patient's case to the Tribunal.

Independent medical examination

With regard to tribunals, any registered medical practitioner authorised by or on behalf of the patient may, at any reasonable time, visit the patient, examine the patient in private, and require the production of and inspect any records relating to the detention or treatment of the patient in any hospital (Section 76).

Applications and references concerning Part III patients

Table 10.2 summarises the Sections of Part III of the Mental Health Act 1983 under which an application may be made to a Mental Health Tribunal by a patient who is subject to compulsion under Part III of the Act, the period during which such application may be made (known as the relevant period), and by whom such application may be made. There is no role for the nearest relative for restricted patients.

Table 10.2 Access to Mental Health Tribunal – Part III patients

Section	Purpose of Section	Relevant period	Who can apply
37	Hospital order	In the second six months	The patient and the nearest relative
37/41	Hospital order with restrictions	In the second six months	The patient
37	Guardianship order	Within first six months	The patient and the nearest relative*
45A	'Hybrid' order	In the second six months	The patient
47	Transfer to hospital of serving prisoner	Within 6 months of the transfer	The patient
47/49	Transfer to hospital of serving prisoner with restrictions	In the second six months	The patient
48	Transfer to hospital of other prisoner	Within 6 months of the transfer	The patient
48/49	Transfer to hospital of other prisoner with restrictions	In the second six months	The patient
20	Renewal of authority	The period for which authority for the patient's compulsion is renewed	The patient (and nearest relative for unrestricted patients)

* the nearest relative can only apply once in the first year

Discharge of patients

Patients detained under Section 2

Under Section 72(1)(a) of the Mental Health Act 1983 (as amended by a remedial order in 2001) a Mental Health Tribunal shall direct the discharge of a patient liable to be detained under Section 2 of the Act (admission for assessment) if it is not satisfied that:

- the patient is suffering from mental disorder or from mental disorder of a nature or degree that warrants his detention in hospital for assessment (or for assessment followed by treatment) for at least a limited period; or
- the detention of the patient is justified in the interests of his health or safety or with a view to the protection of others.

If the grounds for detention are met the Tribunal has a discretionary power to discharge the patient if they wish to do so.

Patients detained under sections other than Section 2 and excluding restricted patients

Under Section 72(1)(b) a Mental Health Tribunal shall direct the discharge of an unrestricted patient liable to be detained under a section of the Act other than Section 2 if it is not satisfied that:

- the patient is suffering from mental disorder or from mental disorder of a nature or degree which makes it appropriate for him to be liable to be detained in hospital for medical treatment; or
- that it is necessary for the health or safety of the patient or for the protection of others that he should receive such treatment; or
- that appropriate medical treatment is available for him; or
- in the case of an application by the nearest relative (against the decision of the Responsible Clinician to bar discharge by the nearest relative) that the patient, if released, would be likely to act in a manner dangerous to others or to himself.

Deferred discharge

Rather than delay a decision, by adjourning the hearing, to allow time for any necessary arrangements relating to discharge to be made (e.g. with respect to care or supervision in the community or to confirm suitable accommodation) a Mental Health Tribunal may, under Section 72(3)(a), direct the discharge of a patient on a future date. Alternatively, the tribunal may:

- with a view to facilitating the patient's discharge on a future date, recommend that the patient be granted leave of absence or transferred to another hospital or into guardianship, or placed on a community treatment order; and
- consider further the patient's case in the event of any such recommendation not being complied with.

Community Treatment Orders

Under Section 72(1)(b) a Mental Health Tribunal shall direct the discharge of a community patient if it is not satisfied:

- that he is then suffering from mental disorder or mental disorder of a nature or degree which makes it appropriate for him to receive medical treatment; or
- that it is necessary for his health or safety or for the protection of other persons that he should receive such treatment; or
- that it is necessary that the responsible clinician should be able to exercise the power under Section 17E(1) to recall the patient to hospital*; or
- that appropriate medical treatment is available for him.

Where the tribunal is hearing an application from the nearest relative because the responsible clinician has barred their discharge order, the tribunal shall direct the discharge of the patient if it is not satisfied that the patient, if discharged, would be likely to act in a manner dangerous to other persons or to himself.

* In determining whether the criterion marked with an asterisk above is met, the tribunal is required to consider, having regard to the patient's history of mental disorder and any other relevant factors, what risk there would be of a deterioration of the patient's condition if he were to continue not to be detained in a hospital (as a result, for example, of his refusing or neglecting to receive the medical treatment he requires for his mental disorder).

Guardianship

Where application is made to a Mental Health Tribunal by or in respect of a patient who is subject to guardianship under the Mental Health Act 1983, under Section 72(4) the tribunal shall direct that the patient be discharged if it is satisfied that:

- the patient is not suffering from mental disorder; or
- it is not necessary in the interests of the welfare of the patient, or for the protection of others, that the patient should remain under such guardianship.

Note that the burden of proof of demonstrating that there is a mental disorder of a nature or degree to warrant guardianship was not amended when the Remedial Order changed the position for detained patients.

Restricted patients

Sections 73, 74 and 75 of the Mental Health Act 1983 deal with the powers of Mental Health Tribunals to discharge restricted patients. The tribunal can leave matters as they are, or order an absolute or a conditional discharge. It cannot lift the restrictions thereby converting the order to an unrestricted hospital order; only the Secretary of State for Justice may do this.

Code of Practice

The English Code of Practice states:

> *32.5 Hospital managers and the local social services authority (LSSA) are under a duty to take steps to ensure that patients understand their rights to apply for a Tribunal hearing. Hospital managers and the LSSA should also advise patients of their entitlement to free legal advice and representation. They should do both whenever:*
>
> - *patients are first detained in hospital, received into guardianship or discharged to SCT;*

- *their detention or guardianship is renewed or SCT is extended; and*
- *their status under the Act changes – for example, if they move from detention under Section 2 to detention under Section 3 or if their community treatment order is revoked.*

32.6 Unless the patient requests otherwise, the information should normally also be given to their nearest relative (subject to the normal considerations about involving nearest relatives...)

32.7 Hospital managers and professionals should enable detained patients to be visited by their legal representatives at any reasonable time. This is particularly important where visits are necessary to discuss a Tribunal application. Where the patient consents, legal representatives and independent doctors should be given prompt access to the patient's medical records. Delays in providing access can hold up Tribunal proceedings and should be avoided.

The Code also reminds authorities of the importance of getting reports in to the tribunal on time. The format for the content of these reports is now set out in the Practice Directions. The detaining authority is required to give basic information on the patient. The clinician's report should cover the patient's medical history including:

(a) full details of the patient's mental state, behaviour and treatment for mental disorder;
(b) in so far as it is within the knowledge of the person writing the report a statement as to whether the patient has ever neglected or harmed himself, or has ever harmed other persons or threatened them with harm, at a time when he was mentally disordered, together with details of any neglect, harm or threats of harm;
(c) an assessment of the extent to which the patient or other persons would be likely to be at risk if the patient is discharged by the Tribunal, and how any such risks could best be managed;
(d) an assessment of the patient's strengths and any other positive factors that the Tribunal should be aware of in coming to a view on whether he should be discharged; and
(e) if appropriate, the reasons why the patient might be treated in the community without continued detention in hospital, but should remain subject to recall on supervised community treatment.

Responsibility for providing a social circumstances report is usually given to a care co-ordinator who is likely to be a nurse or a social worker, but not necessarily an approved mental health professional (AMHP).

References

Department of Health (2008) *Mental Health Act 1983: Code of Practice*. London: TSO.

Tribunals Judiciary (2008) *Practice Direction, Health Education and Social Care Chapter, Mental Health Cases*. London: TSO.

11 Hospital Managers

The term 'hospital managers' as used within the Mental Health Act 1983 can create some confusion. Once the managers have been identified for a particular hospital there are a number of functions for which they are responsible but these are usually delegated to officers or other people. This chapter will set out who the managers are, who can exercise specific functions for them, and how these functions are carried out in practice.

Who are the Hospital Managers?

The first complication is that there are different types of hospital and this determines the identity of the managers. If the hospital is vested in an NHS Trust, then that Trust as a body becomes the hospital managers. If the hospital is vested in an NHS Foundation Trust, then that Foundation Trust becomes the hospital managers. If the hospital is vested in, or the responsibility of, a Primary Care Trust (PCT) then that PCT becomes the hospital managers. Finally, for an independent hospital, the person(s) registered in respect of that hospital by the Care Quality Commission (CQC) (they may be individuals, a company or some other kind of body) becomes the hospital managers. For most decisions, hospital managers do not have to perform their functions personally (e.g. by decision of the board of an NHS Trust), but may delegate them to officers (i.e. members of their staff) and, in some cases, to other people.

It is important to note that the Section 23 power to discharge cannot be exercised by officers or employees. However, the NHS Trust or organisation in charge of the hospital retains responsibility for the performance of the managers' functions so delegated, and therefore, for the competence of those performing them.

The duties of the Hospital Managers

Information for patients and nearest relatives

The managers are required to provide certain information to patients and nearest relatives under Sections 132, 132A and 133. For detained patients the obligation at Section 132 is to:

> *'take such steps as are practicable to ensure that the patient understands:*
>
> *(a) under which of the provisions of this Act he is for the time being detained and the effect of that provision; and*
>
> *(b) what rights of applying to a Mental Health Review Tribunal are available to him in respect of his detention under that provision;*
>
> *and those steps shall be taken as soon as practicable after the commencement of the patient's detention under the provision in question.'*

In many hospitals, this information is given by a nurse on the ward. It has to be given both orally and in writing and it may need to be given on more than one occasion. Similar information has to be given to community treatment orders (CTO) patients. Unless the patient makes a request to the contrary, a copy of the written information should also be given to the patient's nearest relative.

Section 133 states that the managers must inform the nearest relative if a patient is discharged (including where being discharged from hospital on a CTO) unless either the patient or nearest relative has requested otherwise. This information should be given, where practicable, at least seven days before discharge. In most cases, where a CTO is being planned, this requirement should be observed. Part IV of the Regulations covers other occasions when the managers are obliged (unless the patient requests otherwise) to give information to the nearest relative, e.g. on renewal of the patient's detention or his transfer to another hospital, and it sets out how that information is to be given.

There is a requirement under Section 130D to ensure both orally and in writing that 'qualifying patients' understand that help is available from an Independent Mental Health Advocate (IMHA) and how to obtain it. For a detained patient, this is the responsibility of the hospital managers. Again written information given to the patient must be copied to the nearest relative unless the patient requests otherwise.

Information for victims

The Domestic Violence, Crime and Victims Act 2004 was amended by the Mental Health Act 2007 to extend the circumstances in which the victim of a violent or sexual offence should be given information and an opportunity to make representations about the discharge and discharge conditions relating to Part III patients. The provisions used to apply to restricted patients only, but the new provisions also apply to unrestricted patients. The probation service notifies the managers if a victim wishes to be informed or to make representations. Responsible Clinicians and the Tribunal must notify the managers if the patient is to be discharged. The managers' duties are set out in Paragraph 30.29 of the Code of Practice.

> *'This includes liaising with victims in order to:*
>
> - *advise victims if the patient's discharge is being considered or if the patient is about to be discharged;*
> - *forward representations made by victims to people responsible for making decisions on discharge or SCT and for passing information received from those people to the victim;*
> - *inform victims who have asked to be told, if the patient is to go onto SCT and of any conditions on the community treatment order (CTO) relating to contact with them or their family, any variation of the conditions, and the date on which the order will cease; and*
> - *inform responsible clinicians of any representations made by the victim about the conditions attached to the CTO.'*

Other responsibilities

Since April 2010, managers have been under a duty to ensure that the environment of all children and young people admitted for treatment of mental disorder is suitable having regard to their age and subject to their needs.

The managers have an obligation, on a number of occasions, as set out in Section 68, to refer patients automatically to a Mental Health Tribunal. These are also set out in convenient tabular form in the Code of Practice just after Paragraph 30.34.

The managers have the responsibility for ensuring that a detained patient has a responsible clinician (RC) allocated promptly and that this person remains the most appropriate approved clinician (AC) to take on this function as matters change.

There are other issues where the Code of Practice states that managers should draw up policies including: identifying the second professional who has to agree in writing that the criteria for renewal of a patient's detention are met; ensuring that the 72 hour period during which a CTO patient is recalled to hospital is not exceeded; what action should be taken when a detained patient or a CTO patient goes missing.

Managers' hearings

Hospital managers have the power to discharge unrestricted patients, and since November 2008, they have also had the power to discharge CTO patients. Note that the managers did not have the power to discharge patients on the CTO's predecessor, i.e. supervised aftercare. The managers must review the patient if their detention is renewed under Section 20, or if their CTO is extended under Section 20A. They should also consider reviewing the patient if the RC has issued a barring order under Section 25. They may also review a patient's detention, at any time, either at the patient's request or at their discretion. In deciding whether to conduct a review where they have a discretion the Code states at Paragraph 31.12 that they may take into account whether the Tribunal has recently considered the patient's case or is due to do so in the near future.

When exercising the power to discharge, hospital managers must firstly consider whether the criteria for detention under the relevant section continue to be met. So for a patient detained under Section 3 they should ask:

- Is the patient still suffering from mental disorder?
- If so, is the disorder of a nature or degree which makes treatment in a hospital appropriate?
- Is continued detention for medical treatment necessary for the patient's health or safety or for the protection of other people?
- Is appropriate medical treatment available for the patient?

If the review follows the RC's use of the barring order under Section 25 to prevent discharge by the nearest relative, they should then consider whether the patient, if discharged, would be likely to act in a manner dangerous to other people or to themselves. The test for dangerousness is at a higher level than the risk criteria for the original test for detention which refer to the health or safety of the patient or for the protection of others.

The function of reviewing when to discharge patients may not be delegated to employees or officers of the trust. Who may be appointed depends on the status of the hospital. Chapter 13 of this book contains a table which identifies who is allowed to carry out this function. The managers' panel must always consist of at least three qualifying and authorised people. For example, in the case of an NHS foundation trust the trust may authorise three or more people, but they must not include executive directors of the board of the trust, nor employees of the trust.

A majority decision to discharge is not sufficient unless the panel comprises more than three people, and at least three decide in favour of discharge. Managers should be provided with relevant care planning documentation and written reports from the RC and from other appropriate professionals. The patient should normally be given copies of this material.

In response to criticisms that managers' hearings sometimes discharged people against clinical advice, the code now contains the following statement at Paragraph 31.35:

> *'Members of managers' panels will not normally be qualified to form clinical assessments of their own. They must give full weight to the views of all the professionals concerned in the patient's care. If there is a divergence of views among the professionals about whether the patient meets the clinical grounds for continued detention or SCT, managers' panels should consider adjourning to seek further medical or other professional advice.'*

Unlike the position for tribunals there are no formal rules or prescribed procedure for the conduct of managers' hearings. The Code of Practice at 31.23 notes however that:

> *'the exercise of this power is subject to the general law and to public law duties which arise from it. Hospital managers' conduct of reviews must satisfy the fundamental legal requirements of fairness, reasonableness and lawfulness. Managers' panels should therefore:*
>
> - *adopt and apply a procedure which is fair and reasonable;*
> - *not make irrational decisions – that is, decisions which no managers' panel, properly directing itself as to the law and on the available information, could have made; and*
> - *not act unlawfully – that is, contrary to the provisions of the Act and any other legislation (including the Human Rights Act 1998 and relevant equality and anti-discrimination legislation).'*

The Code of Practice (31.32) also suggests the following:

- the patient should be given a full opportunity, and any necessary help, to explain why they should no longer be detained or on supervised community treatment (SCT);
- the patient should be allowed to be accompanied by a representative of their own choosing to help in putting their point of view to the panel;
- the patient should also be allowed to have a relative, friend or advocate attend to support them; and
- the responsible clinician and other professionals should be asked to give their views on whether the patient's continued detention or SCT is justified and to explain the grounds on which those views are based.

In cases where the renewal or extension of a patient's detention or CTO is uncontested, the managers may decide to consider the case on the papers without having a hearing. However, usually at least one of them should first interview the patient.

Once the managers have reached a decision they should give their reasons. These should be fully recorded at the end of the review and given orally and in writing to the patient, to the nearest relative (where relevant) and to the professionals concerned.

References

Department of Health (2008) *Mental Health Act 1983: Code of Practice*. London: TSO.

Department of Health (2008) *Reference Guide to the Mental Health Act 1983*. London: TSO.

Cases

1983 Mental Health Act.
1998 Human Rights Act.
2004 Domestic Violence, Crime and Victims Act.
2007 Mental Health Act.

12 Cross-border arrangements

Part VI of the Mental Health Act

The Mental Health Act applies to England and Wales, while other parts of the UK (Scotland, Northern Ireland, and the Channel Islands and Isle of Man) have their own mental health legislation. Occasionally psychiatric patients who are currently detained in hospital or are under guardianship, may need to be removed or returned within the UK. Part VI of the Act provides the necessary legislation to allow the transfer of such patients across national boundaries within the UK, without any break in the power for confinement. Similarly, provision is also made (under Section 86 of Part VI of the Act) for the removal of psychiatric patients who are aliens. Note also that there are variations (regarding forms, regulations, etc.) which now apply to Wales.

Removal to and from Scotland

Removal to Scotland

Section 80(1) of the Act applies to the case of patients in England and Wales who are liable to detention under the Act (apart from patients remanded for report or treatment or subject to an interim hospital order; that is, excluding Sections 35, 36 and 38, respectively). If it appears to the Secretary of State that it is in the interests of such a patient that he be removed to Scotland, and that arrangements have been made for admitting him to a hospital there, or where he is not to be admitted to a hospital, for his detention in hospital to be authorised by virtue of the Mental Health (Care and Treatment) (Scotland) Act 2003 or the Criminal Procedure (Scotland) Act 1995, then under Section 80 the Secretary of State may authorise the patient's removal to Scotland and may give any necessary directions for his conveyance to his destination.

Restricted patients

Where a person removed under Section 80 was, immediately before his removal, subject to a restriction order or restriction direction of limited duration, the restriction order or restriction direction shall expire on the date on which the first-mentioned order or direction would have expired if he had not been so removed.

Under Section 80A, if it appears to the Secretary of State, in the case of a patient who:

(a) is subject to a restriction order under Section 41 of the Act; and
(b) has been conditionally discharged under Sections 42 or 73,

that a transfer would be in the interests of the patient, the Secretary of State may, with the consent of the Minister exercising corresponding functions in Scotland, transfer responsibility for the patient to that Minister.

Transfer of responsibility for community patients

Under Section 80ZA, if it appears to the appropriate national authority, in the case of a community patient, that the conditions below are met, the authority may authorise the transfer of responsibility for him to Scotland. The conditions are:

(a) a transfer under Section 80ZA is in the patient's interests; and
(b) arrangements have been made for dealing with the patient under enactments in force in Scotland corresponding or similar to those relating to community patients in this Act.

The appropriate national authority may not act under Section 80ZA while the patient is recalled to hospital under Section 17E.

In Section 80ZA, *the appropriate national authority* means, in relation to a community patient in respect of whom the responsible hospital is in England or Wales, the Secretary of State or the Welsh Ministers, respectively.

Removal to England or Wales

Reciprocal arrangements exist between England and Wales and Scotland with respect to psychiatric patients removed from Scotland to England or Wales.

Removal to and from Northern Ireland

Sections 81 and 82 of the Mental Health Act 1983 allow for the transfer of psychiatric patients, who are currently detained in hospital or are under guardianship, between England or Wales and Northern Ireland without any break in the power for confinement.

Unrestricted patients

Section 81(1) of the Mental Health Act 1983 applies to the case of patients in England and Wales who are either liable to detention without restriction on discharge (apart from patients remanded for report or treatment or subject to an interim hospital order; that is, excluding Sections 35, 36 and 38, respectively) or subject to guardianship under the Act. If it appears to the Secretary of State that it is in the interests of such a patient that he be removed to Northern Ireland, and that arrangements have been made for either admitting the patient to a hospital or receiving the patient into guardianship, as required, then under Section 81 of the Mental Health Act 1983 the Secretary of State may authorise the patient's removal to Northern Ireland and may give any necessary directions for his conveyance to his destination. Such a patient is to be treated in Northern Ireland as if subject to the corresponding enactment of the Mental Health (Northern Ireland) Order 1986 (*see* Chapter 29).

Section 81(4) of the Mental Health Act applies to the case of a patient removed to Northern Ireland from England or Wales such that the patient was liable, immediately before removal, to be detained under an order for admission to hospital for assessment under the Act. On admission to a hospital in Northern Ireland, the patient is to be treated as if he had been admitted in pursuance of an application for assessment under Article 4 of the Mental Health (Northern Ireland) Order 1986 (*see* Chapter 29) made on the date of his admission.

Section 81(5) of the Mental Health Act 1983 applies to the case of a patient removed to Northern Ireland from England or Wales such that the patient was liable, immediately before removal, to be detained under an order for admission to hospital for treatment under the Mental Health Act. On admission to a hospital in Northern Ireland, the patient is to be treated as if he or she had been admitted subject to detention for treatment under Part II of the Mental Health (Northern Ireland) Order 1986 by virtue of a report under Article 12(1) of that Order (*see* Chapter 29) made on the date of his admission.

Section 81(6) of the Mental Health Act applies to the case of a patient removed to Northern Ireland from England or Wales such that the patient was subject, immediately before removal, to a transfer direction given while he was serving a sentence of imprisonment (within the meaning of Section 47(5) of the Act) imposed by a court in England or Wales. Such a patient is to be treated as if the sentence had been imposed by a court in Northern Ireland.

Restricted patients

Section 81(7) of the Mental Health Act applies to the case of a patient removed to Northern Ireland from England or Wales such that the patient was subject, immediately before removal, to a restriction direction of limited duration. The date of expiry of the restriction direction is not changed by the removal to Northern Ireland.

Community patients

Section 81ZA allows for the removal of community patients to Northern Ireland from England and Wales. Under Section 81ZA(1), Section 81 applies in the case of a community patient as it applies in the case of a patient who is, for the time being, liable to be detained under the Mental Health Act, as if the community patient were so liable.

Removal to England or Wales

Reciprocal arrangements exist between England and Wales and Northern Ireland with respect to psychiatric patients removed from Northern Ireland to England or Wales. These are covered by Section 82 of the Mental Health Act.

Removal to and from the Channel Islands and Isle of Man

Sections 83 and 85 of the Mental Health Act 1983 allow for the transfer of psychiatric patients, who are currently detained in hospital or are under guardianship, between England or Wales and the Channel Islands or Isle of Man without any break in the power for confinement. Section 84 of the Mental Health Act 1983 allows for the removal to England or Wales of mentally ill offenders from the Channel Islands and Isle of Man.

Removal to the Channel Islands and Isle of Man

Section 83 of the Act applies to the case of patients in England and Wales who are either liable to detention without restriction on discharge (apart from patients remanded for report or treatment or subject to an interim hospital order; that is, excluding Sections 35, 36 and 38, respectively) or subject to guardianship under the Act. If it appears to the Secretary of State that it is in the interests of such a patient that he be removed to the Channel Islands or the Isle of Man, and that arrangements have been made for either admitting the patient to a hospital or receiving the patient into guardianship, as required, then under Section 83 the Secretary of State may authorise his removal to the Channel Islands or the Isle of Man and may give any necessary directions for his conveyance to his destination.

Removal of psychiatric patients who are offenders from the Channel Islands and Isle of Man

Section 84 of the Act allows for the transfer of mentally ill offenders from the Channel Islands and the Isle of Man to England and Wales.

The Secretary of State may, by warrant, direct that any offender found by a court in any of the Channel Islands or in the Isle of Man to be insane or to have been insane at the time of the alleged offence, and ordered to be detained during Her Majesty's pleasure, be removed to a hospital in England and Wales. Such a patient, on reception into the hospital in England or Wales, shall be treated as if he were subject to a hospital order together with a restriction order. Also, the Secretary of State may, by warrant, direct that any such removed patient be returned to the island from which he was so removed, to be dealt with there according to law in all respects as if he had not been removed under this Section.

Removal to England or Wales

Reciprocal arrangements exist between, on the one hand, England and Wales, and, on the other, the Channel Islands and the Isle of Man, with respect to psychiatric patients removed from the Channel Islands and the Isle of Man to England or Wales. These are covered by Section 85 of the Act.

In the case of such a patient who is subject to an order or direction restricting his discharge, he is treated as if subject to a restriction order or restriction direction. While being conveyed to the hospital in England or Wales, such a patient is deemed to be in legal custody. (Under these circumstances, Section 138 applies to the patient as if he or she were in legal custody by virtue of Section 137.)

Responsibility for community patients transferred from the Channel Islands or the Isle of Man to England or Wales is covered under Section 85ZA.

Removal of Aliens

Section 86 of the Act applies to any patient who is:

- not a British citizen;
- not a Commonwealth citizen having the right of abode in the UK by virtue of Section 2(1)(b) of the Immigration Act 1971;
- receiving treatment for mental disorder as an in-patient in a hospital in England or Wales under the Act (other than under Sections 35, 36 or 38) or in Northern Ireland under the Mental Health (Northern Ireland) Order 1986.

If it appears to the Secretary of State that proper arrangements have been made for the removal of such a patient to a country or territory outside the UK, the Isle of Man and the Channel Islands and for his care or treatment there, and that it is in the interests of the patient to remove him, then, only with the approval of a Mental Health Review Tribunal (or, in the case of Northern Ireland, the Mental Health Review Tribunal for Northern Ireland), the Secretary of State may:

(a) by warrant, authorise the removal of the patient from the place where he is receiving treatment;
(b) give directions for the conveyance of the patient to his destination in that country or territory and for his detention in any place or on board any ship or aircraft until his arrival at any specified port or place in any such country or territory.

Application to the Home Office is usually not required in the case of patients who are willing to travel and for whom suitable arrangements have been made.

According to Green and Nayani (2000):

> *'The current arrangements would seem to satisfy the obligations in respect of "persons of unsound mind" arising under Article 5 of the European Convention of Human Rights (the right to liberty and security of the person). The impact of the Human Rights Act 1998 should, therefore, be minimal with regard to the process of repatriation [under Section 86 of the Mental Health Act 1983].'*

In their experience, Green and Nayani (2000) have found that the following steps are required in order to arrange repatriation:

- Contact the relevant embassy.
- Arrange for an interpreter in order to interview the patient (and his or her relatives), if necessary.
- Obtain information regarding previous contact with psychiatric services in the patient's country of origin and establish which hospital in that country should be responsible for their care.
- Obtain specific information regarding the patient's past psychiatric history, including previous diagnosis, treatment, response to treatment and any history of dangerousness.
- Translate correspondence.
- Continue treatment until the patient is fit to travel.
- Consider repatriation (under Section 86, if necessary) and discuss this with the patient.
- Arrange the date and process of transfer.

They suggest the following useful questions to ask embassy staff:

1. Have you been involved in repatriating psychiatric patients?
2. Will you find information about which hospital the patient should return to?
3. Will you liaise directly with the hospital concerned to obtain information regarding the patient's past psychiatric history and to arrange plans for transfer?
4. Will you be able to translate discharge summaries and other correspondence, and will there be a charge for this?
5. If the patient is detained in this country under the Mental Health Act, is there

any process ensuring the patient remains detained from the time they leave England [or Wales] until the time they arrive in the appropriate hospital?

6 Does the patient return directly to his/her local hospital or is he [or she] assessed at a central hospital initially?

7 Who is responsible for the cost of repatriation?

Reference

Green, L., Nayani T (2000) Repatriating psychiatric patients. *Psychiatric Bulletin* **24**, 405–408.

13 The Mental Health Act Code of Practice and the Reference Guide

The revised Code of Practice to the Mental Health Act 1983 came into force in 2008 to coincide with the major changes brought about by the amending 2007 Act. There are in fact two separate codes, as there is a Welsh code approved by the Welsh Assembly but this chapter will concentrate on the English code. It replaced the third edition of the code, which had been in place since 1999. The Code used to be cross-referenced with the Memorandum which provided an easy-to-read guide to the Act. The Memorandum has now been replaced by the Reference Guide which will be discussed towards the end of this chapter.

There was some discussion as to whether the new principles would be in the Act or the Code. As it transpired, the key aspects of the principles are listed in the Act but the detail is in the Code. This is one area where there are significant differences between the English and Welsh codes and staff moving between the countries must be alert to this. There will be a detailed analysis of the principles in this chapter.

The Code is a substantial document of just short of 400 pages. Those seeking an introduction to the Act would be well advised to look at the slightly shorter 'Reference Guide' which is written in a more accessible style. Both are available free on the internet or hard copies can be purchased through the stationery office (TSO).

Purpose of the Code

The introduction to the Code states that it:

> *'provides guidance to registered medical practitioners ("doctors"), approved clinicians, managers and staff of hospitals, and approved mental health professionals on how they should proceed when undertaking duties under*

the Act. It also gives guidance to doctors and other professionals about certain aspects of medical treatment for mental disorder more generally.'

It indicates that others such as the police and ambulance services should also find the Code beneficial. However, it should be noted that it has been a source of irritation to some that the Code does not have a more formal status for these two groups of staff who are essential for any smooth operation of the Act, especially in terms of compulsory admissions.

The introduction continues to state that it is intended 'that the Code will also be helpful to patients, their representatives, carers, families and friends, and others who support them.'

Status of the Code

The Code was prepared in accordance with Section 118 of the Act which states:

> '(1) *The Secretary of State shall prepare, and from time to time revise, a code of practice:*
>
> (a) *for the guidance of registered medical practitioners, approved clinicians, managers and staff of hospitals, independent hospitals and care homes and approved mental health professionals in relation to the admission of patients to hospitals and registered establishments under this Act and to guardianship and aftercare under supervision community patients under this Act; and*
>
> (b) *for the guidance of registered medical practitioners and members of other professions in relation to the medical treatment of patients suffering from mental disorder.'*

Section 118(2D) then states:

> *'In performing functions under this Act persons mentioned in Subsection (1)(a) or (b) shall have regard to the code.'*

The introduction to the Code notes in Paragraph iv that the Act

> *'does not impose a legal duty to comply with the Code, the people listed above to whom the Code is addressed must have regard to the Code. The reasons for any departure should be recorded. Departures from the Code could give rise to legal challenge, and a court, in reviewing any departure from the Code, will scrutinise the reasons for the departure to ensure that there is sufficiently convincing justification in the circumstances.'*

The status of the Code was considered in *R (Munjaz)* v. *Mersey Care NHS Trust* (2005). The House of Lords held that although not having statutory force, the Code was much more than 'mere advice which an addressee is free to follow or not'. It was guidance 'which any hospital should consider with great care and from which it should depart only if it has cogent reasons for doing so.' Staff specified in the introduction to the Code should then be very careful if they depart from the Code and should record their reasons for doing so. (Examples might be a change in case law or a powerful human rights argument). The recent case of *BB* v. *Cygnet Health Care and London Borough of Lewisham* (2008) illustrates the point. The judge said of the ASW that his 'failure to complete an outline report at the hospital in accordance with Paragraph 11.13 of the Code of Practice did not give the court any confidence in his overall ability properly to discharge his responsibilities under the Act.'

Policy requirements

The Code contains a number of policy requirements which are addressed to hospital managers, local social services authorities (LSSAs) and others. These are helpfully grouped together in Annex B to the code and senior staff should ensure that there are policies to cover all the areas that are listed. An example from Paragraph 8.16 of the Code is 'LSSAs should provide clear, practical guidance to help AMHPs decide whether to make an application to the county court for the appointment of an acting nearest relative for a patient and how to proceed.' Some critics would argue that there are areas where the Code should have taken a more prescriptive line in some areas of law and that this would have left less to local variation.

The guiding principles

There have been criticisms that the Mental Health Act principles were relegated to the Code, whilst those for the Mental Capacity Act are in the statute. This is a little misleading. While it is true that the details are in the Code (and expressed somewhat differently in the Welsh and English codes) the basics are set out in Section 118.

Section 118 requires that the following matters be addressed:

'(a) respect for patients' past and present wishes and feelings,
(b) respect for diversity generally including, in particular, diversity of religion, culture and sexual orientation (within the meaning of Section 35 of the Equality Act 2006),
(c) minimising restrictions on liberty,
(d) involvement of patients in planning, developing and delivering care and treatment appropriate to them,
(e) avoidance of unlawful discrimination,
(f) effectiveness of treatment,
(g) views of carers and other interested parties,
(h) patient wellbeing and safety, and
(i) public safety.'

In Section 118(2C) the Secretary of State is also required to have regard to the desirability of ensuring:

'(a) the efficient use of resources, and
(b) the equitable distribution of services.'

The English code groups these 11 points into five principles.

1 The 'purpose principle' addresses points (f), (h) and (i) with a statement that:

'Decisions under the Act must be taken with a view to minimising the undesirable effects of mental disorder, by maximising the safety and wellbeing (mental and physical) of patients, promoting their recovery and protecting other people from harm.'

2 The 'least restriction' principle covers point (c) with the statement:

'People taking action without a patient's consent must attempt to keep to a minimum the restrictions they impose on the patient's liberty, having regard to the purpose for which the restrictions are imposed.'

3 Points (a), (b) and (e) from the list are covered by the 'respect principle':

'People taking decisions under the Act must recognise and respect the diverse needs, values and circumstances of each patient, including their race, religion, culture, gender, age, sexual orientation and any disability. They must consider the patient's views, wishes and feelings (whether expressed at the time or in advance), so far as they are reasonably ascertainable, and follow those wishes wherever practicable and consistent with the purpose of the decision. There must be no unlawful discrimination.'

4 Points (d) and (g) can be found in the 'participation principle':

'Patients must be given the opportunity to be involved, as far as is practicable in the circumstances, in planning, developing and reviewing their own treatment and care to help ensure that it is delivered in a way that is as appropriate and effective for them as possible. The involvement of carers, family members and other people who have an interest in the patient's welfare should be encouraged (unless there are particular reasons to the contrary) and their views taken seriously.'

5 Finally point (e) and the two points from Section 118(2C) are addressed in the 'effectiveness, efficiency and equity principle' which states:

'People taking decisions under the Act must seek to use the resources available to them and to patients in the most effective, efficient and equitable way, to meet the needs of patients and achieve the purpose for which the decision was taken.'

The Welsh code has a more memorable list of principles which all begin with 'E' namely:

- Empowerment
- Equity
- Effectiveness
- Efficiency.

These are based on the Welsh Assembly Government Mental Health Strategy *Adult Mental Health Services for Wales* which established these four underpinning principles to guide everybody involved in planning, commissioning, managing, working in and using mental health services. The Code elaborates on these in significantly more detail than in the equivalent passage in the English code. It will be interesting to see if these two different approaches lead to any practice differences between the two countries. It may well be that in the long term, a growing awareness of the importance of the European Convention on Human Rights (which applies to both countries) will minimise any differences. The English code notes at Paragraph 1.7 that:

'All decisions must, of course, be lawful and informed by good professional practice. Lawfulness necessarily includes compliance with the Human Rights Act 1998.'

Most recent challenges to practice under the Mental Health Act have focused on the links with the European Convention on Human Rights and those covered by the code are carrying out functions of a public nature and are, therefore, required to avoid breaching human rights unless required to do so by primary legislation.

Informal admission

It is unfortunate that Annex A of the Code confuses informal and voluntary patients. In its list of key words and phrases that are used in the Code it states that: **an 'informal patient' is**

> *'someone who is being treated for a mental disorder and who is not detained under the Act. Also sometimes known as a 'voluntary patient'*

This error is not repeated in the Reference Guide which defines an informal patient as follows:

> *'A patient who is not subject to any* **compulsory measure** *under the Act. In other words, a patient who is not a* **detained patient**, *an* **SCT patient**, *a* **guardianship patient** *or a* **conditionally discharged patient.**'

As we shall see, and as the Reference Guide appears to recognise, not all informal patients are voluntary. There is some history to this issue as far as the Code is concerned. The 1993 edition of the Code had a rather contentious definition of what would constitute an informal inpatient in relation to the doctor's holding power under Section 5(2). Essentially, it described an informal patient as:

> *'one who has understood and accepted an offer of a bed, who has freely appeared on the ward and who has co-operated with the admission procedure.'*

Jones (1996, p. 586) noted:

> *'only patients who are both mentally competent and willing to co-operate with the admission process would come within the scope of this definition. As the wording of the Act does not support an approach which would have the effect of excluding patients who do not possess such characteristics from the application of the holding power, a better definition would be: 'An informal patient for the purpose of this section, is one who has arrived on the ward and who has offered no resistance to the admission procedure.'*

This view was specifically contradicted in October 1997 at the Appeal Court stage of the Bournewood case (*HL* v. *UK* (2004)), but it was, in effect, then supported by the Law Lords' ruling in June 1998. The eight-month period in between the two rulings led to some interesting responses. It is instructive to compare Jones' suggestion with the equivalent paragraph in the revised 1999 Code, which was drafted after the Law Lords' judgment and read:

> *'For the purposes of Section 5(2) informal patients are usually voluntary patients, i.e. those who have the capacity to consent and who consent to enter hospital for inpatient treatment. Patients who lack the capacity to consent but do not object to admission for treatment may also be informal patients ... The Section cannot be used for an outpatient attending a hospital's accident and emergency department. Admission procedures*

should not be implemented with the sole intention of then using the power in Section 5(2).'

The European Court judgment on the Bournewood case (*HL* v. *UK* (2004)) led to changes in the Act and the Code. The idea that *'de facto'* detention was acceptable under common law was overturned. This was because under Article 5 of the European Convention of Human Rights (ECHR) any such detention needed a procedure prescribed by law and appeal to the courts. The Mental Capacity Act 2005 then made it explicit that the provisions of Section 5 of that Act could not be used to deprive someone of their liberty. So any patient who lacked the capacity to agree to admission to a psychiatric hospital and be 'voluntary' could only be informal if their stay in hospital fell short of 'deprivation of liberty'. What does the 2008 edition of the Code have to say on this matter?

Paragraph 4.16 of the Code states:

'If admission to hospital for assessment or treatment for mental disorder is necessary for a patient who lacks capacity to consent to it, an application under the Mental Health Act should be made if:

- *providing appropriate care or treatment for the patient will unavoidably involve depriving them of their liberty and the MCA deprivation of liberty safeguards cannot be used; or*
- *for any other reason, the assessment or treatment the patient needs cannot be safely or effectively delivered by relying on the MCA alone.'*

The Code sits uncomfortably with the GJ judgment which is considered elsewhere in the examination of Deprivation of Liberty Safeguards (DOLS) in this book, and rather ignores Paragraph 12 of Schedule 1A to the Mental Capacity Act which essentially requires one to start with the Mental Health Act where a patient is being deprived of his liberty. It is hoped that the next edition of the code addresses this question more coherently. An even better solution would be to reform the law to simplify the issues, for example, by enhancing guardianship to allow for deprivation of liberty within its remit.

Other key areas of code guidance

The Code is a lengthy document and it is referred to in other parts of this book when looking at the Mental Health Act in practice. It is perhaps worth just identifying a couple of other key areas of guidance however. Chapter 4 is an essential chapter for doctors and AMHPs as it covers applications for detention in hospital. The Conflict of Interests Regulations provide very limited protection for patients but in the Code's coverage of this area there is a particularly useful piece of advice at Paragraph 7.15 which states:

'There may be circumstances not covered by these regulations where the assessor feels, nonetheless, that there is (or could be seen to be) a potential conflict of interest. Assessors should work on the principle that in any situation where they believe that the objectivity or independence of their decision is (or could be seen to be) undermined, they should not become involved or should withdraw.'

Chapter 8 on the nearest relative contains some interesting speculation on who the courts might regard to be an 'unsuitable' nearest relative.

Most aspects of the Act are covered in the Code but critics elsewhere have commented:

> *'There may be a degree of frustration at the number of occasions within the Code when guidance is not in fact given but rather reference made to the numerous policies and protocols which will have to be drawn up (usually by managers) to cover a practice issue.'*

(Barber, Brown and Martin, 2009, p. 19).

Indeed, the Code does seem on many occasions to do little more than restate the Act. In this sense, it is sometimes hard to see how it differs from the Reference Guide.

The Reference Guide

There were plans to have separate Reference Guides for England and Wales but it now seems that for some time to come there will only be the English Guide. Readers in Wales may still find the Guide helpful but should be alert to any differences that might apply in Wales. For example the statutory forms referred to are English and there are separate forms which must be used in Wales.

The introduction to the Reference Guide states that it 'is intended as a source of reference for people who want to understand the provisions of the Mental Health Act 1983.' People new to the law certainly seem to find it helpful in making the law accessible. In some difficult areas of law, it sometimes presents a useful way of summarising the provisions.

Table 12.3 in the Reference Guide provides a visual guide for an area of law that many find difficult and it is replicated below:

If the managers are:	The discharge function may be performed on their behalf by:	Who are:
an NHS trust	three or more: • authorised members of the trust board; or • members of an authorised committee or sub-committee of the Trust	not employees of the Trust.
an NHS foundation trust	three or more people authorised by the board of the trust	neither executive directors of the board of the Trust, nor employees of the Trust.
another NHS body (e.g. primary care trust, local health board)	three or more: • authorised members of the body; or • members of an authorised committee or sub-committee of the body	not officers of the body (within the meaning of the NHS Act 2006 or NHS (Wales) Act 2006).
another body of persons (e.g. company)	three or more: • authorised members of the body; or • members of an authorised committee or sub-committee of the body	

The Guide supplements this with:

'12.119 In Table 12.3, "authorised" means that the person, committee or subcommittee (as the case may be) has been authorised by the managers (i.e. the body in question) specifically for this purpose. "Members" of a body include its Chairman.

12.120 Patients can only be discharged when all three people acting on behalf of the managers agree that they should be discharged. A two to one majority decision is not sufficient (R. (on the application of Tagoe –Thompson) re the hospital managers of the Park Royal Centre [2003] EWCA Civ330). If the decision is taken by more than three people, as well as a majority being in favour, the majority must consist of at least three people in favour of discharge before a decision to discharge can be made.'

In many ways, the Reference Guide is not just helpful for newcomers to the Mental Health Act 1983; it is a source of help to some of the key experts in this field, the Mental Health Act Administrators, a sometimes under-appreciated group of staff. This is because the Guide has taken over from the Memorandum in providing guidance for which errors on forms are rectifiable and which would invalidate a detention. Chapter 2 contains some detailed advice in this area which many will find invaluable.

It is interesting that the Code contains no significant guidance on the question of errors. Rather it points to the need for a policy in this area. It does at least reference the relevant passages in the Guide but this is an example of an apparent blurring of the purpose of the two documents. Together they total in excess of 700 pages and it might be thought there would be a briefer way of providing guidance and explanation. When you add the list of policy documents that the Code requires, it is a significant volume of reading for mental health practitioners. In a striking contrast, the ECHR occupies just a few short pages.

References

Barber, P., Brown, R. and Martin, D (2009) *Mental Health Law in England and Wales*. Exeter: Learning Matters.

Department of Health (2008) *Mental Health Act 1983: Code of Practice*. London: TSO.

Department of Health (2008) *The Mental Health (Conflicts of Interest) (England) Regulations 2008* Statutory Instrument No. 1205/2008 (England). London: TSO.

Jones , R (1996) *Mental Health Act Manual*, 8th Edn. London: Sweet and Maxwell.

Welsh Assembly (2008) *Mental Health Act 1983: Code of Practice*. Welsh Assembly Government.

Welsh Assembly (2001) *Adult Mental Health Services for Wales*. Welsh Assembly Government.

Cases

R (Munjaz) v. *Mersey Care NHS Trust* (2005).

BB v. *Cygnet Health Care and London Borough of Lewisham* (2008).

HL v. *UK* (2004).

R. (on the application of Tagoe–Thompson) re the hospital managers of the Park Royal Centre [2003] EWCA Civ330.

14 The Care Quality Commission

The Care Quality Commission (CQC) was established by Section 1 of the Health and Social Care Act 2008. It assumed responsibility for monitoring the use of the Mental Health Act in England in April 2009 when it replaced the Mental Health Act Commission. In Wales, these functions were taken on by the Health Inspectorate for Wales. The CQC also replaced the Commission for Healthcare Audit and Inspection and the Commission for Social Care Inspection. Its functions are, therefore, far wider than the old Mental Health Act Commission including the registration of service providers. In this chapter, we will only be concerned with its functions under the Mental Health Act. This includes the appointment of Second Opinion Appointed Doctors (SOADs) and others to provide certificates for treatment under Sections 57, 58 and 58A and for patients subject to Community Treatment Orders (CTOs). *Monitoring the Use of the Mental Health Act in 2009/10*, the Care Quality Commission's first report on the exercise of its functions in keeping under review the operation of the Mental Health Act 1983, was published in October 2010.

Statutory basis of the Commission

The Care Quality Commission is required by Section 120 of the Mental Health Act 1983 to 'keep under review and, where appropriate, investigate the exercise of the power and the discharge of the duties conferred or imposed by this Act so far as relating to the detention of patients or their reception into guardianship or to relevant patients.' This covers:

- patients liable to be detained under the Act (this includes patients on Section 17 leave as well as those who are currently detained in hospital);
- patients subject to Community Treatment Orders;
- patients subject to guardianship.

The Care Quality Commission is required to authorise people to visit and interview such patients in private. In England, these people are still called Mental Health Act Commissioners and their role will be considered below. Originally, the government was going to use the independent advocacy services to fulfil the visiting and interviewing role but eventually accepted that this was a different function from advocacy.

Section 120 also requires the CQC to investigate any complaints concerning such patients. There is no power to discharge patients.

Section 120(7) gives Commissioners the following powers which may be exercised at any reasonable time:

> '(a) *visit and interview in private any patient in a hospital or regulated establishment,*

(b) *if the authorised person is a registered medical practitioner or approved clinician, examine the patient in private there, and*
(c) *require the production of and inspect any records relating to the detention or treatment of any person who is or has been detained under this Act or who is or has been a community patient or a patient subject to guardianship.'*

The current aim is to visit every psychiatric ward in England where patients are detained at least once every 18 months. The CQC also appoints Second Opinion Appointed Doctors (SOADs) who have a key role in the operation of the consent to treatment provisions of Part IV of the Act which is considered in the chapter on consent to treatment.

Section 120C gave new powers to the CQC to require the provision of records and documents by service providers to the Commission. This can include such matters as: the number of deaths or serious incidents, use of particular powers under the Act, and statistical data on ethnicity, gender etc.

The CQC has inherited the Mental Health Act Commission's powers to make decisions over the withholding of correspondence from certain patients.

The CQC's annual reports draw on the findings of the Mental Health Act Commissioners and SOADs. These reports replace the biennial reports which the Mental Health Act Commission used to publish. It is to be hoped that they will provide a similarly comprehensive review of the Mental Health Act in practice.

Monitoring the use of the Mental Health Act

As well as the Mental Health Act Commissioners and the SOADs, the CQC employs staff members and has a service-user reference panel. This panel consists of 20 people who are, or have been, detained patients. The first annual report (CQC, 2010) contains comments and observations from members of the panel. The CQC is currently looking at ways of broadening its monitoring methodology to consider patients' experiences from initial assessment, through detention or guardianship to after-care. It is also trying to link this work more closely with its wider regulatory framework.

Mental Health Act Commissioners meet with detained patients to discuss their experiences and concerns, to ensure that they understand their rights and to check that staff are using the Act correctly. Commissioners now concentrate on particular patches so they get to know hospitals in greater depth. Many of the visits are unannounced. SOADs check that certain treatments proposed for detained patients are appropriate and that their views and rights have been considered.

Summary of key issues from the first annual report

The CQC's first annual report was published in October 2010 (CQC, 2010) and runs to 120 pages. It considers trends in the use of detention, including the admission of children and adolescents to adult wards. There is a review of police involvement in Section 136. The report provides information on the experience of detained patients and their involvement in planning care. Key areas for special focus include the use of control and restraint, consent to treatment issues, and the use of Community Treatment Orders.

From analysis of these areas, the following areas are identified as needing development and monitoring of good practice:

> '***Assessing people for detention:*** *not keeping medical recommendations in reserve when the assessment is completed and the patient has agreed to go into hospital informally, and making sure that the outcomes of the assessment are communicated to the patient.*
>
> ***Use of Section 136:*** *supporting the police to avoid misuse of Section 136 and ensuring access to hospital-based places of safety.*
>
> ***Production of social circumstances reports:*** *reviewing both the priority given to patients' social circumstance reports and how they are produced; also reviewing the quality of these reports on an ongoing basis.*
>
> ***Assessment and recording of patients' capacity and consent:*** *to ensure this is routinely done and includes evidence of ongoing discussion with patients.*
>
> ***Recording episodes of control and restraint:*** *to ensure that there is a record of the steps that have been taken to de-escalate a situation before other interventions are considered or used, and auditing these records to inform practice development.*
>
> ***Carrying out duties as statutory consultees:*** *ensuring that records are made of conversations with SOADs and indicating that patients have been informed of the outcome of second opinions.*'

Three priority areas are then identified in the report as being in need of improvement.

Involving detained patients in their care and treatment

The report recommends that services focus on ensuring they involve patients in key areas of service planning and delivery: assessment, care planning and review processes, as a basis for developing the patient's personalised care plan; planning the patient's community treatment order where this is relevant; involving the patient as part of assessments of capacity and consent, with these discussions formally recorded on the patient's care plan; ensuring that detained patients are aware of IMHA services and have access to information about them; consulting and informing detained patients about their social circumstances reports.

Practice relating to patients' capacity and consent

Providers should ensure that discussion of these issues with patients are an integral part of treatment planning. The report noted discrepancies between the observations of visiting Commissioners and the patients' recorded consent and their apparent lack of capacity or refusal of consent. Consent to treatment practice is identified as a continuing problem in many mental health services.

Unnecessary restrictions and blanket security measures

While recognising the importance of ensuring the safety of patients, the report urges providers to give more thought to how they can minimise restrictions on detained patients and avoid blanket measures that compromise patients' privacy or dignity, or unnecessarily restrict their autonomy. These are identified as sometimes being counter-therapeutic, as well as a potential breach of human rights principles and are wrong.

Community Treatment Orders

The Mental Health Act Commission expressed some concerns about the use of CTOs in its Biennial Report 2007–2009. At Paragraph 2.68 the report noted:

> *'In the Mental Health Bill debates, the Secretary of State for Health (Patricia Hewitt) stated that SCT was "designed particularly for the so-called 'revolving door patients' – people who are hospitalised, whether under compulsion or voluntarily, who respond to treatment, who are released, and who then fail to maintain their treatment, producing another crisis and yet another hospitalization". Although SCT was thus designed "particularly" for certain patients, it may yet be applied in practice to the generality of cases which fall within its scope. The revised Codes of Practice (Chapter 25.2 in England, 30.3 in Wales) states that the purpose of SCT is "to allow suitable patients to be safely treated in the community rather than under detention in hospital, and to provide a way to prevent relapse … It is intended to help patients to maintain stable mental health outside hospital and to promote recovery". There is no mention of the concept of the "revolving door" in any official guidance on the implementation of SCT and, although grounds must be given on the statutory forms for certifying that the use of SCT is "necessary", there is no explicit requirement to give objective evidence (for instance of past relapse) to show such necessity. We expect that this will be an issue raised at SCT patients' Tribunal hearings, and may yet be subject to further judicial interpretation.'*

The report continues:

> *'It is to be hoped that the use of SCT does not follow a similar pattern [to that of restricted patients], and as such become a usual stage in the detention process of unrestricted patients. The restrictions placed upon Part 3 patients result either from them having criminal convictions and/or being identified as posing a particular danger by the courts. The unrestricted population of detainees under the Act has, in general terms, no such distinguishing features … It will be vital that the AMHPs concerned make a particular effort to ensure that they take an objective view that takes full account of the wider social context in the case, to avoid their teams developing a culture of using SCT as an automatic discharge process.'*

These concerns appear even sharper in the first annual report from the CQC (CQC, 2010). By publication, it was clear that numbers of CTO cases were far higher than had been anticipated by the government. There were 4 107 CTOs made in 2009/10, with a total of 6 241 orders in the 17 months from their introduction in November 2008. This is an average of 367 each month. It is informative to look at the experience of recall and revocation in this period. The recall power was used 1217 times in 2009/10, or 1424 times from the introduction of the power. This means that approximately one in five patients placed under a CTO have been recalled at some point, although it is not possible to be more precise as some patients may have been recalled more than once. A third of all CTOs implemented up to the end of March 2010 had ended at that time: 922 patients (15%) were returned to detention and 1043 (17%) released from compulsion.

Interesting data emerged on the ethnicity of those made subject to CTOs and these tend to reinforce concerns over compulsion being used more frequently with certain black and minority ethnic groups. This is explored further in the chapter on race, culture and mental health.

The report comments:

> *'Surprisingly, given that CTOs are meant to help "revolving door" patients who would otherwise disengage with services, 30% of the patients in our sample did not have a reported history of non-compliance or disengagement. This suggests that the high use of CTOs – much greater than government estimates at the time the law was passed – could be a result of the powers being applied preventatively beyond the group of patients for whom they were primarily designed. It would be an extremely unfortunate distortion of Parliament's intention if CTOs were to become the "normal" route for the discharge of civil detainees from hospital. This is a question that requires more research.'*

Conclusion

There had been some concern that the CQC's monitoring of the Mental Health Act might lack the cutting edge of its smaller, more tightly focused predecessor, the Mental Health Act Commission. The critical tone of the first annual report and the continued existence of specialist Mental Health Act Commissioners and SOADs may be signs that these concerns were unfounded.

References

Care Quality Commission (2010) *Monitoring the Use of the Mental Health Act in 2009/10*. CQC.

Mental Health Act Commission (2009) *Biennial Report 2007–2009*.

Cases

1983 Mental Health Act.

2008 Health and Social Care Act.

15 Consent and Capacity

It is assumed, unless contested, that every adult has the absolute right and the capacity (legal concept) (competence) to decide whether or not he will accept medical treatment, even if refusal risks permanent injury to health or premature death.

For example, in a case in England (*Re B (Adult: Refusal of Medical Treatment) [2002] 2 ALL ER 449*) of a woman with capacity kept alive by a ventilator who wished the machine to be turned off against her doctors' judgement, it was ruled under common law that she had the right for this to be done and she died as a result. As stated by Dame Elizabeth Butler-Schloss in this case:

> ***'A competent patient has an absolute right to refuse to consent to medical treatment for any reason, rational or irrational, or for no reason at all even when that decision may lead to his or her death.'***

Ethical principles and Consent

Introduction

Ethical principles underlie the practice of medicine and provide a guide for difficult and painful decisions about human behaviour. This is particularly relevant in psychiatry as decisions about restricting individual freedom through mental health legislation routinely occur in this specialty. Also, decisions about administering medication to patients who are not thought to be competent to decide on their treatment have to be taken regularly.

Many factors in today's society create conflicting demands on physicians. These include advances in scientific research, civil rights and consumer movements, increased public education, effects of the law on medicine, pressures of economy and moral, religions and ethnic dilemmas. These require a clear understanding of the ethical principles guiding medical practice.

Autonomy

Informed consent is the cornerstone of the ethical theory of autonomy, which is based on the writings of Immanuel Kant. This theory describes the relationship between the physician and a normal adult patient as a relationship between two responsible people rather than between a parent and child. This is the theory that the law tends to recognise and its assumption of the adult's competence, the right to informed consent in treatment and research, the right to refuse treatment, and limitations on a psychiatrist's ability to hospitalise involuntarily can be seen as recognition of an adult's fundamental right to self-determination in medical decision-making. This is, however, sometimes in direct opposition to society's expectations concerning people with mental health problems and their perceived dangerousness.

Adult patients are assumed to have the right to consent or refuse consent to treatment. However, the effects of illness and particularly mental disorder may confuse the issue.

Definition of Consent

Consent is the voluntary permission of the patient to a particular treatment or procedure. This can be withdrawn at any time and is based on information given to the patient for the purpose of the treatment. What it entails, likely effects and side-effects, alternatives to that treatment, and consequences of refusal should all be explained, e.g. amputation of a gangrenous limb and consequences of non-amputation.

Medical treatment

In the context of mental health legislation, medical treatment refers to the broad range of activities aimed at alleviating or preventing a deterioration of a patient's mental disorder. It includes:

- nursing care
- other forms of care
- habilitation
- rehabilitation
- electroconvulsive therapy (ECT)
- administration of drugs
- psychotherapy.

Treatment plans are essential for informal and detained patients alike. Consultant psychiatrists should coordinate the formulation of the treatment plan in consultation with their other professional colleagues and *record* it.

Before an individual can be given medical treatment, his valid consent is required except in cases in which the law provides authority to treat the patient without consent.

Types of consent

There are two main types of consent:

- Implied consent
- Express consent.

Implied consent

Implied consent occurs in the normal course of contact between a clinical professional and the patient. For example, a patient actively indicates consent by holding out his arm for a blood test or rolling up his sleeve to have his blood pressure taken. This form of consent is used where risk is low and there is minimal invasiveness.

Express consent

Express consent is either verbal or written consent and should be obtained for procedures where there is a risk and a degree of invasiveness, such as in operations for hernia, etc.

Treatment without consent

In general, in medicine and psychiatry, treatment may only be given to a patient with his informed consent. Note that there are two components to this: the patient must give his consent and the consent must be informed. Failure to fulfil either part is generally illegal (unless it is covered by common law or by, for example, the Mental Health Act – *see* below) and may constitute battery or negligence.

Battery

Battery is a trespass against the person and occurs if treatment is given to a patient without his consent.

Negligence

It is not sufficient to obtain the consent of a patient to a treatment in the absence of reasonable explanation (*Chatterton* v. *Gerson and another* (1980); such an action may be construed as being negligent.

Reasons why treatment may need to be given without consent

The position is that treatment can be given without consent when the patient is incapable of giving consent because the patient:

- is a child. In this case, the parent or guardian consents (it is the person with parental responsibility who legally consents);
- is unconscious and is in urgent need of treatment to preserve life, health or well-being (unless there is concrete evidence that the patient does not want treatment);
- is suffering from a mental disorder which is manifesting itself in a way that is causing danger to the patient or to others and it is not immediately possible to make use of the Mental Health Act and the treatment is necessary to avert danger;
- is otherwise incapable and in need of medical care in circumstances in which the patient had not declared unwillingness to be treated before he became incapable.

For the three latter points, the Mental Capacity Act 2005 provides the legal authority for treatment. In all of the four cases, the treatment must be in the patient's best interests (*see* below). Note that the common law applies to all patients, informal or detained, who have capacity, except in those situations in which the Mental Health Act specifically overrides it.

Best interests

There can be no statutory guidance on the meaning of 'best interests', as individuals and their individual circumstances determine the results. Decisions taken on behalf of a person lacking capacity require careful thought about that person as an individual. Best interest now also legally falls within the Mental Capacity Act 2005, in particular, Section 4 of that Act.

In the *Re F* case, it was implied that a doctor should act in accordance with an accepted body of medical opinion (Bolam compliance) i.e., if a doctor did so, he was not negligent and was acting in the best interests of an incapable person.

This caused some criticism and the Law Commission suggested that in deciding what is in a person's best interests attention should be paid to the following:

- The known wishes and feelings of the individual and the factors that person would consider if he were able to do so.
- The need to permit maximum participation in decisions affecting him.
- The views of other people whom it is appropriate to consult.
- Any action or decision should be able to be achieved in a manner less restrictive of the person's freedom of action.

Recent case law has gone much further than the *Re F* case, with Bolam being seen as the starting rather than the end point.

Situations requiring consent

The following situations require consent:

- Medical and nursing procedures
- Mental health treatment
- Photography, videoing, filming etc.
- The presence of students for teaching or work experience
- HIV testing
- Genetic testing.

Legal considerations

In England and Wales, it is unlawful to treat without consent, except under the Mental Health Act 1983 Part IV or under the Mental Capacity Act 2005. Legally if a patient is 'medically touched' without consent, this constitutes the civil wrong of battery and possibly the criminal offence of assault, as well as risking referral to the professional's respective governing body, for example, to the General Medical Council (GMC) for medical practitioners.

Consent should be informed and voluntary, which implies that any mental disorder present, such as dementia, does not affect judgement. In practice, a lower threshold for capacity is adopted for patients who consent to treatment compared with those who refuse. Refusal is not the same as lack of capacity to consent. It is important to never threaten to impose treatment if a patient refuses, and always to ensure that a patient is not simply consenting for a 'quiet life'. A distinction is to be made between coercion and a patient's acceptance of the reality of his or her situation.

Valid ethical consent requires competence and information, resulting in understanding. Understanding and voluntariness can then result in an affirmative decision.

Regarding consent being based on *sufficient information*, to date, the standard applied to this in the UK has been predominantly *profession-based* – that is, giving the level of information that is normally given by the profession in that medical situation based on the duty of care. The alternative standard is *patient-based* – that is, the level of information necessary to allow a patient to operate his autonomy. Information should refer to alternative treatments and advice about substantial or unusual risks. No or very little information given may result in the professional being liable to a charge of battery. Inadequate information may result in a doctor being held liable to a charge of negligence (breach of duty of care). 'Informed consent' is a US term and is not specifically enshrined in UK law. Relevant case law in England and Wales includes *Pearce* v. *United Bristol Healthcare NHS Trust.* Healthcare NHS Trust [1998] 48 BMLR, where Lord Woolf stated that if *'there is a significant risk which would affect the judgement of a reasonable patient, then... it is the responsibility of the doctor to inform the patient of that significant risk...'*.

In *R (Burke)* v. *General Medical Council [2005] EWCA Civ 1003*, the GMCs guidance on withholding and withdrawing life-prolonging treatment was endorsed and it upheld the status quo that *'for a doctor to deliberately interrupt life-prolonging treatment in the face of a competent patient's expressed wish to be kept alive, with the intention of thereby terminating the patient's life, would leave the doctor with no answer to a charge of murder'. 'Once a patient has been received into hospital, a duty of care arises – a duty to provide and to go on providing treatment whether the patient is in/competent or un/conscious'.*

A decision about consent may vary over time, and different messages may be given by the patient in different modalities.

A consent form is only evidence as to consent and does not amount to fact of consent.

The UK standard for sufficient information for valid consent is now closer to the US law – the *objective prudent patient test* (what a reasonable patient should be told) rather than the *reasonable doctor medical test* (profession-based) – due mainly to changing GMC guidelines.

Relevant case law from England and Wales includes the following:

- *Sidaway* v. *Board of Governors of Bethlem Royal and Maudsley Hospital* (1985): the majority of the five law lords supported the doctor-based standard of not telling of the 1 per cent risk of damage to the spinal cord, after a neurosurgical procedure on the cervical vertebrae. However, the judgment suggested that if doctors were lax in informing patients, then the courts may intervene.
- *Bolam* v. *Friern Hospital Management Committee* (1957): the 'Bolam test' – a doctor is required to exercise the ordinary skills of a competent practitioner in the field (profession-based standard), that is a doctor is *'not guilty of negligence if he has acted in accordance with a practice accepted as proper by a responsible body of medical men skilled in that particular art.'*

These two cases clearly imply that a doctor should keep up-to-date with current practice and be cautious about using any new or non-established treatment.

- *Maynard* v. *West Midlands RHA (1985* 1 *All ER 635):* even if the body of opinion is a minority, this is still defendable.
- *Bolitho* v. *Hackney Health Authority (1997 All ER 771):* in order to avoid negligence, even if following a 'responsible body' of medical opinion, a doctor needs to convince the court that the amount of information given or omitted can be defended, i.e. the courts ultimately remain the final arbiter.

Courts are reluctant to put a percentage figure of risk of which a patient should be warned, as the individual significance of injury to the individual is also important. Always put a note of warnings given to the patient in the notes and in a letter to the patient's general practitioner (GP) (not the consent form).

Individuals under the age of 16 years can give valid consent if there is sufficient understanding. Parental consent is valid for individuals aged 16–18 years who do not understand.

Consent in English law for adults (aged 18 years) and minors

The following apply to *competent adult patients*:

- The patient may refuse any, including life-saving, treatment (otherwise battery).
- The patient should be given information about the nature of the procedure, any serious side-effects, the likely benefits and alternatives (otherwise negligence).

Note: doctors are under no obligation to treat a consenting patient at his request if the doctor does not think the treatment is in the patient's best interests.

For *incompetent adult patients*, the following principles apply:

- The doctor should act in the best interests of the patient.
- The patient's relatives and friends cannot give or withhold consent (they can only assent), but they may be sources of information regarding best interests.

For *minors*, the following points apply:

- A person under 18 years of age should not be allowed to come to serious harm on the grounds of the minor or the parents refusing consent to necessary and urgent treatment.
- Patients aged 16–17 years are presumed by statute to have the capacity to give consent, unless the contrary is shown. The Mental Capacity Act 2005 applies to over 16s.
- A child under age 16 years who does have capacity ('Gillick competent' (decision-specific) in common law) can give consent, but if the child refuses treatment, consent can be overridden by the people with parental responsibility or a court.
- Courts are unlikely to consider that people aged 13 years or under have capacity.
- For children who are not Gillick-competent, the people with parental responsibility give consent but have a legal obligation to act in the child's best interests.

Although psychiatric disorders can affect a patient's judgement and therefore capacity to consent, this can also occur in medical disorders, albeit less often.

The House of Lords has ruled that doctors have a common law duty (justification of necessity) to act in the best possible interests of the patient, for example, if the patient is physically ill and not competent (e.g. unconscious) or if the patient is permanently unable to consent (e.g. due to severe learning disability) to treatments not covered by the Mental Health Act 1983. This has been incorporated and updated in the Mental Capacity Act 2005.

Patients detained under the Mental Health Act 1983 may be able to give free valid consent to treatment, providing they are not complying simply to get out of hospital. The patient should know the nature and consequences of the proposed treatment, the consequences of not having the treatment, and the risks of the treatment. The Mental Health Act Code of Practice gives guidance in this area.

Although some doctors argue that it would be negligent in the case of patients not consenting if one did not test for medical conditions suspected (i.e. duty of care), this is not accepted legally. Undertaking a human immunodeficiency virus (HIV)/acquired immunodeficiency syndrome (AIDS) test without the patient knowing the nature of such a test, and its personal and social implications, constitutes assault, even if the patient consented to give blood for unspecified or other tests.

Box 15.1 summarises the principles of consent.

Box 15.1: Consent

- Consent requires:
  - Information (knowing) to either profession or patient-based standard.
  - Competency.
  - Voluntariness.
- Competence + information → understanding.
- Understanding + voluntariness → affirmative decision.
- Competence is not an absolute quality and is no longer considered global.
- Competence is not statutorily defined.
- Competence depends on the patient's functioning (e.g. intelligence) and the purpose of the treatment (e.g. complexity of issues). It is decision-specific.
- An incompetent patient is incapable of giving valid consent (capacity is a legal concept).
- The Mental Health Act 1983 competence means 'knowing the nature, purpose and likely effects' of treatment ...
- Treatment without consent is battery. Harm is presumed and does not have to be proven.
- Detention without consent is false imprisonment.
- Consent by proxy (assent) is not legal (c.f. surrogacy in the USA).

Exceptions to usual requirements for consent

- *Implied consent:*
  - By fact of consultation
  - Patient's consent unavailable, but reasonable person would consent, e.g. unconscious patient after overdose.
- *Necessity:*
  - Some level of patient incompetence and serious harm or death likely to occur
  - Doctor owes duty of care.
- *Emergency:* to prevent serious harm to patient or other.
- *Post-suicide attempt:* can reverse effects of suicide attempt (anachronism, as suicide was previously a crime) but cannot stop a suicidal patient from leaving hospital if not detainable under the Mental Health Act 1983.
- *Detention under Mental Health Act 1983.*

Capacity and competency

Capacity is a legal concept. Competency is a clinical concept but is occasionally used legally. The terms mean the ability to know and understand the nature and consequences of legal proceedings, including for medical purposes.

Assessment of capacity

This is required in many branches of medicine, including psychiatry, for example:

- *Old-age psychiatry:*
  - Testamentary capacity
  - Power of attorney.
- *Finances*
  - Social care, e.g. sheltered care home.
- *Forensic psychiatry:*
  - Fitness to plead and stand trial.
- *Liaison psychiatry:*
  - Treatment refusal
  - Leaving hospital without medical consent.

Capacity may vary over time, for example in delirium.

Legal principles relating to capacity

- An imprudent decision is not itself grounds for incapacity (analyse the way decision was made, not the decision itself).
- Capacity is function-specific, not global.
- Standard of proof is on the balance of probabilities.
- There are three stages of assessing capacity (*Re C [1994] All ER 819*):
  - Comprehension and retention of relevant information
  - Ability to believe information (e.g. no delusion interfering)
  - Weigh information and make decision.

Approaches to making decisions for incompetent patients

- Best interests
- Proxy
- Advance decision directive (living will)
- Substituted judgements (e.g. if patient became competent, what treatment would he or she choose?).

The final three of these are available under the Mental Capacity Act 2005.

British Medical Association and Law Society guidelines (1994) on assessing capacity

- Can the patient understand the nature and purpose of the procedure or treatment and why it is being proposed?
- Does the patient understand the principle benefits and risks, the alternatives, and the risks and consequences of not being treated?
- Capacity does not depend on detainability under the Mental Health Act 1983.
- Take into account the patient's anxiety, language problems and cultural and educational background.
- There is no relation to clinical reality, for example, severity of illness if treatment is refused.

The MB test for capacity (1997) (needle phobia)

- Can the patient comprehend and retain information?
- Can the patient weigh information in balance and reach decision?

Patient attempts suicide and then refuses treatment in accident and emergency department

Theoretically, if competent, such a patient can refuse treatment. However, medical defence organisations in the UK comment that competence can be questioned if an individual has harmed him- or herself, and so it maybe defendable to intervene. The common law justification of 'necessity' allows reasonable interventions, including medical treatments, reasonable to the circumstances, where the competence of the individual is unknown.

Case law propositions on medical treatment prior to the Mental Capacity Act 2005

Lord Donaldson MR in Re T (critically ill young woman) (adult: refusal of medical treatment) (1992) 4 All ER 649 CA

Incapacity may be due to the following:

- Long-term mental incapacity or retarded development
- Temporary factors:
  - Unconsciousness
  - Confusion
  - Fatigue
  - Shock
  - Pain
  - Drugs.

Note: in the case of MB (1997), with needle phobia, panic, indecisiveness and irritability were ruled not factors causing incapacity.

Capacity may be reduced, not removed (i.e. could be taught, not simply assessed). The patient's decision must be independent (e.g. from relatives and religious advisors).

Thorpe J, in Re C Adult Refusal of Medical Treatment (1994) 1 All ER 819

Refusal of treatment can be a declaration never to consent or never in some future circumstances, for example, to electroconvulsive therapy (ECT) (equivalent to 'living will').

The Mental Capacity Act 2005 has now superseded such common law propositions. Advance decisions (directives) are now legal under the Mental Capacity Act 2005; for example, the individual may state that, if his or her mental illness relapses again, he or she wants no haloperidol, only risperidone oral antipsychotic medication.

Consent obtained by coercion or duress is invalid

***Freeman* v. *Home Office* (1983) All ER 589**

Freeman claimed that his relationship as a prisoner with the prison doctor prevented valid consent due to his role in influencing disciplinary procedures. Issue was of covert, as opposed to overt, coercion instead of voluntary consent. The case was lost by Freeman.

***Barbara* v. *Home Office* (1984)**

Barbara was injected in prison against his will. The case was won by Barbara.

Too much information may preclude a patient from making a valid judgement

Lord Templeman in *Sidaway* v. *Board of Governors of Bethlem Royal and Maudsley Hospital* (1985).

Medical treatment for mental disorder under Part IV of Mental Health Act 1983

The definition of medical treatment in the Act includes treatment of physical health problems only when it is part of or ancillary to treatment of mental disorder.

Section 63

Consent is not required for medical treatments that do not fall within Sections 57 or 58, for example, nasogastric feeding of a detained patient with borderline personality disorder refusing to eat ruled by Court of Appeal within scope of Section 63 (*B* v. *Croydon Health Authority* (1995) *(1 All ER 683)*. A further example can be wounds self-inflicted as a result of mental disorder.

Section 145

Medical treatment includes nursing, psychological intervention and specialist mental health habilitation, rehabilitation and care.

Wall J, in *Thameside and Glossop Acute Services Trust* v. *UCH* (1996) 1 FLR 792

Induction of labour and possible Caesarean section of a 41-year-old 38-week-pregnant woman with schizophrenia was ruled treatment within scope of Section 63. The woman consented to induction, but medical staff feared that she would change her mind. The decision was obtained on grounds of (i) to prevent deterioration in the patient's mental state, (ii) that a live baby would promote the patient's health, and (iii) that antipsychotic medication was contraindicated during pregnancy. However, the real issue is competence. Such decisions are often made in a rush, with the patient in labour and taking analgesics, so that 'not competent' is accepted. Also such cases are often heard in court, often *ex-parte* with no representation of the individual (which does not prevent liability). Note that the Court of Appeal ruled in 1988 that a foetus is not a person with legal rights.

***Re C (adult refusal of medical treatment)* (1994)**

C's gangrene of his leg secondary to chronic diabetes was ruled not likely to affect his mental condition. C was a detained patient at Broadmoor Special Hospital and was deluded that he was a great doctor. In spite of this, it was ruled he had capacity to decide on his medical treatment. He insisted, against medical advice, on no amputation in the future and, in fact, he recovered.

References

Department of Health (2008) *Mental Health Act 1983: Code of Practice*. London: The Stationery Office.

General Medical Council (2006) *Consent: In Good Medical Practice*, 4th edn. London: General Medical Council.

Lidz, CW, Meisel, A, Zerutavel, E, *et al.* (1984) *Informed Consent*. London: Guilford Press.

Case

Gillick v. *West Norfolk and Wisbech Area Health Authority* [1986] AC 112.

16 The Mental Capacity Act 2005: Principles

Under old common law, if a patient had capacity, treatment required their consent, but if the patient lacked capacity, the clinician was under a duty to give treatment which was necessary to preserve the patient's life, health or well-being and was also in their best interests.

The common law still applies, if a patient has capacity, i.e. treatment still requires the patient's consent. However, if they lack capacity, the Mental Capacity Act 2005 now applies wherever it is intended to give care or treatment to an incapacitated person outside the Mental Health Act.

Thus, for those with a physical disorder and who lack capacity, the Mental Capacity Act applies. For those with mental disorder who lack capacity, the Mental Capacity Act applies only where treatment is not being given under the Mental Health Act 1983 within its rules.

The Mental Capacity Act 2005 provides a statutory framework not only for adults who lack capacity to make decisions but also for those who have capacity and want to make preparations for a time in the future when they may lose capacity.

Capacity under the Mental Capacity Act 2005

A person may lack capacity:

- at the material time;
- if he or she is unable to make a decision for him- or herself in relation to the matter;
- because of an impairment of, or a disturbance in the functioning of, the mind or brain (Section 2).

It does not matter whether the impairment or disturbance is permanent or temporary.

Impairment or disturbance

> '*The impairment or disturbance may occur in a wide range of situations … people who are affected by … alcohol or drug misuse … delirium … following head injury … mental illness … dementia … learning disabilities … long-term effects of brain damage … grave physical conditions producing confusion, drowsiness or loss of consciousness including as a result of treatment*' [from the Code of Practice].

The definition of incapacity under Section 2 emphasises that it is decision-specific and that an individual may lack capacity in one matter but not another, for example a more complex matter. It is also time-specific. Capacity may fluctuate over time and be lost only temporarily. Section 2(3) emphasises that lack of capacity cannot be implied from a person's age, appearance, medical condition or behaviour.

Ability to make a decision

Under Section 3(1), individuals should be able to:

- Understand information relevant to the decision, including potential consequences of different decisions;
- Retain that information for long enough to make a decision (not permanently);
- Use that information to make a decision;
- Communicate the decision, including by gesture or sign language.

A surprising or unwise decision does not of itself indicate lack of capacity.

There is a two-stage test of capacity: *a diagnostic test* and *a functional test* (Code of Practice Paragraph 4.10). This is detailed in Figure 16.1. The assessment of capacity does not have to be undertaken for the purposes of the Mental Capacity Act by a doctor or other healthcare professional. However, the Code of Practice (Paragraph 4.38–4.43) indicates that the more serious the decision the more formal should be the assessment and the more appropriate it is for the assessment to be undertaken by a professional.

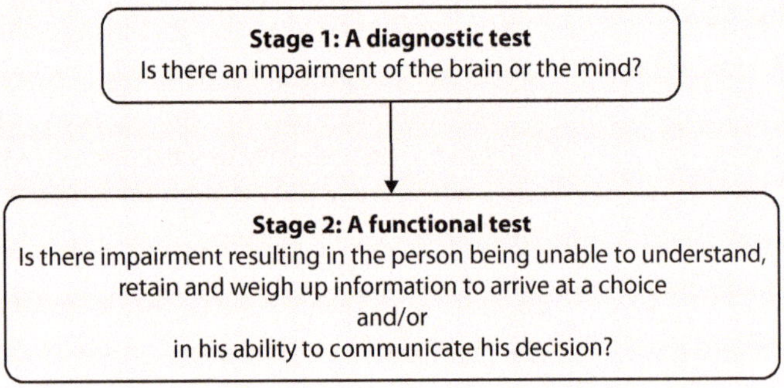

Figure 16.1 Assessment of capacity under the Mental Capacity Act 2005: a two-stage process.

Statutory principles

The statutory principles of the Mental Capacity Act 2005, which are summarised in Figure 16.2, are intended to be supportive of people lacking capacity, not restrictive or excessively controlling of their lives (Code of Practice p. 19). It is intended that these principles should assist in finding solutions to difficult situations.

Under Section 1(1):

- *The presumption of capacity:* everyone is assumed to have capacity, unless shown otherwise (Section 1(2)).
- *Maximising decision-making capacity:* no one is to be treated as unable to make a decision unless all practicable steps to assist have failed (Section 1(3)).
- *Unwise decisions:* a person is not to be treated as lacking capacity only because he or she makes an 'unwise' decision (Section 1(4)).

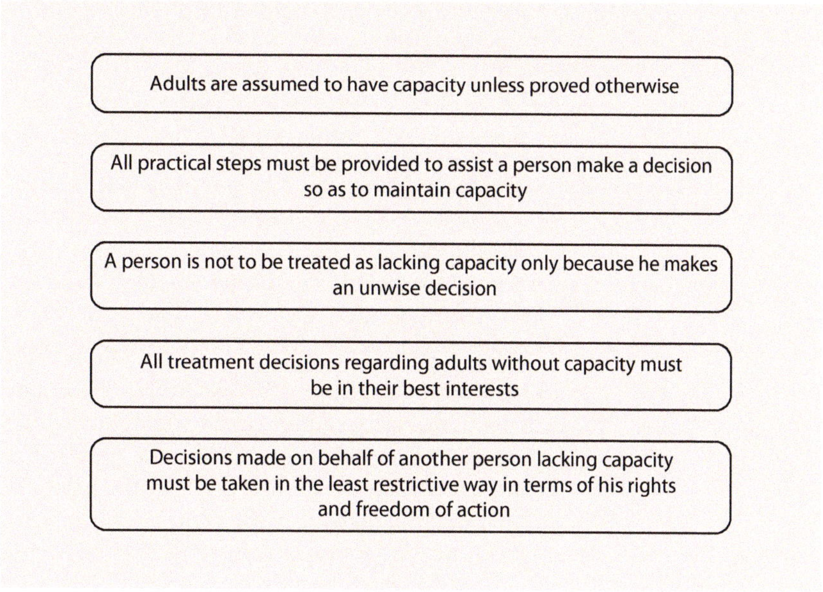

Figure 16.2 Principles of the Mental Capacity Act 2005.

- *Best interests:* any act or decision on behalf of someone who lacks capacity must be done in his or her best interests (Section 1(5)).
- *Least restrictive intervention:* before any act, there must be consideration of whether the objective can be as well achieved in a less restrictive way (Section 1(6)).

Section 4: Best interests

Under Section 4, when determining best interests, a legal concept, one must consider all the relevant circumstances and, in particular:

- Involve the person if possible in any decision.
- Consider other wishes/beliefs, made with capacity, or values that indicate preference.
- Consider anyone already nominated, or any carers, etc., e.g. lasting power of attorney or court-appointed deputy.
- Consider the likelihood of regaining capacity? If so, when?
- Do not seek the subject's death where the decision relates to life-sustaining treatment; consider whether is in the best interests of the person concerned. ('Life-sustaining treatment' is treatment that the provider clinician considers necessary to sustain life.)

Section 4(1) states that best interests should not be based merely on a person's age, appearance, behaviour or particular condition.

Regarding best interests as it relates to life-sustaining treatment, Section 4(5) emphasises that the decision made should not be motivated by a desire to bring about an individual's death. It does not, however, imply that life-sustaining treatment should be provided or continued when it is not in the best interests of the person (Paragraph 5.33).

Section 4(a): A reasonable belief

There is sufficient compliance with the best interests requirements if (having complied with the requirements of Section 4) the person making the determination reasonably believes that what he or she does or decides is in the best interests of the person concerned.

Scope of the Act: exclusions under Section 27

No decision on the following family issues is to be made on behalf of a person:

- Consent to marriage, civil partnership or sexual relations.
- Consent to divorce/dissolution of a civil partnership on the basis of 2 years' separation.
- Consent to a child being placed for adoption or making of an adoption order.
- Discharging parental responsibilities in matters not relating to a child's property.
- Consent under the Human Fertilisation and Embryology Act 1990.

The Mental Capacity Act allows health or social care professionals and informal carers to carry out certain tasks without incurring any legal liability, if reasonable steps have been taken to confirm the person lacks capacity in relation to the matter, and consideration is given to the principles of the Mental Capacity Act and any action taken is in the person's best interests.

Treatment of detained patients under the Mental Health Act 1983 is separate from the Mental Capacity Act and only applies to those with mental disorder. Mental Health Act 1983 consent to treatment provisions then apply.

17 Mental Capacity Act 2005: Provisions

Mental Capacity Act 2005 of England and Wales

The main provisions of the Mental Capacity Act 2005 (MCA) Act are as follows:

- *Designated decision-makers for people who lack capacity:*
  - Lasting powers of attorney (LPAs) – these are like the previous Enduring Power of Attorney (EPAs) but can make health and welfare decisions.
  - Court-appointed deputies – these replace receivership in the Court of Protection. They can make decisions on welfare, healthcare and financial matters, but they cannot refuse consent to life-sustaining treatment.

- *Two new public bodies:*
  - A new Court of Protection
  - A new Public Guardian will:
    - register LPAs and deputies
    - supervise deputies
    - be scrutinised by a Public Guardian Board.

- *Three provisions to protect vulnerable people:*
  - Independent mental capacity advocate (IMCA)
  - Advance decisions to refuse treatment, including, if expressly stated, 'even if life is at risk'
  - New criminal offence of ill-treatment or neglect of a person who lacks capacity.

Introduction into law

- IMCAs became available on 1 April 2007.
- The Code of Practice and the criminal offence of ill-treatment and wilful neglect became law in April 2007.
- From October 2007, all other elements of legislation, including the new Court of Protection, Public Guardian and Office of the Public Guardian became operational.
- Deprivation of liberty safeguards (MCA DOLs) became law in April 2009.

New process for making decisions under the MCA

These include:

- Advance decision (AD)
- Lasting power of attorney (LPA)

- Section 5: Liability for care or treatment
- Court of Protection or Court-Appointed Deputy (CAD).

Advance decisions (AD) (Section 24)

ADs allow those individuals aged 18 and over, who currently have capacity, to refuse specified medical treatment at a future date when they lack capacity to consent to such treatment. Such decisions may be written or oral. The Code of Practice, however, gives guidance about what should be documented and how verbal advance decisions should be recorded. The Court of Protection has the power to rule on the validity and the applicability of an advance decision, but cannot overturn a valid advance decision.

An AD is a decision made by an adult with capacity that if:

- at a later time a specified treatment is proposed to be carried out by a person providing healthcare; *and*
- at that time he or she lacks capacity to consent to that treatment,
- then the specified treatment is not to be carried out or continued.

An AD is not necessarily binding if the following tests are met:

- *Capacity test:* if the person still has capacity to consent to the treatment proposed.
- *Validity test:* if the person withdrew the AD at any time when able to do so, or has done anything clearly inconsistent with the AD.
- *Applicability test:*
  - Not the treatment specified in the AD
  - Any specified circumstances are absent
  - Reasonable grounds for believing that important unforeseen circumstances exist, not anticipated at the time of the AD
  - *Life-sustaining threshold:* an AD is not applicable to life-sustaining treatment unless it is verified by a statement to the effect expressly that it is to apply to that treatment even if life is at risk, and the decision is in writing, signed and witnessed. Where there is doubt, it is prudent for a clinician to err on the side of preservation of life (*Re T* (*adult: refusal of medical treatment)* [1992] *4 ALL ER 649*). Section 62 states that nothing in the MCA affects the law relating to unlawful killing or assisting suicide.

Advance decisions are also discussed further in Chapter 19.

Note: advance decisions to refuse treatment differ from an *Advance Statement* which details a person's views about his future care and preferences, e.g. the type of medical treatment or where they would wish to live in the event of future incapacity. They are not legally binding but can be taken into account when making best interests determinations. The Code of Practice recommends, however, that when an advance statement is not followed, the reasons for this should be recorded (Paragraph 5.43).

Lasting power of attorney (Section 9)

An LPA is a power under which the donor confers on a donee or donees authority to make decisions about:

- his personal welfare or specific aspects thereof; and
- his property and affairs or specified aspects thereof.

An LPA includes authority to make such decisions in circumstances where the donor no longer has capacity. A property and affairs LPA can, however, apply before a donor loses capacity.

The authority conferred by an LPA is subject to:

- any conditions or restrictions specified in the document;
- the provisions of the Mental Capacity Act and, in particular, Section 1 (Principles) and Section 4 (Best Interests).

An LPA thus allows a person over 18 (a donor) to appoint another person or persons (donee or attorney) to act on his behalf should he subsequently lose capacity. It replaces the Enduring Power of Attorney (EPA) as the power of attorney which can operate after a person loses capacity. There are two types of LPA:

1. *A property and affairs LPA*, which relates to decisions about financial and/or property matters and can be used with the donor's consent while the donor has capacity.
2. *A personal welfare LPA*, for use when the donor no longer has the capacity to make a particular decision.

The donor can specify what types of decision can be made on his behalf for either type of LPA and, indeed, can give permission for one or more attorneys to act on his behalf on all issues covered in the LPA. The Court of Protection can give rulings with regard to the meaning and effect of an LPA and, if necessary, remove an attorney who has acted inappropriately.

There is a form for each type of LPA available from the Office of the Public Guardian, which includes a certificate to be signed by an independent person confirming that the donor understands the power he is donating to the attorney and has not been under pressure to agree. The LPA requires registration with the Office of the Public Guardian for a fee before it can be legally used.

Note: EPAs created before the Mental Capacity Act 2005 came into force on 1 October 2007 remain valid.

Section 5: liability for care or treatment

Where the Section 5 conditions are satisfied, someone who does an act 'in connection' with an incapacitated person's care or treatment will incur legal liability only if the act would have been unlawful if it were done with consent; as an example, negligent acts are not protected.

Section 5 conditions are as follows:

- The act is 'in connection with' care or treatment.
- The person doing it takes reasonable steps to establish whether the subject has capacity.
- The person reasonably believes that the subject lacks capacity.
- The person reasonably believes that the act is in the subject's best interests.

- If restraint is used, then the person reasonably believes that it is necessary to do the act in order to prevent harm to the subject *and* that the act is a proportionate response to the likelihood of the subject's suffering harm and the seriousness of that harm.

Under the Mental Capacity Act 2005, restraint is the use of, or threat to use force to do an act 'the person resists', i.e. to achieve an outcome or restriction of liberty of movement, whether or not resisted.

Section 5 does not allow any act which conflicts with a valid advance decision or a valid decision taken by an attorney acting under a Lasting Power of Attorney or a Court of Protection Appointed Deputy. Note that deprivation of liberty, as considered later in this chapter, is more than restraint and is not covered by Sections 5 and 6.

The Court of Protection

The Court of Protection has jurisdiction for the whole of the Mental Capacity Act and is the final arbiter for capacity matters. It is a superior court of record with powers equivalent to the High Court. It has a president, a vice-president, a senior judge and a central Registry (Administration) in London. Cases are heard by specially nominated judges (High-Court, Circuit or District). Hearings take place in a number of locations in England and Wales with a view to being geographically proximate to the individual concerned. Persons lacking capacity, the donor or attorney of an LPA and a Court-Appointed Deputy do not need permission from the Court before making an application to it. Other people do.

The Court has wide-ranging powers, for example, it can make declarations about whether a person has capacity and make orders about those who lack capacity, can appoint deputies to make decisions on behalf of people who lack capacity and remove deputies or attorneys acting under an LPA who act improperly. Serious medical issues such as organ donation, sterilisation, abortion or possible death always have to be heard before the Court of Protection. The Mental Capacity Act Code of Practice provides advice as to the type of cases that should be taken to the Court of Protection.

The Court is assisted by:

- the Public Guardian
- the deputies
- the Court of Protection visitors.

Section 16 powers of the court: where a matter concerns personal welfare or property and affairs, and a person lacks capacity in relation to it, then the court may decide the matter or appoint a deputy (CAD) to make decisions about where the person is to live, contact with others and medical treatment.

Powers of the court over property and affairs include:

- managing, buying and selling property;
- trade, profession, business and partnership matters;
- contracts and debts;
- wills and trust powers;
- legal proceedings.

Court-Appointed Deputies (CADs)

CADs can make decisions on behalf of a person who lacks capacity in his best interests, e.g. where there is no LPA or a dispute among carers. However, the deputy can be a family member or carer or any other person deemed suitable by the Court. The CADs can take decisions on financial welfare and healthcare matters as authorised by the Court. They cannot make a decision if the person has the capacity to make that decision or if it is inconsistent with that of a donee of an LPA. CADs can carry out an act intended to restrain a person (Section 20), so long as certain preconditions are met (similar to Section 6 and LPAs). The deputy cannot refuse to consent to a life-sustaining treatment. The Public Guardian is responsible for the supervision of deputies.

Court of Protection Visitors can be sent by the Court to see people who have attorneys or deputies acting for them and check on their welfare. They report to the Court or the Office of the Public Guardian.

Office of the Public Guardian

The Public Guardian is appointed by the Lord Chancellor and is supported by the Office of the Public Guardian, an executive agency of the Ministry of Justice. Under Section 58, the Public Guardian maintains a register of LPAs, Court of Protection orders appointing deputies, supervises deputies and deals with associated complaints. There is a *Customer Service Unit* which is designed to be the first contact point for advice. The *Public Guardian Board* is appointed by the Lord Chancellor, which includes a judge of the Court of Protection and lay members, and their role is to review the Public Guardian's work and make recommendations.

Independent mental capacity advocacy (IMCA) service (Section 35)

Under Section 36(2) of the Mental Capacity Act, an IMCA should provide support to enable the person to participate as fully as possible in the decision under scrutiny, should obtain and evaluate relevant information, represent the person's wishes, find out about available options and seek further medical opinions if required. The NHS body or local authority involved in decisions about the person must take into account any information or submissions from the IMCA. Indeed, the IMCA can challenge these decision-making authorities on behalf of the person lacking capacity and can also initiate formal complaints and seek referral of a disputed matter to the Court of Protection. The IMCA may be instructed to become involved in accommodation reviews where accommodation has been provided for a person who lacks capacity by an NHS body or local authority. IMCAs may also be instructed to become involved in adult protection cases, if the local authority or the NHS considers this would be of benefit to the person.

The appropriate authority must arrange for IMCAs to be available to support people to whom decisions proposed under Sections 37, 38 and 39 relate:

- *Section 37:* serious medical treatment.

- *Section 38*: accommodation – National Health Service (NHS), when likely to exceed 28 days.
- *Section 39:* accommodation – Local Authority, when likely to exceed 8 weeks.

Examples of serious medical treatments given in the Mental Capacity Act (Department of Constitutional Affairs (2007) *Mental Capacity Act 2005: Code of Practice*. London: TSO.) include chemotherapy and surgery for certain cancers, electroconvulsive therapy, open heart surgery, neurosurgery (other than psychosurgery, which is covered by the Mental Health Act Consent to Treatment Provisions), amputation of an arm or a leg and treatments resulting in loss of hearing or sight.

However, Court of Protection decisions are required for withholding or withdrawing artificial nutrition or hydration for patients in a permanent vegetative state, sterilisation for contraception and organ or bone marrow donation.

Exceptions include where there is:

- a person nominated by the subject (in whatever manner) to be consulted in matters affecting his interests; or
- a deputy appointed by the court (CAD) for the subject; or
- a doner of an EPA created by the subject under earlier legislation.

In such circumstances, the duty to consult an IMCA in relation to decisions under Sections 37–39 does not apply.

A more detailed discussion of IMCAs is given in Chapter 19.

Research

Sections 30–34 give rules governing research involving a person lacking capacity to consent. Research involving people lacking capacity to consent may be lawfully carried out under the Mental Capacity Act if an 'appropriate body' (usually a Research Ethics Committee) agrees the research is safe, applies to the person's condition, cannot be undertaken in those who have mental capacity and produces a benefit to the person that outweighs the risk to them.

Carers and nominated third persons must be consulted and agree that the person would have wanted to participate in such research. The person must be withdrawn from the research if they show any signs of resistance.

A more detailed discussion of the limitations on research as a result of the Mental Capacity Act is given in Chapter 19.

A new offence of ill-treatment or neglect

A new offence of ill-treatment or neglect of a person lacking capacity was introduced in the Mental Capacity Act 2005. A person found guilty of such an offence is liable to up to five years imprisonment. This is discussed further in Chapter 19.

Children and young persons

The MCA does not generally apply to children under 16 years of age, whose care and treatment are generally covered by common law. However, the Court of Protection has the power to make decisions about property or finances on behalf of under-16s when the child is likely to lack capacity when they reach 18 years. The criminal offence of ill-treatment and neglect applies to victims under 16 years.

Only people aged 18 and over can make LPAs or advance decisions and can be the subject of a statutory will authorised by the Court of Protection.

Voting

The Mental Capacity Act does not allow voting on behalf of a person who lacks capacity.

The Code of Practice (MCA CoP)

The MCA Code of Practice (MCA CoP), detailed in Chapter 20, has statutory force regarding its guidance in relation to the Mental Capacity Act. Reasons should be given when practice departs from the Code. Indeed, this applies even to those not under a legal duty resulting from the Mental Capacity Act. Failure to comply with the Code is used in evidence in civil legal proceedings.

Relationship with the Mental Health Act 1983

Detainability under 'the Mental Health Act 1983 should be considered first and has primacy' over the provisions of the MCA. However, the MCA can apply to patients detained under the Mental Health Act if they lack capacity to make a decision regarding treatment for a physical condition unrelated to the mental disorder or in making financial decisions.

Deprivation of liberty safeguards

The Mental Health Act 2007, which updated existing mental health legislation, was also used as a vehicle for introducing the deprivation of liberty safeguards into the Mental Capacity Act 2005. The new safeguards provide a framework for the lawful deprivation of liberty of people who lack capacity to consent to arrangements made for their care or treatment in either a care home or hospital, and who need to be deprived of liberty in their own best interests in order to protect them from harm. The conditions for deprivation of liberty are detailed in Table 17.1.

The Mental Capacity Act 2005 Deprivation of Liberty Safeguards (MCA DOLS) was a response to a European Court of Human Rights (ECtHR) judgment in October 2004 in the Bournewood case of *HL* v. *UK* (2004) 40 E.H.R.R. 761.

Table 17.1 What constitutes Deprivation of Liberty

'Objective Condition': Person confined in a restricted space 'for a not negligible length of time' (Storck)
'Subjective Condition': If person has not validly consented or lacks capacity to consent to confinement (HL, Storck)
The difference between deprivation of liberty and restriction of liberty is one of degree or intensity, not one of nature (Ashingdane, Guzzardi)
Do professionals exercise 'complete and effective control' over the person, so that he is under continuous supervision and control and is not free to leave (HL, Storck and DE)
However, consider whole range of factors arising in a particular case
Cases
Ashingdane v. *UK* (1985) 7 E.H.R.R. 528 *JE* v. *DE and Surrey County Council* [2006] E.W.H.C. 3459 (Fam) *Guzzardi* v. *Italy* (1980) 3 E.H.R.R. 33 *HL* v. *UK* (2004) 40 E.H.R.R. 761 *Storck* v. *Germany* (2006) 43 E.H.R.R. 6

The Court found that a man with autism and a learning disability, who lacked the capacity to decide about his residence and medical treatment, and who had been admitted informally to Bournewood Hospital, was unlawfully deprived of his liberty in breach of Article 5 of the European Convention on Human Rights (ECtHR). A key fact in the case was that if the patient had attempted to leave hospital, his consultant stated he would have been detained under the Mental Health Act 1983.

The MCA DOLS remedy to the breach of the ECtHR was perceived to have been a major step towards better protecting the rights of vulnerable individuals in hospitals and care homes. They have made a big difference to the people in care, who have no or only limited choice about their life. However, there is no doubt that implementing the safeguards has been challenging for care homes, primary care trusts (PCTs) and NHS trusts.

In the main, people covered by the safeguards will be those with severe learning disabilities, older people with one of a range of dementias, and people with neurological conditions such as brain injury. The safeguards generally apply only to those people not covered by the Mental Health Act 1983. (More precisely, the safeguards do not apply to those already detained in hospital under the Mental Health Act or who should be so detained, but not necessarily to all those who are detainable, nor who are already subject to the Mental Health Act where they are in the community).

The safeguards apply to people in hospitals, including independent hospitals, and care homes registered under the Care Standards Act 2000, whether they have been placed there by a PCT or a local authority or through private arrangements.

The MCA DOLS apply to people in hospitals and care homes who meet all of the following criteria. The person must:

- be aged 18 years or over;
- have a mental disorder as defined in Section 1 Mental Health Act 1983, e.g. dementia or a learning disability;
- lack capacity to expressly consent to accommodation in the relevant care home/hospital for the provision of care/treatment;
- need to have their liberty taken away in their own best interests in order to protect them from harm.

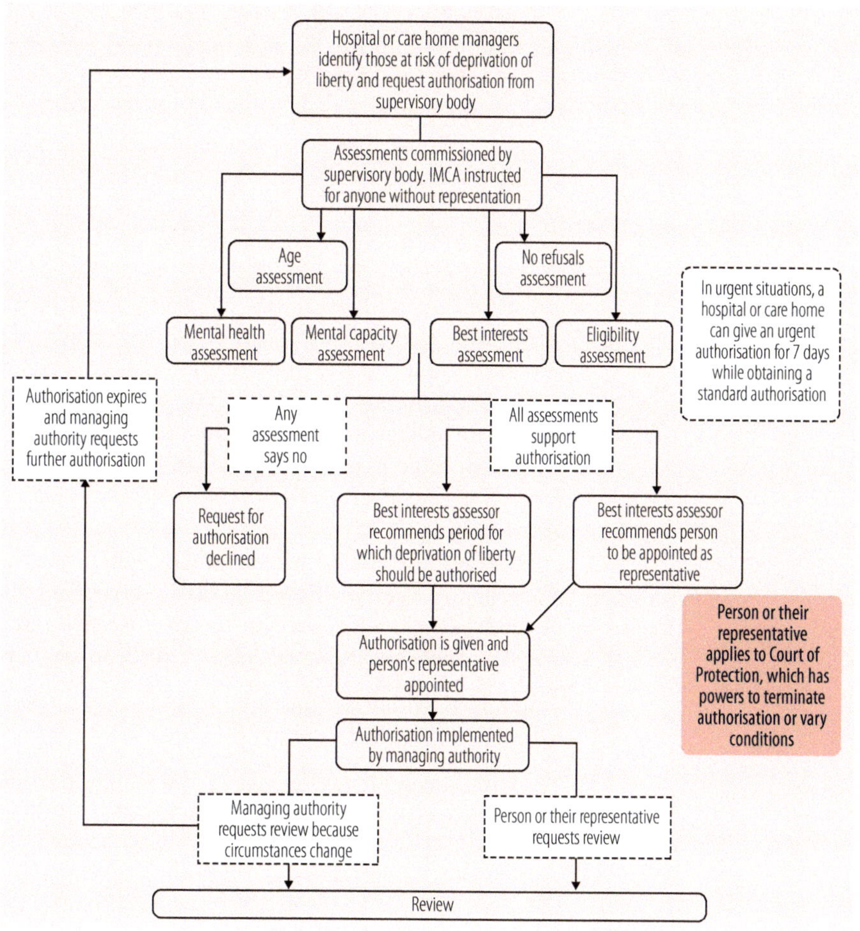

Figure 17-1 Overview of the deprivation of liberty safeguards (DOLS) process

Figure 17.1 gives an overview of the deprivation of liberty safeguards process. Deprivation of liberty with regard to Article 5(1) of the European Convention on Human Rights does not provide protection from liability unless authorised by the Court of Protection, or under the Deprivation of Liberty Safeguards or is in order to provide life-sustaining treatment, or is otherwise essential while a decision is sought from the Court of Protection.

Registered medical practitioners need to be approved as DOLS assessors. Once approved, they can undertake mental capacity, mental health and eligibility assessments. For the latter, they must also be Mental Health Act 1983 Section 12(2) approved.

Social workers, mental health or learning disability nurses, clinical psychologists and occupational therapists can become Best Interests Assessors (BIAs) if also approved as DOLS assessors. BIAs can undertake any assessment except the mental health assessment. They must, however, also be an Approved Mental Health Professionals (AMHPs) to undertake an eligibility assessment. There are also differences between the above for England and the situation in Wales regarding the criteria for approval of DOLS and for becoming an eligibility assessor.

Some guidance on when to use the DOLS provision and when to detain under the Mental Health Act has been given in the case of *G.J.* v. *The Foundation Trust and Ors* [2009] EWHC 2972 (Family). G.J. suffered from vascular dementia, Korsakoff's psychosis and alcohol-related amnesia, as well as insulin-dependent diabetes mellitus. The latter was managed by his wife and when she died, he was unable to cope. In brief, the court decided that it was appropriate for Mr G.J. to be deprived of his liberty under DOLS, rather be detained under the Mental Health Act. If he had needed to be detained only to receive a package of physical treatment for his physical illnesses, he would not have needed to be detained under the Mental Health Act. However, as stated in the judgment, detainability under *'The Mental Health Act should be considered first and has primacy.'*

A supplement to the MCA COP has been developed which covers and gives guidance regarding the DOLS. The safeguards apply to all hospitals and care homes, including public or private facilities, but not to a person's own home or other supported living arrangements, other than a care home. Only the Court of Protection can deprive a person of his liberty in his own home or such other living arrangements.

There is a distinction between DOL, which is unlawful unless authorised, and restriction of liberty, which is lawful if carried out in accordance with other parts of the MCA (as illustrated in the case Re MIG and MEG [2010] EWHC 785 (FAM)). There are two mechanisms for depriving a person of his liberty:

- Standard Authorisations
- Urgent Authorisations.

The latter can apply, if required, before Standard Authorisations can be completed.

For a *Standard Authorisation*, the relevant hospital or care home, known as the *managing authority*, must complete an application form when it appears likely that someone will need to be deprived of his liberty during the next 28 days. The form must be sent to the appropriate *Supervisory Body* (the commissioning PCT for hospitals in England, the Welsh Ministers or local health board for hospitals in Wales or the local authority for care homes). The Supervisory Body must then appoint a minimum of two independent assessors, one of whom must be a doctor with experience in mental disorder, to assess whether the criteria for DOL are satisfied. To this end, the Supervisory Body must secure six types of assessments detailed below. If it is concluded that the person meets the criteria, the Supervisory Body issues a Standard Authorisation which can last up to 12 months, the maximum length being decided by the Best Interests Assessor (the Supervisory Body could go for a shorter period).

The six assessments detailed in Table 17.2 are:

- Age assessment. To confirm a person is over 18 years.
- Mental health assessment. To establish the presence of mental disorder within the meaning of the Mental Health Act 1983, but not excluding learning disability. The assessing doctor must be approved under Section 12 of the Mental Health Act 1983 or have at least three years' post-registration experience in psychiatry.
- Mental capacity assessment.
- Best Interests assessment. This is crucial.
- Eligibility assessment. To ensure a person cannot be dealt with more appropriately under the Mental Health Act 1983.
- No refusals assessment. To ensure DOL is not inconsistent with an advanced decision, a lasting power of attorney or a decision made by a deputy appointed by the Court of Protection.

Table 17.2 Qualifying Requirements for DOLS

Type of Assessment	Comments
1 Age Requirement	Person is aged 18 or over, i.e. not children
2 Mental Health Requirement	Person suffers from mental disorder within meaning of Mental Health Act 1983, but disregarding any exclusion for persons with learning disability. Best interests assessor needs to be advised of outcome
3 Mental Capacity Requirement	Person lacks capacity to decide whether or not to reside in care home or hospital
4 Best Interests Requirement	Person is or will be detained in their best interests in order to prevent harm to them and whose detention is a proportionate response to the risk of such harm
5 Eligibility Requirement	To confirm not ineligible to be deprived of liberty by the Mental Capacity Act, e.g. if is being or should be dealt with under the Mental Health Act 1983 e.g. detained under Sections 2 or 3, or subject to community treatment order
6 No Refusals Requirement	No conflict with an advance decision, decisions of LPA donee or deputy

The Supervisory Body must give a standard authorisation if all six assessments conclude the person meets the qualifying requirements.

Urgent Authorisations should not be used where there is no expectation of a Standard Authorisation or where it is anticipated that the person will be in a particular environment for a short period, e.g. an Accident and Emergency department. They can last up to seven days, pending the completion of a Standard Authorisation, though it can be extended for a further seven days by the Supervisory Body.

Figure 17.2 illustrates the mechanisms for depriving a person of his liberty by Standard or Urgent Authorisations.

Once a Standard Authorisation has been given, the Supervisory Body must appoint a representative for the person to support the individual. The representative has the right to require a review, use the complaints procedure or appeal to the Court of Protection on the person's behalf. In the absence of a representative, the Supervisory Body must appoint an IMCA to undertake this function.

Reviews of DOL must be undertaken by the Supervisory Body if requested by the person, his representative or the managing authority. The grounds for review

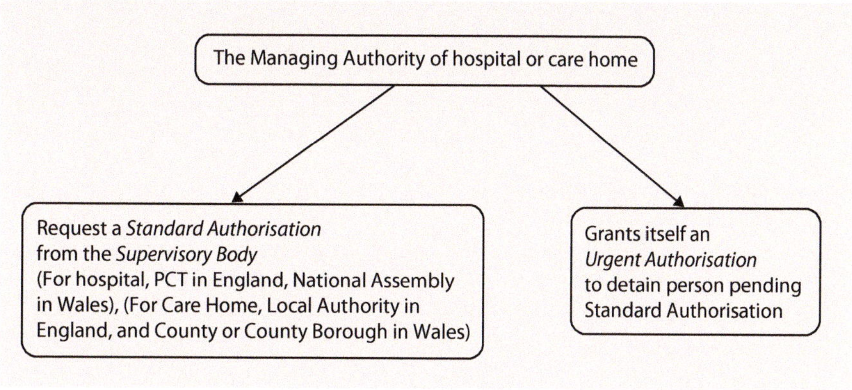

Figure 17.2 Mechanisms for depriving a person of liberty

include that the person no longer meets one of the six requirements for DOL, or it is appropriate to make changes to the conditions of the Authorisation, or that the reasons given in the Authorisation are now different but still qualify for DOL.

There is a right of appeal to the Court of Protection before an Authorisation is given or after a Standard or Urgent Authorisation has been given.

People subject to DOLS are not eligible for after-care services under Section 117 of the Mental Health Act 1983 unless entitled on other grounds.

References

Department of Constitutional Affairs (2007). *Mental Capacity Act 2005: Code of Practice*. London: TSO.

18 Assessment of Capacity

Prior to the Mental Capacity Act 2005 of England and Wales, there was no legal procedure that could enable a decision to be made on behalf of an adult who was unable to do so because of lack of capacity, to take the appropriate care of the person without risking a charge for assault.

In the 1990s, the Law Commission Document No 231 highlighted the need for such a legal framework. At that time, the High Court responded individually to major problems which arose such as Re C and Re MB, but it was impractical to go to court as small problems arose, and so this did not provide sufficient protection for people who lacked capacity, or for the people who looked after them. The Mental Capacity Act 2005 Code of Practice was published to provide good practice in assessing capacity.

Principles

(1) A person is deemed to have capacity unless it is established that he lacks capacity.
(2) A person is not to be treated as unable to make a decision unless all practicable steps to help him to do so have been taken without success.
(3) A person is not treated as unable to make a decision merely because he makes an unusual decision.
(4) An act done, or decision made, under this Act for, or on behalf of, a person who lacks capacity must be done, or made, in his best interests.
(5) Before the act is done, or the decision is made, regard must be had to whether the purpose for which it is needed can be effectively achieved and in a way that is less restrictive of the person's rights and freedom of action.

According to the Code of Practice of the Mental Capacity Act 2005, a person's capacity (or lack of capacity) refers to their capacity to make a ***particular decision at the time it needs to be made*** in the following steps (*see* Figure 18.1):

- Establish that the person is an adult over the age of 18, because there are existing laws regarding decision-making in relation to children and young people (Children Act 1989 and the Act in relation to young people aged 16 and 17).
- Presumption of capacity: this is here to help us remember that all people have the right and ability to make their own decisions. It also reminds us that if someone has lacked capacity previously it does not follow that they will not be able to make the decision in question. Capacity is time- and situation-specific.
- Do everything to support the person to make their own decision, including taking 'practicable steps' to help him to do so.

Practicable steps are not defined but examples of 'practicable steps' suggest that we provide any relevant information in whatever form is suitable for that person such as leaflets, DVDs etc. Explain the purpose and effect of any treatment proposed, describe the risks and benefits and explain any possible choices. It is suggested that this communication is done with understandably simple language and using an interpreter or advocate as necessary. It is also necessary to be aware of any relevant cultural or religious factors. The person should be made to feel at their ease and the best time to assess them is when they are at their most alert. They should have anyone they wish to support them present. It is also advisable to wait until any medical condition which may be increasing their confusion is treated, such as a urinary tract infection.

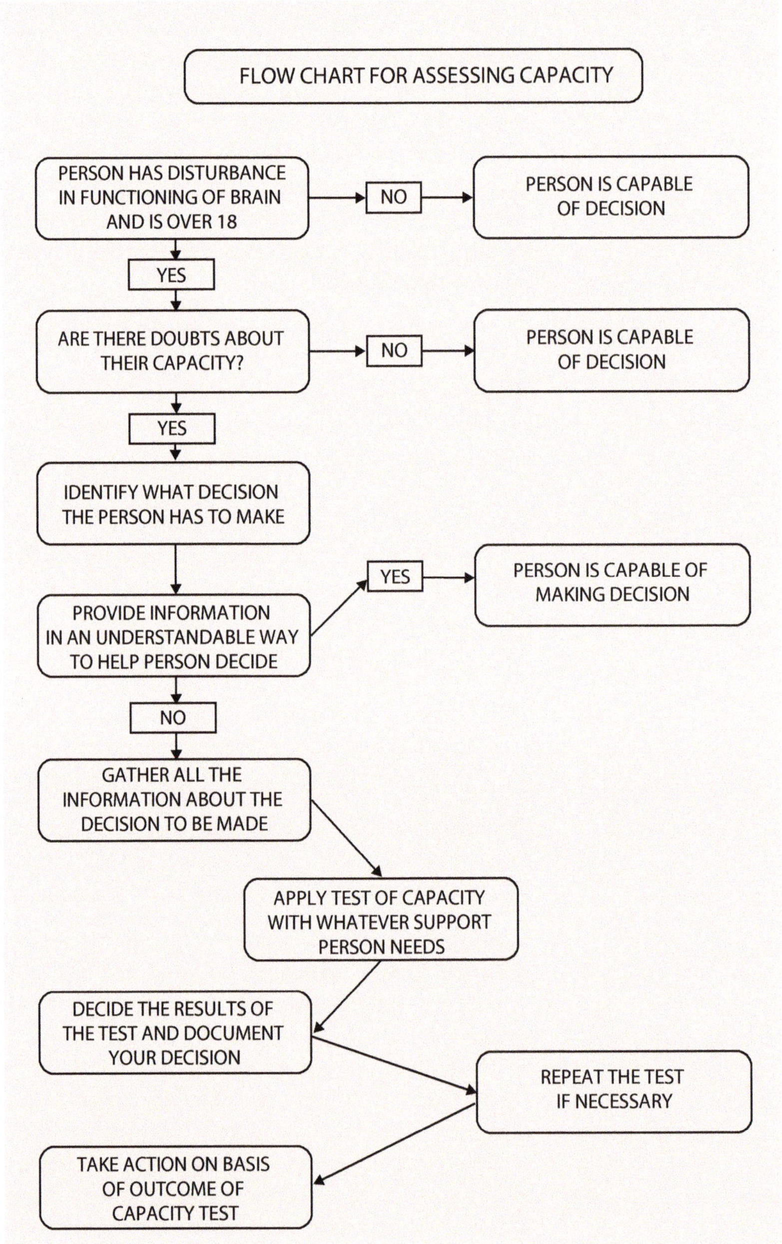

Figure 18.1 Flow chart for assessing capacity

Scenario. Using practicable steps to assist understanding of a decision

Matthew has learning difficulties and he has been having trouble with toothache. His dentist thinks that he may require some treatment but he is very frightened and does not want to go to see the dentist.

His key worker talks to him about it and explains that the dentist would like to look at his teeth. She finds a picture book which depicts a person visiting a dentist with a successful outcome. He agrees to visit the dentist and, after a couple of visits, he feels confident enough and understands what treatment of his toothache would entail and allows it to occur.

- Be aware that a person can make an unwise decision. Even though a decision may seem to be unreasonable, irrational or eccentric, it may make sense in the context of the person's belief systems and they should not be judged as lacking capacity. However, if the person repeatedly makes unwise decisions which put them at risk of exploitation or make a decision which is out of character, this may mean that they do lack capacity and they should be assessed accordingly.
- Do not judge a person's ability to make competent decisions by their age, appearance or behaviour. This ensures that people are not treated less favourably because of any preconceptions and prejudices such as extreme age, skin colour or dress, physical disabilities or behaviour.

Scenario: Principle of equal consideration

Mrs Smith is a fit 97-year-old who has developed a hernia which needs treatment. She asks to see a doctor about it and is taken there by her daughter-in-law. The doctor asks her questions and explains the problem to her. Her daughter-in law becomes very annoyed and demands that the doctor talks to her instead as her mother-in-law is 'too old for these things'. The doctor explains that her mother-in-law understands the problem and has capacity and is the one who should consent to any remedial process.

Assess Capacity

This step will be carried out if the person's ability to make a decision seems questionable. ANYONE assessing a person's capacity to make a decision for themselves, should use a two-stage test of the person's capacity.

- Does the person have an impairment of the mind or brain, or is there a disturbance affecting the way their mind or brain works?
- If so, does that impairment or disturbance make the person unable to make the decision in question at the time it needs to be made?

Impairment/disturbance of the mind includes dementia, long-term effects of brain damage whether due to accident, illness, and disease, learning difficulties or conditions associated with mental illness. The second stage establishes whether he is deemed unable to make a decision as set out below.

In the Mental Capacity Act 2005, a person is described as being unable to make decisions if he is unable:

1

(a) to understand the information relevant to the decision

(b) to retain that information
(c) to use or weigh that information as part of the process of making the decision, or
(d) to communicate his decision (whether by talking, using sign language, writing or by any other means).

2 A person is not to be regarded as unable to understand the information relevant to a decision if he is able to understand an explanation given to him in a way that is appropriate to his circumstances (using simple language, visual aids or any other means).

3 The fact that a person is able to retain the information for a short period only does not prevent him from being regarded as able to make a decision.

4 The information relevant to a decision includes information about foreseeable consequences of:
(a) deciding one way or another, or
(b) failing to make the decision.

- **To understand the information relevant to a decision** the person must understand the nature of the decision, information about why the decision is necessary and the reasonable foreseeable consequences of deciding one way or another or of failing to arrive at a decision. The information should be presented, as stated above, in simple form without any jargon, using the most effective way of communicating for that person. It should be repeated as often as necessary. The more serious the consequence of the decision, such as a proposed amputation, the more important it is to spend time so that the person is given the best chance to understand the information relevant to that decision.
- **To retain the information** a person can be said to retain the information in order to weigh it up, if he can hold it in his mind long enough to use it to make an effective decision. The Act specifically points out that a person should not be prevented from being regarded as able to make a decision just because he can only retain the information for a short time. The Code also encourages the use of aids to retention such as notebooks, videos, photographs and recorders and repetition will also assist in arriving at a conclusion. However, some people will have such short-memory spans that they will not be able to retain the information long enough to do anything with it and will not remember what the information is, if it is written down.

Scenario: Assessing a person's ability to retain information

Mary is an elderly widow with dementia and has a poor short-term memory. She has no close relatives but has a very good neighbour. She cannot remember her neighbour's name but recognises her at once and appears to trust her.

She decides that she wants to buy her neighbour a Christmas present and decides to buy her a watch. Her neighbour is concerned about this and suggests that Mary ask her solicitor who manages her financial affairs if it would be wise. The solicitor assesses her capacity to make this decision and believes that Mary has the capacity to give this gift.

- **To use or weigh up that information as part of the process of making a decision**

For a person to have capacity to make the decision in question he must be able to weigh up all the relevant information that has been given to him and arrive at a decision. People may understand what they are told but brain impairment can stop them from using that information or they can arrive at a decision without either understanding or using the information, or they do not believe the information in the case of paranoia. Examples of the former happening occur in eating disorders, where the person understands the need for nutrition but is unable to eat because he believes that food will make him fat and similarly, people with dementia will make decisions that they have made before in other circumstances, without understanding any of the information that they are currently given and without having weighed it up.

- **Inability to communicate the decision**

This does not apply very often but it can apply to people who are unconscious or comatose. It can also apply to people who have 'locked in syndrome' where they are conscious but are often unable to move anything except for their eyes. They can often be taught by speech and language therapists to communicate by moving their eyes and thus to spell out their wishes. These people illustrate the importance of making every effort to facilitate everyone to communicate their wishes as others may believe that they are totally unable to decide on important issues and make decisions which that person would not want.

- **Fluctuating capacity**

People may have fluctuating capacity such as when they have a problem that occasionally worsens. This can happen in a person with a bipolar illness who may have temporary manic phases which can cause them to lack capacity to make financial decisions and to spend money imprudently.

- **Other legal tests of Capacity**

There are several common laws that have been produced following judgments in court. These are:

- Capacity to make a will
- Capacity to make a gift
- Capacity to enter a contract
- Capacity to litigate
- Capacity to enter marriage.

The Mental Capacity Act 2005 is in line with the tests used to draw up these and does not replace them.

- **Prove lack of capacity**

The person making a claim that someone lacks capacity has to prove that this is the case. This usually occurs in the setting of a caring situation. The legal test of proof is on the balance of probabilities. i.e., being able to show that it is more likely than not that a person lacks capacity to make the decision in question.

19 Safeguards under the Mental Capacity Act 2005

The introduction of the Mental Capacity Act 2005 provided a statutory framework for decision-making on behalf of people who lack the capacity to consent to their care or treatment. It also allowed for capacitated adults to make preparations for a time when they might lack capacity in the future. Before this Act, people who lacked capacity were mainly dealt with under the common law doctrine of necessity, which provided for the care or treatment of incapacitated adults in their 'best interests'. It was generally regarded that this was lacking in safeguards for those who lacked capacity. This chapter will look in more detail at four specific safeguards briefly described in Chapter 17 that have been introduced by the Mental Capacity Act 2005: Independent Mental Capacity Advocates; offences of ill-treatment or neglect; advanced decisions to refuse treatment; and, limitations on research. Chapter 17 covered the specific safeguards against inappropriate deprivation of liberty with an overview of the Deprivation of Liberty Safeguards (DOLS), including the role of the Best Interests Assessor and the Medical Assessor also covered in Chapter 17.

Independent Mental Capacity Advocates (IMCAs)

The Mental Capacity Act was drafted with the expectation that most people who would lack capacity to make an important decision (for example, about medical treatment or where to live) would have family members or friends who could be consulted by any decision-maker. This process would be governed by the best interests checklist in Section 4 of the Act. Section 40 states that if someone has been nominated by the person (when they had capacity to do so) to be consulted in matters affecting their interests, there will be no requirement to instruct an IMCA. This will also be the case if there is a donee of a lasting power of attorney or a deputy appointed by the Court of Protection for the person. Essentially, the IMCA service was created for people who lack family, friends or an appointed person to help represent their best interests.

Section 35 of the Mental Capacity Act sets out the responsibilities of local authorities in England, and Health Boards in Wales, when they are commissioning relevant advocacy services.

The Code of Practice (Chapter 10) states that the role of the IMCA is:

> *'to help particularly vulnerable people who lack the capacity to make important decisions about serious medical treatment and changes of*

accommodation, and who have no family or friends that it would be appropriate to consult about those decisions. IMCAs will work with and support people who lack capacity, and represent their views to those who are working out their best interests.'

The IMCA should support and represent the person concerned, to discover their wishes and feelings and to check that the Mental Capacity Act's principles and Section 4 best interests checklist are followed. Although the IMCA cannot veto certain decisions, the relevant authority must take into account any information or submissions provided by the IMCA. Where an IMCA is particularly concerned that a person's best interests are not being observed, they could challenge any decision by referring the case to the Court of Protection.

Serious medical treatment

Section 37 requires an NHS body to instruct an IMCA to represent a person if:

'(i) it is proposing to provide serious medical treatment for that person;
(ii) the person lacks capacity to consent to the treatment, and
(iii) it is satisfied that there is no-one, other than one engaged in providing care or treatment for them in a professional capacity or for remuneration, whom it would be appropriate to consult in determining what would be in the person's best interests.'

As noted above, this would therefore apply to someone who had no suitable family or friends to consult and where the person had not appointed someone with a Lasting Power of Attorney.

'Serious medical treatment' as referred to here means treatment which involves providing, withholding or withdrawing treatment of a kind prescribed by regulations made by the appropriate authority. The Mental Capacity Act 2005 (Independent Mental Capacity Advocates) (General) Regulations (2006, No. 1832) at 4(2) describes serious medical treatment as:

'treatment which involves providing, withdrawing or withholding treatment in circumstances where:

(a) in a case where a single treatment is being proposed, there is a fine balance between its benefits to the patient and the burdens and risks it is likely to entail for him,
(b) in a case where there is a choice of treatments, a decision as to which one to use is finely balanced, or
(c) what is proposed would be likely to involve serious consequences for the patient.'

Provision of accommodation by the NHS

An NHS body is required by Section 38 to instruct an IMCA to represent a person, if they propose to make arrangements:

> *'(i) for the provision of accommodation in a hospital or care home for a person who lacks capacity to agree to the arrangements; or*
> *(ii) for a change in their accommodation to another hospital or care home; and*
> *(iii) it is satisfied that there is no person, other than one engaged in providing care or treatment for them in a professional capacity or for remuneration, whom it would be appropriate for it to consult in determining what would be in the person's best interests.'*

This refers to any accommodation which is likely to last for more than 28 days in a hospital or 8 weeks in a care home. The IMCA's role will be to support and represent the person concerned and the relevant authority must take into account any views expressed by the IMCA.

Provision of accommodation by a Local Authority

Section 39 requires a local authority to instruct an IMCA to represent a person if they propose to make arrangements:

> *'(i) for the provision of residential accommodation for a person who lacks capacity to agree to the arrangements; or*
> *(ii) for a change in the person's residential accommodation; and*
> *(iii) it is satisfied that there is no person, other than one engaged in providing care or treatment for them in a professional capacity or for remuneration, whom it would be appropriate for it to consult in determining what would be in the person's best interests.'*

This section applies to any accommodation which is likely to last for more than 8 weeks, but arrangements can be made in an emergency. The IMCA's role here is the same as for accommodation provided by the NHS.

Key functions of the IMCA

The IMCA is expected to provide support to the person whom he has been instructed to represent so that they may participate as fully as possible in any relevant decision. To do this, the IMCA will need to: obtain and evaluate relevant information; ascertain what the person's wishes and feelings would be likely to be, and the beliefs and values that would be likely to influence them, if they had capacity; ascertain what alternative courses of action are available; and obtain a further medical opinion where treatment is proposed and the advocate thinks that one should be obtained. The Act confers certain powers on the IMCA to enable them to carry out these tasks effectively. Section 35(6) states that:

> *'For the purpose of enabling him to carry out his functions, an independent mental capacity advocate:*
>
> *(a) may interview, in private, the person whom he has been instructed to represent, and*
> *(b) may, at all reasonable times, examine and take copies of:*

> (i) *any health record,*
> (ii) *any record of, or held by, a local authority and compiled in connection with a social services function, and*
> (iii) *any record held by a person registered under Part 2 of the Care Standards Act 2000 (c. 14),*
>
> *which the person holding the record considers may be relevant to the independent mental capacity advocate's investigation.'*

Offences of ill-treatment or neglect

Section 44 of the Mental Capacity Act creates offences of ill-treatment or neglect, carrying a maximum sentence of five years' imprisonment. In practice, any ill-treatment must be either deliberately or recklessly undertaken, whether or not actual harm was caused. The Code of Practice states that wilful neglect usually means that a person has deliberately failed to carry out an act they knew they had a duty to do.

The offence can be committed by: a person having care of someone who lacks or whom he reasonably believes to lack capacity; a person appointed under a Lasting Power of Attorney or an Enduring Power of Attorney created by the victim; or a deputy appointed by the Court of Protection for the victim.

Advance decisions

Advance decisions can be made by capacitated adults who are aged 18 and over. It should be noted that most of the Act applies to people of 16 or more. Advance decisions need not be in writing unless they concern life-sustaining treatment, in which case, they must be in writing, and they should be verified and witnessed. All advance decisions need to state what treatment cannot be given, and under what circumstances. There is no provision to make statements of preferred treatments, so for practical purposes advance decisions are in effect always advanced refusals of treatment.

Advance decisions will only be effective if they are recognised as both valid and applicable. Thus, they are only effective if the specific treatment is proposed and the person at that point lacks capacity in relation to the treatment decision. They only cover the refusal of medical treatment and so cannot affect decisions about social care. In this sense, they are very different from Lasting Powers of Attorney which can grant the attorney decision-making powers in social matters as well as healthcare. In most instances, an advance decision can be nullified where a patient is detained under a section of the Mental Health Act 1983 to which Part IV applies. The exception here is the new safeguards for people who make advance refusals of ECT, to ensure that their refusal is respected, unless certain emergency criteria are met.

Limitations on research

New safeguards in relation to research projects involving persons who lack capacity to agree to such research are provided by Sections 30 to 34. Research would include direct medical interventions for research purposes, as well as broader research such as asking patients for their views about health and social care services, observing them in a social care setting or undertaking research on medical notes.

Any 'intrusive research' carried out on or in relation to a person who lacks capacity is unlawful unless it is part of an approved research project and complies with the provisions relating to consultation and other safeguards contained in the Act. Research would need to be approved by a recognised Research Ethics Committee. Clinical trials which are subject to the provisions of the Medicines for Human Use (Clinical Trials) Regulations 2004, do not come within the provisions of the Mental Capacity Act.

Section 31 sets out conditions which would need to be met before approval could be given for a research project. For example, there must be reasonable grounds for believing that research of comparable effectiveness cannot be carried out if it has to be confined to people who have capacity to consent. The research must either have the potential to benefit the person lacking capacity (without imposing on him a burden disproportionate to the potential benefit) or be intended to provide knowledge of the causes or treatment of, or of the care of persons affected by, the same or a similar condition.

Chapter 11 of the Code of Practice gives examples of potential benefits of research for a person who lacks capacity. These could be: developing more effective ways of treating a person or managing his condition; improving the quality of healthcare, social care or other services to which he has access; discovering the cause of his condition; or reducing the risk of his being harmed, excluded or disadvantaged.

Section 32 sets out a consultation requirement. Before enrolling a person into an approved research project, the researcher must take reasonable steps to identify someone with whom he can consult. This must be someone interested in the person's welfare but not somebody professionally involved with the care of the person, nor a paid carer. An attorney appointed under an LPA or a deputy appointed by the court could fulfil this role. If the researcher is unable to identify such a person, he must nominate somebody who is not connected with the research project. If the consultee advises that, in their opinion, the person would not have wished to take part in the research project, the researcher must ensure that he does not participate. If the person is already participating, he must be withdrawn from it unless the researcher believes on reasonable grounds, that to do so would pose a significant risk to the person's health.

Section 33 places further restrictions on what can be done to a person lacking capacity who has been enrolled in an approved research project. There is a presumption in favour of the interests of the person lacking capacity outweighing those of science and society. Additionally, a researcher must not do anything to which the person appears to object unless it is necessary to do so to protect him from harm or reduce pain or discomfort suffered by him. In addition, the researcher must withdraw the person from the project if he indicates, in any way, that he wishes to be withdrawn. If the person has made a valid and applicable advance decision or any other form of statement refusing consent to anything being done or proposed to be done to him during the research project the researcher may not proceed.

There are various sets of regulations related to this part of the Act which anyone should consult if they are planning research with patients who may lack capacity to consent.

References

1983 Mental Health Act.

2000 Care Standards Act.

2005 Mental Capacity Act.

2005 Mental Capacity Act (Independent Mental Capacity Advocates) (General) Regulations (2006, No. 1832).

2005 Mental Capacity Act (Independent Mental Capacity Advocates) (Expansion of Role) Regulations (SI 2006, No 2883).

2005 Mental Capacity Act Loss of Capacity during Research Project (England) Regulations (SI 2007, No 679).

20 The Mental Capacity Act Codes of Practice

There are two Codes of Practice to the Mental Capacity Act 2005. The first 'green' code was laid before Parliament to coincide with the implementation of the Act in two stages in 2007. It was broadly welcomed and provided clear guidance to working within the provisions of the Act just as it came into effect. The second 'blue' code is a supplement to the first code and was written to provide guidance to the workings of the Deprivation of Liberty Safeguards (DOLS) which were introduced by amendments to the Mental Capacity Act made by the Mental Health Act 2007. DOLS and the 'blue' code were introduced in 2008. The DOLS code was, in some ways, even more welcome than the first Code. In stark contrast with the main body of the Act (which was a model of clear drafting) the Schedules introduced to cover DOLS are poorly drafted, obtuse and defeat many professionals' attempts to read and understand them. The Code provides a coherent way in to the legislation.

Status of the Codes

The publication of the Codes is a requirement of Section 42 of the Act which provides a list of areas that the Codes must cover. Subsection 4 makes it

> *'the duty of a person to have regard to any relevant code, if he is acting in relation to a person who lacks capacity and is doing so in one or more of the following ways:*
>
> *(a) as the donee of a lasting power of attorney*
> *(b) as a deputy appointed by the court*
> *(c) as a person carrying out research in reliance on any provision made by or under this Act (see Sections 30 to 34)*
> *(d) as an independent mental capacity advocate*
> *(da) in the exercise of functions under schedule A1*
> *(db) as a representative appointed under Part 10 of Schedule A1*
> *(e) in a professional capacity*
> *(f) for remuneration.'*

Schedule A1 refers to DOLS.

The introduction to the main code confirms this list of people who must have regard to the Code but then notes that:

> *'the Act applies more generally to everyone who looks after, or cares for, someone who lacks capacity to make particular decisions for themselves. This includes family carers or other carers. Although these carers are not*

legally required to have regard to the Code of Practice, the guidance given in the Code will help them to understand the Act and apply it. They should follow the guidance in the Code as far as they are aware of it.'

Although the Code is very long, it is written in an easy style and contains many examples so it should be accessible to anyone working within the provisions of the Mental Capacity Act.

Another situation that staff working with the Mental Capacity Act should be aware of, is that Section 42(5) makes the Code relevant to some court and tribunal situations. It states:

> *'If it appears to a court or tribunal conducting any criminal or civil proceedings that:*
>
> *(a) a provision of a code, or*
> *(b) a failure to comply with a code,*
>
> *is relevant to a question arising in the proceedings, the provision or failure must be taken into account in deciding the question.'*

This parallels the position with the Mental Health Act Code with which staff will be familiar but it states this in the Act itself rather than just in the Code.

What does the main Code cover?

The following list is a breakdown of the Code's chapters and what they contain. For those who do not have their own copy of the Code, it is available free of charge on the internet at: www.publicguardian.gov.uk

Use of this list should allow quick access to the relevant passages of the Code.

Chapter 1 introduces the Mental Capacity Act 2005.

Chapter 2 sets out the five statutory principles behind the Act and the way they affect how it is put in practice.

Chapter 3 explains how the Act makes sure that people are given the right help and support to make their own decisions.

Chapter 4 explains how the Act defines 'a person who lacks capacity to make a decision' and sets out a single clear test for assessing whether a person lacks capacity to make a particular decision at a particular time.

Chapter 5 explains what the Act means by acting in the best interests of someone lacking capacity to make a decision for themselves, and describes the checklist set out in the Act for working out what is in someone's best interests.

Chapter 6 explains how the Act protects people providing care or treatment for someone who lacks the capacity to consent to the action being taken.

Chapter 7 shows how people who wish to plan ahead for the possibility that they might lack the capacity to make particular decisions for themselves in the future are able to grant Lasting Powers of Attorney (LPAs) to named individuals to make certain decisions on their behalf, and how attorneys appointed under an LPA should act.

Chapter 8 describes the role of the new Court of Protection, established under the Act, to make a decision or appoint a decision-maker on someone's behalf in cases where there is no other way of resolving a matter affecting a person who lacks capacity to make the decision in question.

Chapter 9 explains the procedures that must be followed if someone wishes to make an advance decision to refuse medical treatment to come into effect when they lack capacity to refuse the specified treatment.

Chapter 10 describes the role of Independent Mental Capacity Advocates appointed under the Act to help and represent particularly vulnerable people who lack capacity to make certain significant decisions. It also sets out when they should be instructed.

Chapter 11 provides guidance on how the Act sets out specific safeguards and controls for research involving, or in relation to, people lacking capacity to consent to their participation.

Chapter 12 explains those parts of the Act which can apply to children and young people and how these relate to other laws affecting them.

Chapter 13 explains how the Act relates to the Mental Health Act 1983.

Chapter 14 sets out the role of the Public Guardian, a new public office established by the Act to oversee attorneys and deputies and to act as a single-point-of-contact for referring allegations of abuse in relation to attorneys and deputies to other relevant agencies.

Chapter 15 examines the various ways that disputes over decisions made under the Act or otherwise affecting people lacking capacity to make relevant decisions can be resolved.

Chapter 17 summarises how the laws about data protection and freedom of information relate to the provisions of the Act.

What does the DOLS Code cover?

Again, the following list is a breakdown of the Code's chapters and what they contain.

1 **What are the deprivation of liberty safeguards and why were they introduced?** What are the safeguards? Who is covered? When can someone be deprived of their liberty? Are there any cultural considerations in implementing the safeguards? Where do the safeguards apply? How do they relate to the rest of the Mental Capacity Act 2005?

2 **What is deprivation of liberty?** What does case law say to date? How can deprivation of liberty be identified? What practical steps can be taken to reduce the risk of unlawful deprivation of liberty occurring? What does the Act mean by 'restraint'? How does the use of restraint apply within a hospital or when taking someone to a hospital or a care home? Examples of case law.

3 **How and when can deprivation of liberty be applied for and authorised?** How can deprivation of liberty be authorised? How should managing authorities decide whether to apply for an authorisation? What is the application process? Who should be informed that an application has been made? What action does the supervisory body need to take when it receives an application for authorisation? Can an application for authorisation be made in advance? What happens when the managing authority and the supervisory body are the same organisation? When should an IMCA be instructed?

4 **What is the assessment process for a standard authorisation of deprivation of liberty?** What assessments are required before giving a standard authorisation? When must assessments take place? How should assessors be selected? What

is the assessment process? What guidelines are there relating to the work of assessors?

5 **What should happen once the assessments are complete?** What action should the supervisory body take if the assessments conclude that the person meets the requirements for authorisation? How long can an authorisation last? What restrictions exist on authorisations? Can a person be moved to a different location under a standard authorisation? What happens if an assessment concludes that one of the requirements is not met? What are the responsibilities of the managing authority and the commissioners of care if a request for an authorisation is turned down?

6 **When can urgent authorisations of deprivation of liberty be given?** When can an urgent authorisation be given? What records should be kept about urgent authorisations? Who should be consulted before giving an urgent authorisation? Can a person be moved into care under an urgent authorisation? What happens at the end of an urgent authorisation period? How and when can an urgent authorisation be extended?

7 **What is the role of the relevant person's representative?** What is the role of the relevant person's representative? How should managing authorities work with this person? Who can be a representative? When should they be identified? How should they be selected? How should they be appointed? How should their work be supported and monitored? When can the appointment be terminated? What happens when there is no representative available? When should an IMCA be instructed?

8 **When should an authorisation be reviewed and what happens when it ends?** When should a standard authorisation be reviewed? What happens when a review is going to take place? How should standard authorisations be reviewed? What happens if any of the requirements are not met? Is a review necessary when the relevant person's capacity fluctuates? What happens when an authorisation ends?

9 **What happens if someone thinks a person is being deprived of their liberty without authorisation?** What action should someone take if they think a person is being deprived of their liberty without authorisation? What happens if somebody informs the supervisory body directly that they think a person is being deprived of their liberty without authorisation? How will the assessment of unlawful deprivation of liberty be conducted? What happens once the assessment has been conducted?

10 **What is the Court of Protection and when can people apply to it?** When can people apply to the Court of Protection about the deprivation of liberty safeguards and who can apply? How should people apply to the Court of Protection? What orders can the Court of Protection make? What is the role of the Court of Protection in respect of people lacking capacity who are deprived of their liberty in settings other than hospitals or care homes? Is legal aid available to support applications to the Court of Protection in deprivation of liberty safeguards cases?

11 **How will the safeguards be monitored?** Who will monitor the safeguards? What will the inspection bodies do and what powers will they have?

The DOLS code is also available at: www.publicguardian.gov.uk

Unlike the Mental Health Act codes, where there are separate versions for England and Wales, both countries use the same codes. They are available in English and in Welsh.

Checklists

Both codes contain useful checklists. In the DOLS Code these are more accessible as they are together at the end of the Code before the annexes. There are three and they cover key points for care homes and hospitals (managing authorities) and for local authorities and NHS bodies (supervisory bodies) with regard to DOLS. They are clear and invaluable for those who are unfamiliar with the details of the provisions. There are lists in the 'green' code on such matters as the best interests checklist and key factors in determining when there is a deprivation of liberty but these have to be looked for in the relevant chapters.

21 Human Rights Act 1998 in mental health legislation in the UK

The Human Rights Act 1998 came into force in October 2000. The Act aims to ensure everyone's basic human rights in their contact with the legal system, government and public bodies and organisations.

The rights conferred by the Human Rights Act 1998 are the rights drawn up in 1951 in an international treaty after the atrocities of the Second World War by the European Convention on Human Rights (ECHR).

Before the Human Rights Act 1998 the standards of the Convention could only be accessed on application to the Strasbourg Court and anyone who felt that their rights had been breached had to take the case to Strasbourg which was expensive and took a long time.

Under the Human Rights Act 1998, human rights standards are now applied from the beginning and public authorities must act compatibly with the human rights standards. In the event of someone believing that their human rights have been unlawfully interfered with, the very first court or tribunal before which a case is heard must take human rights into consideration and ensure that whatever decision is reached does not interfere with these rights.

The ECHR reflects on three basic principles such as right to life, and the right not to be subjected to torture, to ensure that people are given a fair hearing in court, the protection of privacy and full expression and protection from discrimination.

The European Convention rights included in the Human Rights Act 1998 and which affect mental health legislation are:

- Article 2: **The right to life** – When the Convention was drawn up most of the countries in the Council of Europe used the death penalty but now none of them do. Excessive force by police or security services or failure to protect someone whose life might be in danger in community or prison could count as a breach of Article 2.
- Article 3: **Freedom from torture and inhuman or degrading treatment or punishment** – This could apply to interrogation techniques or inadequate or insanitary prison conditions, corporal punishment to children and includes deportation back to a country where the person will face torture or be subjected to inhuman and degrading treatment.
- Article 5: **The right to liberty** – No one should be deprived of liberty except in

defined circumstances, such as prison sentence after conviction by a properly regulated court. Anyone who is arrested or detained must be informed why they have been so treated and have a prompt and speedy trial.

- Article 6: **The right to a fair trial** – There is an obligation to ensure fairness between parties to a case (civil or criminal).
- Article 8: **The right to respect for privacy and family life – the home and correspondence** – This article protects an individual's right to privacy and prevents public authorities from intruding disproportionately in someone's private live, e.g. surveillance, telephone bugging or newspaper accounts of private life. It also protects the right to have a family life. Custody and adoption cases must take account of family life for all involved.
- Article 9: **The right to freedom of thought, conscience and religion** – This article protects the rights of people to practise their chosen religion.
- Article 10: **The right to freedom of expression** – This article guarantees everyone's right to express their views and opinions without interference of the authorities.
- Article 12: **The right to marry and have a family** – This article guarantees the right of a man or woman of marriageable age to marry.

There has now developed a body of case law which has helped define the role of the Human Rights Act 1998 and mental health legislation.

Article 2: This article is concerned with the most fundamental provisions on the Convention. It cannot be interpreted as conferring the right to die: nor can it give an individual the right to choose death rather than life [*Pretty* v. *United Kingdom* (2000) *35 E.H.R.R.1* at Paragraph 39).

- In mental health *Osman* v. *United Kingdom* (2000) *29 E.H.R.R. 245* it was stated that there is an obligation on the authorities to protect those at risk from the criminal acts of another person. The authorities knew and should have known of the existence of a real and immediate risk to life in this case and failed to take measures to avoid the risk. The Osman case places professionals operating under the Mental Health Act 1983 under an obligation to take appropriate preventative measures in respect of patients known to be dangerous and to prevent them from threatening the lives of others.

Article 3: This article prohibits people being subjected to inhuman or degrading treatment or punishment and can include some psychiatric treatments and seclusion. It must also be remembered that mentally ill persons are often vulnerable and in some cases unable to complain coherently.

- *Keenan* v. *United Kingdom* (2001) *33 E.H.R.R. 38* Paragraph 110. Here the court stated that the 'treatment of a mentally ill person may be incompatible with the standards imposed by Article 3 in the protection of fundamental human dignity'.
- Also in *S* v. *Airedale National Health Service Trust* (2002) *E.W.A.C. Admin* 1780 when Stanley Burnton J found that the seclusion of a mental disorder person can amount to an infringement of Articles 3 and 5.
- *R* v. *Secretary of State for Home Department* (2001). In this case the Home Secretary applied to deport an immigrant whose leave to remain had been refused. The immigrant was receiving treatment for schizophrenia in hospital. He applied for a judicial review of the decision to deport him but this was dismissed and he appealed. He said that to move him would increase his risk of

self harm and give rise to deterioration in his mental health and Article 3 would be breached. The Court held that the proposed removal by a tribunal heard under Section 8 of the Act could not be described as inhuman or degrading treatment and it could proceed.

Article 5 – This is the chief area where infringement can occur in mental health legislation.

The Human Rights Act 1998 states that no one can be deprived of his liberty except in the following cases:

1

- (a) lawful detention of a person after conviction by a competent court;
- (b) lawful arrest or detention of a person for non-compliance with the lawful order of a court etc;
- (c) the lawful arrest of someone to bring them before the competent legal authority;
- (d) the detention of a minor for the purpose of educational supervision;
- (e) lawful detention of persons for prevention of spreading infectious diseases;
- (f) the lawful arrest or detention of a person to prevent his affecting an unauthorised entry into the country or one where action is being taken with a view to deportation or extradition.

2 Everyone who is arrested shall be informed promptly, in a language which he understands, of the reasons for his arrest and of any charge against him.

3 Everyone arrested or detained in accordance with the provisions of paragraph 1(c) of the Article shall be brought promptly before a judge or other officer authorised by law to exercise judicial power and shall be entitled to trial within a reasonable time or to release pending trial. Release may be conditioned by guarantees to appear for trial.

4 Everyone who is deprived of his liberty by arrest or detention shall be entitled to take proceedings to assess the lawfulness of his arrest or detention speedily by a court and his release ordered if the detention is not lawful.

5 Everyone who has been wrongfully detained in contravention of the provision of this Article shall have an enforceable right to compensation.

- In the famous case of *Winterwerp* v. *Netherlands* (1979) *2 E.H.RH.R. 387* Paragraph 45 the Court observed that 'unsound mind' is a term whose meaning is continually evolving as research in psychiatry progresses. The Article embraces the detention and release but not the right to treatment.

  The Court has heard that it is essential that the detaining authority helps that person to maintain contact with his close family, *see Messina* v. *Italy (No 2)* 28 September 2000.
- Concerning meaning of 'deprivation of liberty' in *Ashingdane* v. *United Kingdom* (1985) *7 E.H.H.R. 528* Paragraph 41. This states that in the established law of court Article 5 1(e) is not wholly concerned with their restriction of liberty of movement but must also look at a whole range of things such as type, duration, effects and manner of implementation of the measure in question. The distinction between deprivation and restriction upon liberty is merely one of degree.

  In the above case the applicant was on a restriction order and was found to be detained even though he was in an open ward after his transfer from Broadmoor to a local hospital. As the restriction order had been continued he could only leave the hospital as a privilege conferred by the authorities.

- In *Johnson* v. *United Kingdom* (1999) *27 E.H.H.R. 296* the Mental Health Review Tribunal had deferred a conditional discharge of the above applicant pending suitable arrangements for his discharge to be made. Unfortunately a suitable hostel could not be found and the Court held that the applicant's release from detention was unreasonably delayed. Detention only lasts from the time when the detention is authorised and to the time when it is officially lifted.

Article 5 as stated in Ashingdane is not concerned with suitable treatment or conditions. However, if the absence of suitable treatment has a severe effect on the patient it might be possible to argue that this constitutes a violation of Article 3.

Speedily – With regard to Article 5(4) 'in the Court's view this concept cannot be defended in the abstract: the matter must be determined in the light of the circumstances of each case'.

- In *R* v. *Mental Health Review Tribunal London South and West Region* (2001) *EWCA Civ 1110 [2002] 1W.L.R. 176* the Court of Appeal established that routinely delaying the hearings by eight weeks was unacceptable.
- The case of *R* v. *MHRT North and East London Region* (2001) resulted in a declaration that Sections 72 and 73 of the Mental health Act 1983 were incompatible with the European Convention on Human Rights because rather than requiring that the lawfulness of continuing detention should be proven before a mental health review tribunal, these sections effectively reversed the burden of proof by requiring that the patient prove that the conditions for detention were no longer satisfied.

Article 8: This Article is concerned with the Right to Respect for Private and Family Life.

Compulsory administration of treatment which would otherwise require consent is invariably an infringement of Article 8 of the Convention. It can be justified when it is given in accordance with the law and where it is proportionate to a legitimate aim such as the reduction of risk posed by a person's mental disorder.

- In *Goodwin* v. *United Kingdom* (2002) *35 E.H.H.R. 18* the issue came before the Court as to whether the UK government had failed to comply with a positive obligation to ensure that the applicant, a transsexual person who was post operative after a male to female reassignment, had a right to respect for her private life including legal recognition being given to her gender reassignment. It was found that there had been a breach.
- In the question of 'home' in *R* v. *North and East Devon Health Authority Ex Parte Coughlan* (1994) *2 CCLC 285* the Court of Appeal held that the enforced move of an elderly lady from accommodation that had been promised as a 'home for life', when it shut down was emotionally devastating and seriously anti-therapeutic and it was found that there had been a breach of Article 8.

22 Mental Health, medication and the law

The reason for administration of medication to a patient suffering from a mental disorder is similar to the administration of medication for any other disorder. That is, to alleviate or control the suffering which the person is experiencing, and to cure the underlying condition that is causing the patient to suffer. The patient should have the capacity to consent to taking the medication. He or she should have been provided with information in sufficient detail to enable him to make a decision, based on an adequate knowledge of the nature, purpose, likely effects and risks of that medication, including the likelihood of its success and any alternatives to it. The patient is also free to refuse the medication if he wishes.

There is, however, a difference in the case of a patient detained under the Mental Health Act 1983 when they may not, because of their symptoms, accept the need for medication and therefore do not consent to receive it. Many detained patients are, nevertheless, capable of consenting to take medication but there are some who are incapable of doing so.

Mental Heath Act 1983

The administration of medication to detained patients is subject to Parts IV and 4A of the Act. Sections 57, 58 and 58A of the Act set out the types of medical treatment to which special rules and procedures apply, including the need for certificates from a second opinion appointed doctor (SOAD) approving the treatment. The certificate states which psychotropic medications are to be given and whether the doses conform to the British National Formulary (BNF) guideline doses.

The following Table shows a summary of treatments covered by Sections 57, 58 and 58A.

Section	Form of treatment covered
57	Neurosurgery for mental disorder
	Surgical implantation of hormones to reduce male sex drive
58	Medication after a three month period except as part of ECT
58A	ECT and medication administered as part of ECT

Section 58 of the Mental Health Act 1983 applies to the administration of medication for a mental disorder. However, it only applies after three months have passed from the day on which any form of medication was first administered to the patient, during their current period of detention under the Act, and does not cover medication delivered as part of electroconvulsive therapy (ECT).

Section 58 applies only to detained patients and can only be given if the approved clinician in charge of the treatment, or a SOAD, certifies that the patient has the capacity to consent and has done so, or the SOAD certifies that the treatment is appropriate and the patient has capacity to consent or that the patient has capacity to consent but refuses to do so.

In *urgent cases* Section 64G applies and Sections 57, 58 and 58A do not apply where treatment is immediately necessary in the following circumstances:

- To save life.
- To prevent serious deterioration of the patient's condition, and the treatment does not have unfavourable physical or psychological consequences which cannot be reversed.
- To alleviate suffering by the patient, and the treatment does not have unfavourable physical or psychological consequences which cannot be reversed and does not entail significant physical hazard.
- To prevent the patient from behaving violently or being a danger to themselves or others, and the treatment represents the minimum interference necessary for that purpose, does not have unfavourable physical or psychological consequences which cannot be reversed, and does not entail significant physical hazard.

If the treatment is ECT, the first two categories only apply.

Supervised Community Treatment (SCT) is to allow suitable patients to be safely treated in the community rather than under detention in hospital. SCT of patients not recalled to hospital (Part 4A of the Act) is operated under different rules. The rules differ depending on whether the patient has the capacity to consent to the treatment in question; If Part 4A patients have the capacity to consent to a treatment they cannot be given the treatment unless they consent to it. There are no exceptions to this rule, even in emergencies.

Part 4A patients who lack the capacity to consent to a treatment may nevertheless be given it, if their attorney or deputy or the Court of Protection consents to the treatment on their behalf.

Part 4A patients who lack the capacity to consent to treatment may also be given it, without anyone's consent, by or under the direction of the approved clinician in charge of the treatment. Certificate requirement applies to any treatment for which a certificate would be necessary under Sections 58 or 58A of the Act, were the patient to be detained.

Emergency treatment can also be given to Part 4A patients who lack capacity and have not been recalled to hospital in the case of an emergency but only if treatment is necessary in the following circumstances:

- To save life.
- To prevent serious deterioration of the patient's condition, and the treatment does not have unfavourable physical or psychological consequences which cannot be reversed.
- To alleviate suffering by the patient, and the treatment does not have unfavourable physical or psychological consequences which cannot be reversed and does not entail significant physical hazard.
- To prevent the patient from behaving violently or being a danger to themselves

or others, and the treatment represents the minimum interference necessary for that purpose, does not have unfavourable physical or psychological consequences which cannot be reversed and does not entail significant physical hazard.

The Act requires healthcare professionals to understand if the patient has capacity to consent to, or refuse a particular form of medical treatment, and if so know that the patient, in actual fact, consents to it.

The criteria for capacity to consent are as defined by the Mental Capacity Act 2005 and state that:

1. People must be assumed to have capacity until it is established that they do not have capacity.
2. All practicable steps to help them to have capacity must have been taken.
3. People should not be treated as unable to make a decision just because they make an unwise decision.

The Mental Capacity Act 2005 states that a person lacks capacity in relation to a matter if, at the material time, he is unable to make a decision for himself in relation to the matter because of an impairment of, or a disturbance in the functioning of, the mind or brain.

However, some patients can be detained in hospital and not be covered by these rules. This includes emergency application under Section 4, only in very limited circumstances: when the criteria for Section 2 are met, and the patient's detention is required as a matter of urgent necessity, and obtaining a second medical recommendation would cause undesirable delay. Patients detained on the emergency basis of emergency applications may not be treated without their consent under Part 4 of the Act, unless a second medical recommendation is received.

Patients held under Sections 5(2) and 5(4), as well as Sections 135/136 can be detained for up to 72 hours for assessment but the sections do not confer any power under the Act to treat the patients without their consent.

The rules in Part 4 of the Act do not apply and treatment cannot be given under the Act without the patient's consent in a prison healthcare centre as it is not regarded as a hospital within the meaning of the Act. Patients temporarily detained in hospital under Section 35 of the Act for a report, cannot be treated unless they give consent or, in the case of someone who is over 16 and lacks capacity to consent, they can be treated in accordance with the Mental Capacity Act 2005. A hospital order, with or without restrictions, diverts the person from punishment to treatment and the period of detention will be determined by the disorder.

There have been challenges under the **Human Rights Act 1998** concerning detention and treatment such as in the case of *Winterwerp* v. *Netherlands 6301/73* (1979) *ECHR 4*. The Court made clear that the individual should not be deprived of their liberty unless he has been reliably shown to be of 'unsound mind'. Further, the validity of continued confinement depends upon the persistence of such a disorder. In *Aerts* v. *Belgium* the ECHR found a violation of Article 5(1)(e) because Mr Aerts received no treatment required by the condition that gave rise to his detention. Accordingly, the courts have shown that in the light of the Human Rights Act 1989 treatment should only be given in the absence of consent, if the proposed treatment is in the patient's best interests, and has been convincingly shown to be medically necessary.

Misuse of Drugs Regulations 2004

The Misuse of Drugs Act 1971 led to the Misuse of Drugs Regulations 1985. They governed how controlled drugs are supplied and stored. Nine amendments to the regulations were consolidated into the Misuse of Drugs Regulations 2001, with the earlier legislation being revoked. Following the Shipman enquiry, the regulations were revised in 2004, with new measures relating to record-keeping and collection procedures.

A comprehensive guide to the regulations is available on the National Prescribing Centre (NPC) website. (www.npc.co.uk)

Schedule 1

Schedule 1 controlled drugs include the hallucinogenic drugs ecstasy, LSD and cannabis. A Home Office licence is required for legal possession of these drugs. Currently, the only exemption occurs when a professional removes the drug from a person for the purpose of destruction or handing to the police; this should be witnessed by another professional and documented.

Some cannabis derivatives are being used in clinical trials; the relevant centres have Home Office licences to cover this work. Any resulting products are likely to be Schedule 2 controlled drugs.

Schedule 2

Schedule 2 drugs include the opiates, major stimulants, and secobarbital. All except secobarbital require specified secure storage. Words and figures are required on prescriptions. The method of destruction and the witnesses required for this are laid out in the regulations.

Schedule 3

Schedule 3 drugs include most of the barbiturates (except secobarbital, which is in Schedule 2), buprenorphine, flunitrazepam, temazepam and others. Words and figures are required when writing a prescription for all of them except temazepam and phenobarbital. There are safe-storage requirements for buprenorphine and temazepam but registers are not legally required.

Some hospitals opt to use registers for Schedule 3 drugs to avoid confusion.

Schedule 4

Schedule 4 drugs include the remaining benzodiazepines and various hormonal products that are prone to abuse. These may be prescribed and stored in the same way as ordinary prescribed medications.

Schedule 5

Schedule 5 drugs include preparations such as kaolin and morphine mixture and codeine tablets. Their abuse potential is lessened by their formulation, and they are treated as ordinary medications.

Prescription and collection of controlled drugs

An example of a prescription for controlled drugs can be found at the front of the BNF, describing how the prescription is to be written with the quantity in words and figures. It no longer needs to be in the prescriber's own handwriting, but it must be in ink or otherwise indelible. Words and figures are not required for hospital in-patient drug charts if the drug required is stock on the ward. A ward register is not required by these guidelines, but is required by DoH guidelines. Records (e.g. registers) may now be kept electronically using approved software.

Private prescriptions for drugs in Schedules 2 and 3 must now be written on a standard form (similar to an FP10) and, once dispensed, this has to be sent to a national centre for collation and storage. For Schedule 2 drugs, the prescription is now only valid for 28 days. For Schedule 2 drugs, the person collecting the drugs from the pharmacy must provide proof of identity, and their details must be recorded in the register. They must sign for collection.

Controlled Drugs Supplementary Legislation

This comprises the Health Act 2006, The Controlled Drugs (Supervision of Management and Use) Regulations 2006, and the Misuse of Drugs (Safe Custody) (Amendment) Regulations 2007.

They stipulate who in an organisation is responsible for aspects of use of controlled drugs, and make minor changes such as moving Midazolam from Schedules 4 to 3.

Details can be seen on the NPC website.

Legal liability

All clinicians have a duty of care to their patients. Anyone who fails in this care and is found to be negligent, could be pursued through the courts using criminal or civil law.

To bring a successful action, the claimant must establish (i) that a duty of care was owed to him, (ii) that the duty was breached, and (iii) he suffered injury or harm caused by that breach.

A doctor or other health professional is required by law to exercise the care and skill of a reasonable professional. Negligence is a failure to reach that standard. *(Bolam* v. *Friern Hospital Management Committee* (1957) *2 ALLER 118 [1957] 1 WLR 582 (McNair J)).*

The law only makes a doctor liable if his negligent act or omission resulted in injury to the patient. Criminal law requires a greater burden of proof than civil law. The former requires that the cause of the harm was the prescriber's breach of duty and the burden of proof is 'beyond reasonable doubt' whereas, in a civil case, the burden of proof required is 'on the balance of probabilities'.

There are a number of ways in which harm may occur to a patient in the course of drug administration.

1 Errors on the prescription sheet

Wrong drug
Wrong dose
Drug prescribed leads to side effects or drug interactions
Patient is allergic to drug
Writing is illegible.

2 Dispensing errors

Wrong drug dispensed
Wrong patient (similar name)

Wrong dose
Failure to note dangerous drug interaction
Difficulty due to illegible writing.

3 Error in administration

Wrong patient, not checked with prescription card
Wrong amount of drug given
Wrong drug
Wrong route of administration
Drug not given.

It is estimated that there are 850 000 incidents per annum (National Patient Safety Agency) in Hospitals in the UK. These occur for a variety of reasons.

Errors of prescribing can occur if the wrong drug is written, or the correct drug in the wrong dose, e.g. heparin 25 000 units when 2500 units were intended. Another source of prescribing error occurs when a drug is added to a patient's drugs which will interact dangerously with an existing drug, e.g. adding a tricyclic antidepressant when the patient is already taking a monoamine-oxidase inhibitor (MAOI).

There is scope for the prescription to be misinterpreted if it is not written carefully enough. The heparin error above has also occurred when the doctor wrote 2500 u and the nurse administering it misread the u as a zero. (The BNF recommends that the word 'units' should always be written in full for this reason). Also, doses smaller than 1 mg should be written in micrograms, e.g. digoxin 62.5 micrograms, not 0.0625 mgms. There have been numerous incidents of the doctor writing 0.625 mg by mistake or of the nurse miscalculating the conversion.

Abbreviations can also be misinterpreted, e.g. ISDN 10 mgms (isosorbide mononitrate) has been dispensed as Istin 10 mg (the commercial name for Amlodopine 10 mg AZT (Ziovudine) has been misinterpreted as Azothiaprine with fatal consequences.

Dispensing errors can occur if the pharmacist selects the wrong drug from the shelf because of similar names or similar packaging. The correct drug can be supplied labelled with the wrong dose. Also, the correct drug and dose but the wrong patient's name can be on the label.

Errors in administration can occur when a drug is given to the wrong patient. The wrong amount can also be given due to the miscalculation of the volume of the liquid as the amount of medication per ml is not standardised and has to be worked out for each substance. Intravenous administration and intrathecal administration have been confused in the case of vincristine with tragic results.

National Patient Safety Agency

This is an independent NHS body created to promote safety in patient care.

Incidents or potential incidents are reported to the National Patient Safety Agency (NPSA) who analyse the data, producing reports, and issuing guidance and alerts as appropriate. The aim is to promote an open and fair culture within the NHS, with the emphasis on improvement rather than blame. Their website is www.npsa.nhs.uk.

Using licenced drugs for unlicenced purposes

The efficacy of each drug is tested in a clinical trial. The manufacturer can then apply for a licence to produce the drug. A summary of the process can be found at www.ukmi.nhs.uk/Med_info/licensing-process. The licence specifies how the drug can be used, the details of which are listed in the Summary of Product Characteristics (SPC), which includes indications for use, dose, contra-indication and precautions for use. The SPC will also include details of any monitoring required, e.g. monitoring of white cell count in patients on Clozapine. Product licences for generic drugs may differ between manufacturers, e.g. indications for use may differ.

If a product is used within the terms of its licence and a patient suffers from a serious side effect, they may sue the manufacturer for any damage sustained. If a product is used outside its licence, then the clinician must be able to justify that use, otherwise liability is with the clinician. For example, if Clozapine was used without monitoring of white cell count, the clinician would be liable. Documentation of such monitoring having been done is crucial. Usage outside the product licence is common in certain areas, particularly in paediatrics as most medicines are only licensed for use in adults. Using medicines within what the body of medical opinion deems appropriate will then give the clinician legal protection. Some Trusts now have a mechanism for logging the use of unlicensed drugs and some Trusts have documentation. This should be incorporated in the patient's notes to identify unlicensed use. If such a form does not exist, it would be good practice to record the decision in the notes, with a statement that the patient has been informed. This is required in some Trusts if higher than BNF doses of psychiatric medicines are used.

Clinical trials

Trials have to be carried out on any new drug at each stage of its development for various reasons. The trials with which clinicians are most familiar are in phase three of their development, just prior to the licence application being prepared. The results of these trials will establish the drug's place in therapy of the relevant disease. They will further previous knowledge on side-effects, interactions and doses for specific patient groups.

If a manufacturer is organising the trial, they should ensure that the clinical trial certificate exemption has been obtained from the licensing authority, and should inform the clinician that this has been done. If a manufacturer is not involved, the Local Research Ethics Committee can advise on what is needed. For a trial involving several centres, the manufacturers will obtain overall ethics approval, but each area will need to gain approval from their local ethics committee.

The trial itself can take a number of forms: An open study is one where both the clinician and the patient know what is being taken. Usually, this will be the active drug. The purpose of such a study will be to obtain further information on the drug, e.g. side-effects or effect of long-term use.

In a single-blind study, the clinician will know what is being taken, but the patient themselves will not know which option has been assigned to them. These studies usually compare one or more doses of the drug being tested with placebo. Sometimes, there are clinical or ethical reasons why a placebo cannot be used, so the new drug will be compared with an exiting one that is known to be efficacious in the same field.

In a double-blind study, the items used are the same as for a single-blind one, but the clinician is also unaware of which drug has been assigned to which patient, i.e. both the clinician and the patient are 'blinded'. This eliminates bias if the clinician is involved in assessing the patient's response to a given drug. Blindness can be lost if there are certain side-effects and, in this case, the manufacturers may suggest that two clinicians be involved (one to administer the medication and another to assess the patient's symptoms).

The outward appearance of both drugs should be the same and, if this is not possible, then each person should have two tablets and one will be active and another not. This is known as a 'double dummy'.

In certain situations, such as depression or epilepsy, it would not be ethically acceptable to leave a patient on only placebo or to use a comparison with an existing drug. This problem is overcome by giving the new drug or placebo, in addition to an established therapy. This is called an 'add on' study.

The trial has to continue for as long as it takes the treatment to work. In the case of depression, it would be unrealistic to expect a full effect in less than three weeks.

If the trial is comparing two drugs, it should use equivalent doses of both drugs, e.g. in the comparison of painkillers it would be unreasonable to compare a single daily dose of Aspirin with two paracetamol four times a day.

In testing a new drug, the number of patients being treated should be enough for any difference to be clearly seen.

This will vary according to the condition being treated.

For clinical reasons, it is sometimes useful to run a trial involving just one patient (an 'n=1 trial'). The patient will be asked to use one treatment for a period of time then to use another treatment of placebo for a similar time. The response during each phase is monitored.

Clinical trial phases

Phase 1

Safety – clinical pharmacology for safety and kinetics

Phase 2

Clinical efficacy and further pharmacology for dose regime
Efficacy in the patient population and side-effects
Detailed pharmacology

Phase 3

Place in therapy of the disease for comparison with other drugs
Increased patient exposure, e.g. less common side-effects
Interactions
Doses for varying patient types
Geriatric/paediatric applications?
General Practitioner use?
Further pharmacology and mode of action
Driving skills

Not all of the above are required prior to registration.

Phase 4

Post-marketing targeted studies in a wider setting.

Patient group directions

These were described in HSC 2000/026, which replaces HSC 1998/051 and is entitled *'A Report on the Supply and Administration of Medicines under Group Protocols'*. A good guide to these is available on the Medicines Health Regulation Authority (MHRA) website www.mhra.gov.uk – search 'patient group directions'.

This allows a medicine to be supplied for a patient by a specific health professional without a prescription written by a doctor. The professional involved must work to a protocol drawn up by a doctor or dentist, a senior pharmacist, and a member of the profession, who will be giving the supply to the patient and must be signed by them before being authorised by the PCO, Trust or other relevant organisation. Only named individuals can make the supply, and they must be trained in the application of the protocol.

The largest PGD at the moment has concerned pharmacists in some health authorities who have supplied emergency hormonal contraception from retail pharmacy by this means. Day surgery units have also found the mechanism useful where standard antibiotic cover or analgesia to take home is used in specific procedures. The administration of anticholinesterases to demented patients would lend itself to this type of policy.

Non-medical prescribing

Non-medical healthcare professionals may now train to become prescribers. Nurses, pharmacists, and optometrists may become Independent Prescribers who can prescribe without the involvement of a doctor. Other groups such as physiotherapists and radiographers can become Supplementary Prescribers. At present, Independent Prescribers have legal limits as to which Controlled Drugs they can prescribe, though these limits are being reviewed. Otherwise, they can prescribe within their own competency. They will agree with their medical colleagues what their role will be within a particular workplace.

Independent Prescribers can respond to changing or unexpected situations and can deal with long-term or acute episodes of care. Supplementary Prescribers are only allowed to prescribe according to a Clinical Management Plan (CMP) which is agreed with the relevant doctor and the patient. All three parties agree to the plan. Supplementary prescribing is of use in long-term conditions such as Lithium or Clozapine clinics where the doctor sees the patient at intervals according to clinical need, with the supplementary prescriber makes intermediate dose adjustments. The Trust must be involved with the setting up of the CMP, and only staff registered with their professional body as prescribers can work in this way.

There is information on non-medical prescribers on the National Prescribing Centre website www.npc.co.uk.

Local research ethics committees

This is found in HSG (19)5 which states that each health area should have a local research ethics committee (LREC) to advise NHS bodies on the ethical acceptability of research proposals involving human subjects.

An LREC should have 8 to 12 members to allow for a sufficiently broad range of experience and expertise so that the scientific and medical aspects of a research project can be reconciled with the welfare of the research subjects and any broader ethical implications.

It is suggested that members be drawn from a wide range of people including:

- hospital medical staff
- nursing staff
- general practitioners
- two or more lay persons.

Legal liability

LREC members may be concerned that they may be legally liable for injury caused to patients participating in research projects but legal advice from the Department of Health is that there is little prospect of a successful claim against an LREC member for a mishap arising from a project approved by them.

Proposals for research where capacity to consent is impaired need special consideration by the LREC. They balance the benefits, discomforts and risks for the individual and the need to advance knowledge so that people with mental disorder may benefit.

The presence of a mental disorder does not imply incapacity nor does detention under the Mental Health Act 1983.

23 Research ethics

IRAS

In the UK, at the time of writing, there is one system used for applying for the permissions and approvals needed to conduct health, social care and community care research. This is known as the Integrated Research Application System, or IRAS for short. It involves an on-line application via its website, which is at www.myresearchproject.org.uk.

Question 7 of the initial project filter requires the applicant to answer in the affirmative, if it is possible that the intended research project could at any stage include adults (that is, those aged 16 years or over) who are unable to consent for themselves owing to physical or mental incapacity. Detailed guidance on ethical review of applications involving adults unable to consent for themselves is available on the NRES website at: http://www.nres.npsa.nhs.uk/docs/guidance/AWI_Guidance.pdf.

If the intended research is a clinical trial of an investigational medicinal product, then the inclusion of adults unable to consent for themselves in any part of the UK is governed by the Medicines for Human Use (Clinical Trials) Regulations 2004; the Mental Capacity Act 2005 has no application here. The ethical review will consider whether the trial is justified having regard to the conditions and principles specified in these Regulations, and includes provision for informed consent by the subject's legal representative. Further details are available at: http://www.nres.npsa.nhs.uk/recs/guidance/guidance.htm#consent. Applicants need to give information about the inclusion of adults unable to consent in Part B of the IRAS application form.

If the intended research is not a clinical trial of an investigational medicinal product, then the inclusion of adults unable to consent for themselves in England and Wales requires approval by an 'appropriate body' under the Mental Capacity Act 2005, Section 30, and this approval must be given by an NHS research ethics committee (REC) (even if the intended research does not involve NHS patients). In Scotland, approval is required under Section 51 of the Adults with Incapacity (Scotland) Act 2000 (with approval being sought from the Scotland A REC), while in Northern Ireland, at the time of writing, inclusion in research of adults unable to consent for themselves is governed by common law (with application being made to any Health and Social Care (HSC) REC in Northern Ireland, in the case of research that is intended to take place only in Northern Ireland).

Ministry of Justice

In the case of research intended to take place in prisons or probation services in England and Wales, approval is required from the National Offender Management Service (NOMS). Further details are available from the Offender Health Research Network website at http://www.ohrn.nhs.uk.

In making an IRAS application, additional information may need to be provided for the Ministry of Justice, as appropriate, for example in relation to risk registers.

Human Tissue Act

The Human Tissue Act 2004 makes provision with respect to activities involving human tissue. Parts of it apply only to England, Wales and Northern Ireland. Schedule 1 (Scheduled purposes) Part 1 (Purposes requiring consent: general) covers the following seven areas:

1. Anatomical examination.
2. Determining the cause of death.
3. Establishing after a person's death the efficacy of any drug or other treatment administered to him.
4. Obtaining scientific or medical information about a living or deceased person which may be relevant to any other person (including a future person).
5. Public display.
6. Research in connection with disorders, or the functioning, of the human body.
7. Transplantation.

Thus, the use of human tissue for research requires informed consent from the donor; this is a legal requirement. Consent is not required if the human tissue is anonymous so far as the researcher is concerned *and* also the corresponding research study has ethical approval. Similarly, consent is not required if the human tissue was an existing holding as on 1 September 2006; but the researcher must be able to prove that this was so.

The following materials, derived from humans, are included within the term human tissue within the Human Tissue Act 2004:

- Blood
- Bone marrow
- Embryonic stem cells
- Human tissues samples containing cells
- Non-blood derived stem cells
- Primary or cultured cell lines (where the cell line contains cells from the original sample)
- Saliva swabs
- Slides or tissue blocks containing cells
- Stem cells created inside the human body
- Umbilical cord blood stem cells
- Urine.

The Act seeks to enforce good practice through the use of standard operating procedures which cover the acquisition, importing, use, exporting and disposal of human tissue as defined above. For each research institution, there needs to be a *designated individual* who should ensure that policies, systems and procedures are in place to comply with the law, *persons designated*, who act as focal points of knowledge in individual research groups, and a *licence holder*. Compliance with the Act is audited by the Human Tissue Authority.

Section 1 of the Human Tissue Act 2004 includes the following activities as being lawful if done with appropriate consent:

(d) the storage for use for a purpose specified in Part 1 of Schedule 1 of any relevant material which has come from a human body;
(f) the use for a purpose specified in Part 1 of Schedule 1 of any relevant material which has come from a human body.

Section 6 of the Human Tissue Act 2004 covers activities involving material from adults who lack capacity to consent and states that where—

(a) an activity of a kind mentioned in Section 1(1)(d) or (f) involves material from the body of a person who:
    (i) is an adult, and
    (ii) lacks capacity to consent to the activity, and
(b) neither a decision of his to consent to the activity, nor a decision of his not to consent to it, is in force, there shall for the purposes of this Part be deemed to be consent of his to the activity if it is done in circumstances of a kind specified by regulations made by the Secretary of State.

Royal College of Psychiatrists

The Royal College of Psychiatrists has issued Council Report CR82 (Guidelines for Researchers and for Research Ethics Committees on Psychiatric Research Involving Human Participants). In 2011, its Academic Faculty issued a statement on the ethics of psychiatric research, in which it stated that the following issues merit particular emphasis:

1. Research can bring major benefits to individuals, health services, and to society at large. Arguably, there is a greater need for research in psychiatry than in any other medical specialty. Whenever and wherever possible, ethically sound, high quality research should be facilitated.
2. Patients have the right to know about ethically approved and high quality research for which they may be eligible and offered the opportunity to take part.
3. The principles underlying the ethical conduct of research in psychiatry are the same as apply to other branches of medicine. Research in psychiatry must be held to the same high ethical standards as other medical research. It is important that additional barriers are not placed in the way of the conduct of research in this area.
4. The capacity to give consent to participate in research is task and time specific. Although certain individuals with psychiatric disorders may at times lack the capacity to consent, the vast majority of people with a mental illness have the right to decide for themselves whether or not they wish to take part in a study.
5. There are specific groups of individuals in psychiatric research who require additional safeguards – those with learning difficulties, detained patients, prisoners, children or vulnerable groups such as refugees, are examples. It is important that there is no actual or perceived coercion to participate.
6. Whenever possible, patients should be empowered to participate in research if they wish to do so.

7 Work must be done to foster an active and positive research culture in mental health services. It is important to challenge the common, but erroneous and stigmatising, view that research in psychiatry entails greater risk and has less potential benefit than research in other areas of medicine.
8 In order to avoid erroneous and stigmatising assumptions, the deliberations of ethics committees should be facilitated by direct advice from those experienced in clinical work and research in the relevant area(s).

References

2004 Human Tissue Act.
2007 Mental Health Act.

24 Child mental health law

Children are recognised both within international and UK law as deserving of special protection and specialised services. Most children presenting with complex mental health disorders will require multi-agency services and be subject to a number of legal frameworks. Thus, it is important that mental health professionals working with children are knowledgeable about relevant child welfare and criminal justice legislation.

Who can make decisions for children concerning their treatment including for mental disorder? The framework for such decisions is complex and contained in both statute and common law as well as in many policy initiatives and good practice guidance, all of which can be interlinked and overlapping. The overriding principle for mental health professionals in decision-making about the care and treatment of children is that the best interests of the child should be the primary consideration.

Overview of chapter

Legal frameworks applying to children

United Nations Convention on the Rights of the Child and the Human Rights Act

The tenets of the HRA and UNCRC underlie UK legislation including the Children Act 1989 and 2004 and NHS policy.

The Children Act 1989	Principles
	Orders
	Secure Accommodation Order
	Children in Need
	Concept of Significant Harm
	Parental Responsibility
The Mental Health Act 1983	Principles
	Age appropriate environment
	Mental Health Review Tribunals
	Duty of the Local Authority

Mental Health Act or Children Act 1989?

Fitness to Plead/Effective Participation in children

Consent, Capacity and Confidentiality

Consent & Capacity – general principles

Treatment decisions in children aged 16–17 years

Mental Capacity Act 2005
– general principles
– limitations for 16 and 17 year olds

Treatment decisions in children aged under 16 years

– Gillick Competence
– children who are not Gillick competent

Legal frameworks applying to children

Definition of a child

The definition of a child is subject to a legal framework. The Children Act 1989 Section 105 defines a child as less than 18 years. However, the Code of Practice of the Mental Health Act 1983 distinguishes between children who it describes as less than 16 years old and young people who are 16 and 17 years old; the Mental Capacity Act applies to all adults who are defined as over 16 years. The Criminal Law and criminal justice system frequently treats children as adults. In England and Wales, the age of criminal responsibility is set at 10 years (Children and Young Persons Act 1933, Section 50) this is low in comparison with other countries in Europe, where the median age is 14–15 years.

Human Rights Act

Since 2 October 2000 the principles of the European Convention on Human Rights have been incorporated into domestic law by the Human Rights Act. Every public body and court of law is required to make decisions in compliance with the principles of the Convention.

United Nations Convention on the Rights of the Child (UNCRC)

The United Nations Convention on the Rights of the Child (UNCRC) is an international human rights treaty that grants all children and young people under the age of 18 years (Article 1) a comprehensive set of rights. On 20 November 1989, the governments represented at the UN General Assembly, including the UK, agreed to adopt the UNCRC into international law. The UK signed the Convention on 19 April 1990, ratified it on 16 December 1991, and it came into force in the UK on 15 January 1992. It is the most widely ratified international human rights treaty with all UN member states except for the United States and Somalia (which has signalled its intention to ratify) having now ratified the Convention.

The Convention comprises 54 substantive 'articles': Articles 1–41 detail children's social, economic, cultural, civil and political rights; Article 42 requires the state to publicise the Convention, while Articles 43–54 set out how governments must implement the Convention.

The rights include:

- The best interests must be a top priority in all actions concerning children (Article 3).
- Governments must respect the rights and responsibilities of parents to guide and advise their child so that, as they grow, they learn to apply their rights properly (Article 5).
- Every child has the right to say what they think in all matters affecting them and to have their view taken seriously (Article 12).

- Every child has the right to privacy. The law should protect the child's private, family and home life (Article 16).
- Both parents share responsibility for bringing up their child and should always consider what is best for their child (Article 18).
- The right to education (Article 28) and leisure, play and culture (Article 31).

Children Act 1989

The Children Act 1989 implemented for the most part on 14 October 1991 introduced comprehensive changes to legislation in England and Wales affecting the welfare of children. Its main provisions apply to all individuals aged less than 18 years of age. It brings together private and public law. Although the Act has been amended since 1989 (most importantly by the **Adoption and Children Act 2002**, the **Children Act 2004** and the **Children and Adoption Act 2006**), the original framework remains intact.

Working Together to Safeguard Children (2010) sets out how organisations and individuals should work together to safeguard and promote the welfare of children and young people in accordance with the **Children Act 1989** and **Children Act 2004**.

The **Children Act 1989** is arranged in 12 parts and 15 schedules. For a comprehensive account the reader is advised to look at the Act itself. In this chapter we describe key aspects and the most recent guidance from Working Together most relevant to mental health workers.

Principles of the Children Act 1989:

- The child's welfare is paramount.
- The concept of parental responsibility (*see* below) was introduced to replace 'parental rights'.
- The Act allows children to be parties to proceedings in their own right, separate from their parents.
- Identification of children in need and safeguarding and promoting their welfare are identified explicitly as duties for local authorities in partnership with others (especially parents).
- The Act and its guidance include duties and powers for local authorities to provide certain services for children and families.
- The welfare checklist was introduced into courts as a mandatory part of the decision-making process.
- The no-order principle directs courts and others involved in proceedings to make sure that any order made is better for the child than making no order at all.
- There is an explicit assumption that delay in deciding questions concerning children is prejudicial to their welfare and that in all proceedings this will be minimised.

Courts must have regard, in opposed applications for a Section 8 order and in care proceedings, to the Welfare Checklist concerning the child's circumstances as set out in Section 1(3), including:

- the ascertainable wishes and feelings of the child (considered in the light of his age and understanding);
- physical, emotional and educational needs of the child;
- likely effect on the child of any change in circumstances;
- age, sex, background and any characteristics which the court considers relevant;

- any harm that the child has suffered or is at risk of suffering;
- the capability of each of the child's parents, and any other person in relation to whom the court considers the question to be relevant, of meeting his needs; and
- the range of powers available to the court in the proceedings in question.

A wider list of matters relating to circumstances in which adoption is being considered is contained in the Adoption and Children Act 2002.

Orders under the Children Act 1989

The main Public law orders are:

Section Care order 31
Section Interim care order 38
Section Contact with children in care 34
Section Supervision order 31
Section Education supervision order 36
Section Interim supervision order 38
Section Child assessment order 43
Section Emergency protection order 44–45
Section Recovery order 50

The most important of the Private law orders are known as Section 8 orders and are:

- Residence order
- Contact order
- Specific issues order
- Prohibited steps order.

Secure Accommodation Order

Section 25 of the Children Act 1989 sets out the criteria, which must be fulfilled before a young person is placed in secure accommodation by a Local Authority:

- S/he has a history of absconding and is likely to abscond from any other type of accommodation AND
- If s/he absconds s/he is likely to suffer significant harm OR
- If s/he is kept in any other type of accommodation s/he is likely to injure her/himself or other persons.

Children under the age of 13 years cannot be placed in secure accommodation without the prior approval of the Secretary of State. In an emergency where the criteria are met and an immediate placement is needed a Directors Order can be obtained for a period of up to 72 hours. Subsequently a court can authorise detention for up to a period of three months initially, which can be renewed for up to six months at a time.

For a child not on a Care Order parental agreement is needed. If parents withhold consent consideration of application for an Interim Care Order, along with a secure accommodation order needs to be made. For those young people who are aged 16 who are accommodated, an interim or full Care Order should be considered. A Secure Accommodation Order provides the legal justification for detaining the child in a particular setting but it does not provide legal justification for compulsory treatment of the child.

Children can be remanded into secure accommodation in criminal proceedings and the criteria are different.

Key concepts from the Children Act 1989

Children in Need

Many young people with complex mental health problems are children in need. Children who are defined as being 'in need', under Section 17 of the **Children Act 1989**, are those whose vulnerability is such that they are unlikely to reach or maintain a satisfactory level of health or development, or their health and development will be significantly impaired, without the provision of services (Section 17(10) of the **Children Act 1989**), plus those who are disabled. The critical factors to be taken into account in deciding whether a child is in need under the **Children Act 1989** are:

- what will happen to a child's health or development without services being provided; and
- the likely effect the services will have on the child's standard of health and development.

Local authorities have a duty to safeguard and promote the welfare of 'children in need'. (*Working Together* 2010 Section 1.25)

The concept of Significant Harm

The Children Act 1989 introduced the concept of significant harm as the threshold that justifies compulsory intervention in family life in the best interests of children, and gives local authorities a duty to make enquiries to decide whether they should take action to safeguard or promote the welfare of a child who is suffering, or likely to suffer, significant harm.

A court may make a care order (committing the child to the care of the local authority) or supervision order (putting the child under the supervision of a social worker or a probation officer) in respect of a child if it is satisfied that:

- the child is suffering, or is likely to suffer, significant harm; and
- the harm, or likelihood of harm, is attributable to a lack of adequate parental care or control (Section 31).

Working Together to Safeguard Children highlights that

> *'There are no absolute criteria on which to rely when judging what constitutes significant harm. Consideration of the severity of ill-treatment may include the degree and the extent of physical harm, the duration and frequency of abuse and neglect, the extent of premeditation, and the presence or degree of threat, coercion, sadism and bizarre or unusual elements. Each of these elements has been associated with more severe effects on the child, and/or relatively greater difficulty in helping the child overcome the adverse impact of the maltreatment. Sometimes, a single traumatic event may constitute significant harm, for example, a violent assault, suffocation or poisoning. More often, significant harm is a compilation of significant events, both acute and long-standing, which interrupt, change or damage the child's physical and psychological development. Some children live in family and social circumstances where their health and development are neglected. For them, it is the corrosiveness*

of long-term emotional, physical or sexual abuse that causes impairment to the extent of constituting significant harm. In each case, it is necessary to consider any maltreatment alongside the child's own assessment of his or her safety and welfare, the family's strengths and supports, as well as an assessment of the likelihood and capacity for change and improvements in parenting and the care of children and young people'.

Parental Responsibility

When assessing or treating a child services must establish who has parental responsibility for the child. Sometimes it may be necessary to request copies of relevant court orders.

Parental responsibility is defined in Section 3 of the Children Act 1989 as:

'All the rights, duties, powers, responsibilities and authority which by law a parent of a child has in relation to the child and his property.'

Who has parental responsibility?

- A mother retains parental responsibility for her child unless the child is adopted.
- A father has parental responsibility if he is married to the mother when the child is born or marries the mother after the birth and since 1 December 2003 by jointly registering the birth of the child with the mother. He can acquire parental responsibility by co-signing a 'parental responsibility agreement' with the mother and submitting it to the court or by a parental responsibility order, made by a court.
- Step parents: may acquire parental responsibility through a parental responsibility agreement or a court parental responsibility order.
- Guardian: where the person(s) with parental responsibilities have died, a guardian can be appointed by a court order or by the person(s) with parental responsibilities, in writing, that is, in a will.
- Residence Order: this is an order of the court that sets out who the child or young person is to live with and gives that person parental responsibility. Such orders may be made in favour of any person, or persons, and may provide for the child or young person to live with one person at one time and other people at other times (CA 1989).
- Care Order: this places the child or young person under the care of the local authority (Section 33 CA 1989). The court will only make this order if satisfied that the child or young person is suffering or likely to suffer significant harm as described above. Care orders cannot be made for those aged 17 or over, or 16 if the person is married (Section 33 CA 1989).
- Under Section 33(3) of the Children Act 1989 if a child is subject to a Care Order the local authority has parental responsibility for the child and the power to determine the extent to which a parent of the child may meet his or her parental responsibility for the child.
- Special Guardianship Order: introduced by the Adoption and Children Act 2002, Special Guardianship is intended to provide another option for legal permanence for children who cannot grow up with their birth families. It gives the special guardian legal parental responsibility for the child which is expected to last until the child is 18. But, unlike Adoption Orders, these orders do not remove parental responsibility from the child's birth parents, although their ability to exercise it is extremely limited.

Adoption

- Adoption Orders are irrevocable, whereas Care Orders, Residence Orders and Special Guardianship Orders can be varied or discharged by the court.
- Wardship Orders: these are orders made by the High Court under its inherent jurisdiction. Since the introduction of the CA 1989, the use of wardship has dramatically declined.
- A person who has care of the child (but not parental responsibility) may do 'what is reasonable in all the circumstances of the case for the purpose of safeguarding or promoting the child's welfare' (Section 3(5) CA 1989). Whether the intervention is reasonable or not will depend upon the urgency and gravity of what is required and the extent to which it is practicable to consult a person with parental responsibility.

Section 2(7) of the Children Act 1989 states:

> *'Where more than one person has parental responsibility for a child, each of them may act alone and without the other (or others) in meeting that responsibility.'*

However, case-law has established that in certain circumstances those with parental responsibility are under a legal duty to consult each other. The consensus is that the following matters require the consent of all those who have parental responsibility for the child:

- Change of surname.
- Removing the child from the jurisdiction (i.e. England and Wales) for more than one month.
- Serious medical treatment except in an emergency.
- Decisions about education.

The MHA Code 36.5 advises:

> *'It is good practice to involve both parents and others close to the child or young person in the decision-making process. However, if one person with parental responsibility strongly disagreed with the decision to treat and was likely to challenge it in court, it might be appropriate to seek authorization from the court before relying on the consent of another person with parental responsibility.'*

Mental Health Act 1983 as amended by the MHA 2007

The Mental Health Act has no lower age limit. In this chapter we explore aspects particularly relevant to working with children. The Code of Practice states that those responsible for the care and treatment of children and young people should be child specialists. Where this is not possible, it is good practice for the clinical staff to have regular access to and make use of a CAMHS specialist for advice and consultation.

The Code of Practice identifies a number of principles which should be borne in mind when taking decisions under the Act about children and young people.

- The best interests of the child or young person must always be a significant consideration.

- Children and young people should always be kept as fully informed as possible, just as an adult would be, and should receive clear and detailed information concerning their care and treatment, explained in a way they can understand and in a format that is appropriate to their age.
- The child or young person's views, wishes and feelings should always be considered.
- Any intervention in the life of a child or young person that is considered necessary by reason of their mental disorder should be the option that is least restrictive and least likely to expose them to the risk of any stigmatisation, consistent with effective care and treatment, and it should also result in the least possible separation from family, carers, friends and community or interruption of their education, as is consistent with their wellbeing.
- All children and young people should receive the same access to educational provision as their peers.
- Children and young people have as much right to expect their dignity to be respected as anyone else.
- Children and young people have as much right to privacy and confidentiality as anyone else.

Age appropriate environment

The age appropriate environment duty is set out in Section 131A of the Mental Health Act and came into operation in April 2010. It requires hospital managers to ensure that: 'the patient's environment in the hospital is suitable having regard to his age (subject to his needs)'. This duty applies to all patients under 18, admitted to hospital.

The Code of Practice to the Mental Health Act 1983 for England (2008) highlights the factors to be considered when deciding whether the ward environment is suitable for the child or young person concerned.

They should have:

- Appropriate physical facilities.
- Staff with the right training, skills and knowledge to understand and address their specific needs as children and young people.
- A hospital routine that will allow their personal, social and educational development to continue as normally as possible.
- Equal access to educational opportunities as their peers, in so far as they are able to make use of them, considering their mental state.

The Code of Practice identifies situations when young people might be admitted to adult facilities. These are in an emergency when the important thing is that the patient is in a safe environment or when an assessment concludes that the best place for a young person is an adult ward.

As from 1 December 2008 Government policy is that no child under 16 is to be placed on an adult mental health ward. Any such admissions are treated as Serious Untoward Incidents (Department Health, June 2007) and must be reported to the Strategic Health Authority.

The age appropriate environment duty is underpinned by the following core duties of public bodies, including Local Authorities and NHS bodies:

- Duty to put in place arrangements to safeguard and promote the welfare of children and young people: this is set out in Section 11 of the Children Act 2004.

- When carrying out their statutory functions, organisations should take into account the United Nations Convention on the Rights of the Child. Article 37C states: '...every child deprived of liberty shall be separated from adults unless it is considered in the child's best interests not to do so...'.

The Royal College of Psychiatrists website contains further information about providing an age appropriate environment.

Mental Health Review Tribunal – Rights to apply

Young people have rights as other patients to apply to the Tribunal. Where older patients must be referred after a three-year period without a Tribunal hearing, children and young people must be referred after one year.

Duty of the Local authority when children are in hospital

The MHA Code of Practice and the Pan London Child Protection guidelines highlight duties of local authorities in relation to children in hospital which include ensuring that they receive visits. When a child has been or is planned to be in hospital for more than three months, under Section 85 of the Children Act 1989 the hospital is required to notify the child's home authority, that is, the local authority for the area where the child is ordinarily resident.

Mental Health Act 1983 or Children Act 1989?

In practice, this is a key issue and may be determined by ethics/clinical practice of individual clinicians. The decision-making process may also have significant implications for resources of agencies. Mental health provision within secure accommodation is very variable. The Code of Practice provides some guidance regarding this:

> 36.17 However, where the child or young person with a mental disorder needs to be detained, but the primary purpose is not to provide medical treatment for mental disorder, consideration should be given to using Section 25 of the Children Act 1989.
>
> 36.18 For example, if a child or young person is seriously mentally ill, they may require to be admitted for treatment under the Mental Health Act. But if they are behaviourally disturbed, and there is no need for them to be hospitalised, their needs might be more appropriately met within secure accommodation under the Children Act.

Fitness to Plead/Effective Participation in children

Unless a child is found unfit to plead the expectation is that they will participate in court proceedings. The Pritchard Criteria operate as with adults. The legal statute regarding Fitness to Plead does not operate in youth court. If a court considers that a prosecution is an abuse of process it may stay the proceedings (i.e. prevent the prosecution continuing). The test is can the defendant receive a fair trial. In cases where the youth, cognitive deficits or emotional immaturity of a defendant mean that s/he cannot participate effectively in the proceedings the judge may find that it is an abuse of process to proceed with criminal charges.

Article 6 of the Human Rights Act guarantees the right of an accused to participate effectively in his or her own trial. With child defendants, the European Court of Human Rights has emphasised that this includes a developmental perspective. In *T* v. *United Kingdom: V* v. *United Kingdom* [1999] the court found that notwithstanding the special arrangements made to help ensure that the youths could properly participate in the trial process in the Crown Court, 'it is highly unlikely that either applicant would have felt sufficiently uninhibited, in the tense court room and under public scrutiny, to have consulted with their legal representatives during the trial or, indeed, that, given their immaturity and disturbed emotional state, they would have been capable outside the court room of co-operating with their lawyers and giving them information for the purpose of their defense'.

It therefore followed, in the view of the Court, that the applicants had been denied a fair hearing in breach of Article 6(1).

In its ruling the court said that 'it is essential that a child charged with an offence is dealt with in a manner which takes full account of his age, level of maturity and intellectual and emotional capacities and that steps are taken to promote his ability to understand and participate in the proceedings.'

In response to this ruling, the Lord Chief Justice issued a Practice Direction which suggests ways in which the trial procedure might be modified for a child defendant to promote understanding and participation. The suggestions include allowing the child to sit with his or her family and legal advisers, the removal of wigs and gowns, simplification of the language used in court and taking regular breaks.

In America, the MacArthur Foundation Research Network for Adolescent Development and Juvenile Justice compared the response of youths and adults in a series of hypothetical legal situations. Nearly one-third of 11 to 13-year-olds and one-fifth of 14 to 15-year-olds had deficits that the court might see as serious enough to question their ability to proceed in a trial. The network next assessed relevant emotional aspects of maturity including the ability to take into consideration long-term consequences, perceive and comprehend risk, deflect peer influence and weigh whether to comply with authority figures. In general the youngest young people were more likely to endorse decisions that comply with what an authority seem to want as measured by their willingness to confess and plea bargain. They were significantly less likely to recognise the inherent risks in various decisions and they were less likely to comprehend the long-term consequences of these decisions. The study found no differences by age in the effects of peer pressure on decision-making. Those with low IQs performed more poorly on all items.

The Youth Rehabilitation Order

The Youth Rehabilitation Order (YRO), a generic community sentence for children, came into force on 1 November 2009 and can have a Mental Health Treatment Requirement.

A YRO with a Mental Health Treatment Requirement requires a young person to submit, during the periods specified in the order, to treatment by or under the direction of a registered medical practitioner or a registered psychologist (a person registered in the part of the register maintained under the Health Professions Order 2001 which relates to practitioner psychologists) with a view to improving their mental condition.

A court may not attach a Mental Health Treatment Requirement to a YRO unless:

- The court is satisfied, on the evidence of a registered medical practitioner approved under Section 12 of the Mental Health Act 1983, that the mental condition of the young person is such that it requires and may be susceptible to treatment, but is not such as to warrant the making of a Hospital Order or Guardianship Order under that Act.
- The court is also satisfied that arrangements have been or can be made for the treatment that they intend to specify in the order, this includes where the young person is required to submit to the treatment as a resident patient, and arrangements for the reception of the young person.

For a YRO with a Mental Health Treatment Requirement to be made, the young person must have expressed a willingness to comply with it.

Consent and Capacity

Consent in children – general principles

Increasing weight is given to respecting children's autonomous decisions as they mature and in the course of normal development, children are encouraged to make more complex and important decisions for themselves. Legal frameworks impose arbitrary cutoffs based on chronological age, however decision-making continues to develop even into adulthood with adults' beliefs and values changing over time.

Treatment decisions in children aged 16 and 17 years of age

Since the passing of the **Family Law Reform Act 1969** it has been recognised that a person aged 16 may give consent to treatment in the same way as an adult. The Act provides that:

> *'the consent of a minor who has attained the age of 16 years to any surgical, medical or dental treatment which, in the absence of consent, would constitute a trespass to his person, shall be as effective as it would be if he were of full age; and where a minor has by virtue of this section given an effective consent to any treatment it shall not be necessary to obtain any consent for it from his parent or guardian.'*

Mental Capacity Act (MCA) 2005

The Mental Capacity Act is dealt with in detail in Chapters 16–20. The Mental Capacity Act concerns 'adults' who are defined in the Act as people 16 years of age and over.

For those individuals who are 16 years of age or over and who lack the mental capacity to make a particular decision for themselves, the Mental Capacity Act 2005 provides the legal framework for acting and making decisions on their behalf. The underlying philosophy of the Act is to ensure that any decision made, or action taken, on behalf of someone who lacks the capacity to make the decision or act for themselves is made in their best interests.

The five statutory principles are outlined below with issues to consider when applying them to adolescents highlighted:

1. *A person must be assumed to have capacity unless it is established that they lack capacity.*

The Act's starting point is to confirm in legislation that it should be assumed that an adult (aged 16 or over) has full legal capacity to make decisions for themselves (the right to autonomy) unless it can be shown that they lack capacity to make a decision for themselves at the time the decision needs to be made. This is known as the 'presumption of capacity'. Guidance in both the MCA 2005 Code of Practice and the MHA Code reflects that not all young people who are unable to make a decision will lack capacity within the meaning of the MCA. In order to fall within the remit of the MCA the decision-making difficulties must arise from an 'impairment of or disturbance in the functioning of the mind or brain' rather than developmental immaturity, i.e. a young person will not lack capacity if they are unable to make a decision due to immaturity related appropriately to their chronological age and the nature of the decision. In many such instances treatment decisions are made without problem as the young person is in agreement with the decision made by the person or agency with parental responsibility. Where the young person contests the decision, in an emergency treatment can be given in their best interests. In less urgent cases treatment may be postponed, modified or withheld.

2. *A person is not to be treated as unable to make a decision unless all practicable steps to help him to do so have been taken without success.*

The Act states that people must be given all appropriate help and support to enable them to make their own decisions or to maximise their participation in any decision-making process. This emphasises the need to provide age appropriate information for young people that is presented in language that is accessible and in a format that engages them.

3. *A person is not to be treated as unable to make a decision merely because he makes an unwise decision.*

Capacity is decision-specific and does not imply that the decision made needs to be considered a wise or 'good' decision. This maybe problematic in adolescents, who may be more likely to take decisions that do not reflect the full complexities able to be considered by a more developmentally mature adult. Adolescent decision-making is characterised by increased tendency to be more impulsive and risk taking and a lesser likelihood to fully consider the long-term implications of their decision. How much weight is given to such issues should depend on the importance and outcome of the decision being made, although this too will be a matter of judgment for the parents, carers and professionals involved.

4. *An act done, or decision made, under this Act for or on behalf of a person who lacks capacity must be done, or made, in his best interests.*

Decisions made on behalf of a young person who is deemed to lack capacity must be made in the 'best interests' of the young person. 'Best interests' do not necessarily equate to 'medical best interests' and will depend on questions of values and culture as well as facts. Best interests are not defined in the Act but must take into account the young person's known past and wishes and feelings, so entails discussions with others who know the person. In 16- and 17-year-olds, this would ideally mean the person with parental responsibility. Independent Mental Capacity Advocates (IMCAs) support people who lack capacity when decisions are being made about serious medical treatments or long-term change in accommodation. They are invoked when a person lacks friends or relatives. In a 16- or 17-year-old who lacks friends or relatives it would be good practice to involve social services.

5. *Before the act is done, or the decision is made, regard must be had to whether the purpose for which it is needed can be as effectively achieved in a way that is less restrictive of the person's rights and freedom of action.*

To maximise continued healthy development of children and young people it is important to ensure that any treatment or decision will impact as little as possible in their participation in normal developmental tasks and activities.

Treatment decisions made under the Mental Capacity Act may include the use of restraint but only if the professional believes that it is necessary to prevent harm to the person who lacks capacity and that the restraint is proportionate to the likelihood and seriousness of harm. (MCA Section 6)

Limitation to the MCA for 16- and 17-year-olds

Lasting Power of Attorney

16- and 17-years-olds cannot make advance decisions to refuse treatment or a lasting power of attorney.

Deprivation of Liberty Safeguards (DOLS)

The Deprivation of Liberty Safeguards were introduced into the Mental Capacity Act 2005 through the Mental Health Act 2007. These safeguards were formerly known as the Bournewood safeguards and act to ensure that people with mental disorder or disability of mind are cared for the in the least restrictive regimes and are not arbitrarily deprived of their liberty. DOLS only apply to those over 18 years of age; safeguards for 16- and 17-year-olds should be ensured through the Children Act.

Treatment decisions in children aged less than 16 years of age

Gillick (Fraser) competence and treatment decisions

Gillick competence arises from case law and establishes that a child less than 16 years of age can give valid consent to treatment for medical matters. The 'Gillick competent' child is defined as – 'A child who has attained sufficient understanding and intelligence to be able to understand fully what is involved in the proposed intervention will be regarded as competent to consent to a particular intervention, such as admission to hospital or proposed treatment.'

Assessing competence in a child or young person requires understanding the individual's stage of developmental maturity in the context of the specific decision required. Serious and complex decisions (such as consent to admission or medication) would require a higher level of understanding than consent to attend an out-patient appointment for counselling. As with the assessment of capacity in adults, it is decision-specific and may fluctuate over time.

Children under 16 years of age who are not Gillick competent

Young children will commonly have decisions about medical treatment or treatment for mental disorder made by their parents. This 'Parental Consent' is not usually problematic, however consent for some treatments such as for electro-convulsive therapy (ECT) is outside the zone of parental control. The Mental Health Act Code of Practice states that relying on parental consent for admission to hospital for treatment is not advisable. This reflects the increasing emphasis on greater autonomy for children and young people in making their own health decisions and provides greater legal safeguards for children admitted to hospital either informally or under the Mental Health Act.

Difficulties will sometimes arise when there is disagreement between parents and doctors over whether treatment is appropriate or not.

How is decision-making resolved when parents and doctors disagree? Negotiation is the initial way forward, recognising that medical best interests do not necessarily reflect best interests from the perspective of the child and the family. Education about the proposed treatment and alternatives as well as options such as speaking to other families who have experienced similar treatment may provide a way forward. A compromise position such as delaying the onset of treatment or adapting treatment may be achieved. If no such agreement or compromise can be reached then there is recourse for the medical team to the courts as a final arbiter.

Summary of Consent to Treatment for Mental Disorder in Children not involving the Mental Health Act

The majority of decisions made concerning treatment for children with mental disorders will be made on an 'informal' basis, i.e. the provisions of the Mental Health Act do not apply. This will include decisions around admission to hospital as well as medication and other forms of psychological and medical treatment and occurs:

- When the child is able to decide and has consented (Family Law Reform Act for children over 16 years and the Gillick competent child under 16 years of age).
- With parental consent (for child who has not been able to decide, i.e. not Gillick competent and is under 16 years).

- For a child 16 years or over who lacks capacity the treatment can take place under MCA if treatment in **their best interests and the care regime does not amount to a deprivation of liberty.**
- On application to the Court.

Treatment of children without consent

If the failure to treat is likely to lead to death or serious harm then a child or young person can be treated without consent. Situations where this may arise are:

- where a child is able to decide but refuses;
- the person with Parental Responsibility could consent but is unavailable; or
- the person with Parental Responsibility does not consent

and there is no time to seek a decision from the Court.

Treatment in such circumstances is limited to that which is immediately necessary to stablise a condition and must be in the child or young person's best interests and must be reviewed when the condition stabilised.

Confidentiality

The right to confidentiality extends to children and young people where a child or young person is assessed as being capable of making decisions about information sharing of their personal and medical details. This can include decisions not to share information with their parents/carers.

Limits to confidentiality

In consultations with children and young people practitioners need to be clear about the limitations of confidentiality.

General Medical Council (GMC) Guidance – principles of confidentiality in 0–18 years – reminds practitioners that if a child or young person lacks capacity there is a duty to act in their best interests and this may require the sharing of information with parents or appropriate authorities.

Section 49 of the GMC Guidance states that if a child or young person refuses consent, or if it is not practical to ask for consent, the practitioner should consider the benefits and possible harms that may arise from disclosure. Any views given by the child or young person on why you information should not be disclosed should be taken into account. Information can be disclosed if this is necessary to protect the child or young person, or someone else, from risk of death or serious harm. Potential scenarios are of three different types:

(a) *Safeguarding children:* a child or young person is at risk of neglect or sexual, physical or emotional abuse.
(b) *Public protection:* the information would help in the prevention, detection or prosecution of serious crime, usually crime against the person.
(c) *Duty of care:* a child or young person is involved in behaviour that might put them or others at risk of serious harm.

It is important to record reasons for disclosure and disclose only the information relevant for the purpose identified, promptly to the appropriate person or authority. If you judge that disclosure is not justified, you should record your reasons for not disclosing.

It is good practice to explore the reasons behind the child or young person's request not to share information. If the clinician considers it would be beneficial to treatment to involve parents/carers in the young person's care then exploration of whether there is anything that can be done to alter the decision may be indicated. Even where consent to share information is not given, in some contexts it may be possible to obtain information from parents/carers without breaching confidentiality, provided that information is not revealed which the parent or carer would not reasonably be expected to know already.

Conclusion

Decision-making about the care and treatment for children with mental disorders is a complex area, with increasing weight given to respecting children's autonomous decision-making. Where children are not able to decide for themselves, health and social care professionals have a duty to act in the child's best interests. In order to do so all professionals need to be aware of the complex legal framework covering the care of children. In complex cases it will be important that professionals discuss decisions with peers and sometimes seek advice from Trust solicitors.

References

Children Act 1989 and Guidance (particularly Volumes 1, 4, 6 and 7).

Department of Constitutional Affairs (2007) *Mental Capacity Act 2005 Code of Practice*. London: TSO.

Department of Health (2008) *Mental Health Act 1983: Code of Practice*. London: TSO.

General Medical Council. *0–18 Years: Guidance for All Doctors*.

HM Government (2010) *Working Together to Safeguard Children*.

National Institute for Mental Health in England (2009) *The Legal Aspects of the Care and Treatment of Children and Young People with Mental Disorder*.

Cases

1969 Family Law Reform Act

2005 Mental Capacity Act

25 Race, culture and mental health

Since April 2001, all public bodies have had a general duty to work towards the elimination of unlawful racial discrimination and to promote equality of opportunity and good relations between different racial groups (*see* Section 1 of the 2000 Act). This duty applied to all those working under the remit of the Mental Health Act 1983. There are also important links with the Human Rights Act 1998, which will be considered below. The Equality Act 2010 has brought together and harmonised discrimination law, including race, and an overview of this new law is also included in this chapter.

The Race Relations Act of 1976 had been designed to strengthen the law against racial discrimination and it established a single new statutory body, the Commission for Racial Equality, which combined law enforcement and promotional responsibilities in place of the Race Relations Board and Community Relations Commission. In turn, this body has now been replaced by the Equality and Human Rights Commission which was established by the Equality Act 2010.

Under the 1976 Act, discrimination was made unlawful in employment, education, housing and the provision of goods, facilities and services (including clubs). The provisions were more comprehensive than those of the previous legislation. In particular, the definition of racial discrimination was extended to cover nationality, and it included not only direct discrimination but also the application of unjustifiable requirements and conditions that are formally neutral as between different racial groups but that are, in practice, discriminatory in effect (referred to as 'indirect discrimination'). Racial discrimination became a civil wrong for which the normal forms of civil redress were available. Aggrieved individuals were able to seek redress directly in designated county courts or, for employment cases, in industrial tribunals.

Human Rights Act 1998

Article 14 of the European Convention on Human Rights requires that 'the enjoyment of the rights and freedoms set forth in this Convention shall be secured without discrimination on any ground such as sex, race, colour, language, religion, political or other opinion, national or social origin, association with a national minority, property, birth or other status'. It does not provide a free-standing prohibition on discrimination but applies only in relation to the enjoyment of the rights contained in the other relevant articles. However, Section 6 of the Act makes it unlawful for a public authority to act in a way which is incompatible with a Convention right unless it is required to do so by primary legislation or inevitably incompatible secondary legislation.

International Conventions

As well as the protection of the European Convention on Human Rights, people from ethnic minorities have the 'International Convention on the Elimination of All Forms of Racial Discrimination' to support them. The Convention has its own monitoring body. This and other human rights treaties are explored by Larry Gostin and Lance Gable in a thorough review of principles of mental health law and policy (Gostin et al., 2010). The Human Rights Committee of the United Nations defines racial discrimination as 'any distinction, exclusion, restriction or preference based on race, colour, descent, or national or ethnic origin which has the purpose or effect of nullifying or impairing the recognition, enjoyment or exercise, on an equal footing, of human rights and fundamental freedoms in the political, economic, social, cultural or any other field of public life.'

Equality Act 2010

The Equality Act is an attempt to harmonise discrimination law, and to strengthen the law to support what the government saw as progress on equality. It extends the circumstances in which a person is protected against discrimination, harassment or victimisation because of a 'protected characteristic'. These characteristics include race as well as religion or belief, age, disability, gender reassignment, marriage and civil partnership, pregnancy and maternity, sex and sexual orientation.

The Act extends the circumstances in which a person is protected against discrimination by allowing them to make a claim if they are directly discriminated against because of a combination of two relevant protected characteristics. It also creates a duty on listed public bodies when carrying out their functions (and on other persons when carrying out public functions) to have due regard when carrying out their functions to:

- the need to eliminate conduct which the Act prohibits;
- the need to advance equality of opportunity between persons who share a relevant protected characteristic and those who do not; and
- the need to foster good relations between people who share a relevant protected characteristic and people who do not.

The practical effect is that listed public bodies will have to consider how their policies, programmes and service delivery will affect people with the protected characteristics. In mental health, some critics would argue that there is significant progress to be made.

The Explanatory Notes to the Act provide helpful explanations on how the Act will operate with regard to race and religion, starting with a commentary on Section 47:

> *'For the purposes of the Act, "race" includes colour, nationality and ethnic or national origins.*
>
> *48. The section explains that people who have or share characteristics of colour, nationality or ethnic or national origins can be described as belonging to a particular racial group. A racial group can be made up of two or more different racial groups.*
>
> *49. The section also enables a Minister of the Crown to amend the Act by order so as to add 'caste' to the current definition of 'race'. When*

exercising this power, the Minister may amend the Act, for example, by including exceptions for caste, or making particular provisions of the Act apply in relation to caste in some but not other circumstances. The term 'caste' denotes a hereditary, endogamous (marrying within the group) community associated with a traditional occupation and ranked accordingly on a perceived scale of ritual purity. It is generally (but not exclusively) associated with South Asia, particularly India, and its diaspora. It can encompass the four classes (varnas) of Hindu tradition (the Brahmin, Kshatriya, Vaishya and Shudra communities); the thousands of regional Hindu, Sikh, Christian, Muslim or other religious groups known as jatis; and groups amongst South Asian Muslims called biradaris. Some jatis regarded as below the varna hierarchy (once termed 'untouchable') are known as Dalit.

50. This section replaces similar provisions in the Race Relations Act 1976. However, the power to add caste to the definition of race is a new provision.

Colour includes being black or white.

Nationality includes being a British, Australian or Swiss citizen.

Ethnic or national origins include being from a Roma background or of Chinese heritage.

A racial group could be 'black Britons' which would encompass those people who are both black and who are British citizens.

Religion or belief

51. This section defines the protected characteristic of religion or religious or philosophical belief, which is stated to include, for this purpose, a lack of religion or belief. It is a broad definition in line with the freedom of thought, conscience and religion guaranteed by Article 9 of the European Convention on Human Rights. The main limitation for the purposes of Article 9 is that the religion must have a clear structure and belief system. Denominations or sects within a religion can be considered to be a religion or belief, such as Protestants and Catholics within Christianity.

52. The criteria for determining what is a 'philosophical belief' are that it must be genuinely held; be a belief and not an opinion or viewpoint based on the present state of information available; be a belief as to a weighty and substantial aspect of human life and behaviour; attain a certain level of cogency, seriousness, cohesion and importance; and be worthy of respect in a democratic society, compatible with human dignity and not conflict with the fundamental rights of others. So, for example, any cult involved in illegal activities would not satisfy these criteria. The section provides that people who are of the same religion or belief share the protected characteristic of religion or belief. Depending on the context, this could mean people who, for example, share the characteristic of being Protestant or people who share the characteristic of being Christian.

53. This section replaces similar provisions in the Employment Equality (Religion or Belief) Regulations 2003 and the Equality Act 2006.

The Baha'i faith, Buddhism, Christianity, Hinduism, Islam, Jainism, Judaism, Rastafarianism, Sikhism and Zoroastrianism are all religions for the purposes of this provision.

Beliefs such as humanism and atheism would be beliefs for the purposes of this provision but adherence to a particular football team would not be.'

Race and the Mental Health Act 1983

The Care Quality Commission's (CQC's) first annual report *Monitoring the Use of the Mental Health Act in 2009/10* found that the proportion of Black and minority ethnic patients who were subject to Community Treatment Orders was larger than might be expected from census findings on the detained population liable to be placed on a CTO (i.e. those on unrestricted treatment detention orders). These groups are already frequently over-represented in the detained population so this is an especially disappointing finding.

A similar pattern emerges when looking at consent to treatment issues among detained patients. In a breakdown of the ethnicity of patients who, after three months' treatment, remained incapacitated by their illness, or refused consent for further treatment, the proportion of this detained group who were from Black and minority ethnic groups was higher than in the general detained population.

The CQC recommends that further research on the possible race equality impact of CTOs is carried out. Some will be disappointed that the CQC's own important research into ethnicity issues in the form of the 'Count Me In' studies has come to an end. It is hoped that the requirements of the Equality Act will lead to better information gathering by public authorities.

Conclusion

There is a history of concern over the relationship between race and the use of compulsion under the Mental Health Act. After the death, in a medium secure facility, of David 'Rocky' Bennett in 1998 there were several initiatives from the Department of Health to address race issues in mental health. These problems clearly interact with wider social factors and at the moment it is hard to see signs of significant progress in this area.

References

Gostin, L., McHale, J., Fennell, P. et al. (2010) *Principles of Mental Health Law and Policy*: Oxford. Oxford University Press.

Care Quality Commission (2010) *Monitoring the Use of the Mental Health Act in 2009/10*. CQC.

26 Suicidal patients

Suicide is defined in the Oxford English Dictionary as the 'intentional killing of oneself'. The practical and emotional consequences of this are felt by family and friends particularly but also colleagues, professionals and all who were closely involved with the deceased.

Epidemiology

Suicide is an important public health issue but whenever figures on suicide are presented or discussed there is always the question of their reliability since, in some instances, suicide as a reason for death can be hidden. Therefore, the real figures may be higher. The National Clinical Survey carried out by Professor Louis Appelby published in the *British Journal of Psychiatry* in 2006 as part of the National Confidential Inquiry into Suicide and Homicide by People with Mental Illness from 1996–2000 in England and Wales received notification of 20 927 deaths including 14 048 deaths with coroner's verdicts of suicide and 6 879 open verdict deaths from undetermined cause. Of these, 5 099 were confirmed to have been in contact with mental health services in the year prior to death. In order to get an idea of how significant suicide is as a cause of death, it is useful to compare these figures with other commonly perceived causes of death. Approximately 2 000 people die from asthma and a further 2 000 from cervical cancer over a similar period.

There has been a striking change in the world picture with regards to age. In some places, one can still find suicide rates between six and eight times higher among the elderly, as compared with young people but overall in the UK, currently more young people than elderly people are dying from suicide. Historically, older men used to have the highest suicide rate, but now this appears to have been eclipsed by younger men as the suicide rate in younger people is increasing at a greater pace than it is in the elderly. Suicide and accidents are the commonest cause of death in men under 35 years of age.

The suicide rate varies from country to country, and the rate also varies in different cultures and religions. The Baltic States appear to have the highest number of completed suicides worldwide, although this is also true of island countries such as Cuba, Japan, Mauritius and Sri Lanka. The lowest rates, as a whole, are found in the Eastern Mediterranean Region which comprises countries that follow Islamic traditions.

There is a constant predominance of male over female suicide rates with the exception of China where suicide rates in females are consistently higher than suicide rates in males, particularly in rural areas.

The social factors which appear to influence the successful completion of suicide include male sex, living alone, mental illness, unemployment, and homelessness.

Health issues such as depression, substance misuse and previous self harm and serious illnesses also appear to be important.

The incidence of completed suicides also seems to vary with different occupations. Some studies suggest that farmers, vets, pharmacists, doctors and social workers are at greater risk perhaps because of stress and access to lethal means of suicide.

The methods of suicide appear to depend upon the availability of an appropriate lethal method such as bridges over rivers, tall buildings, railway lines and self-poisoning with substances such as paracetamol. Hanging was very common in the group studied by the national patient survey, followed by jumping. Women tend to use less violent means compared with men, such as overdose of medication or attaching a hosepipe to a car exhaust pipe.

History of suicide attitudes and legislation

The morality of suicide has provoked many strong emotions over the centuries. Aristotle and Plato felt that it was 'an offence against all the gods of all the State'.

In common law, suicide was seen as a form of felonious homicide that offended both God and the king. It offended God because the person in question rushed into His presence when 'uncalled for' and offended the king because he 'hath interest in the preservation of all his subjects'. A person who completed suicide successfully had all his estate seized and the body was placed at the crossroads of two highways and a stake driven through it. In France, the body was hung, drawn and quartered. This attitude prevailed until 1823 when it was relaxed a little, but the body of a suicide could still not be buried in consecrated ground.

However, there have always been conflicting feelings about suicide. The Roman Stoics condoned suicide and felt that 'it was a lawful and rational exercise of individual freedom and even wise in the cases of old age'.

As it was difficult to prosecute people who had killed themselves and were dead, the law concentrated on prosecuting people who attempted suicide.

The Suicide Act 1961

Section 1 of the Suicide Act 1961 stated that to commit suicide was no longer to be considered a crime. The attitude of society in general had ameliorated before this legislation became law but suicide still retained a stigma of disgrace.

Section 2(1) states that anyone who aids, abets, counsels or procures the suicide of another, or an attempt by another to commit suicide, is liable upon conviction on indictment for a term not exceeding 14 years.

This clause created a new offence of complicity in suicide: there is nothing like it elsewhere in the law. It became a crime to assist with something that was not itself a crime. The effect of Section 2(1) is to protect the vulnerable, the terminally ill, the frail and elderly from manipulation, exploitation or coercion by anyone to end their life after suicide ceased to be a crime without financial sanctions.

This section has been considered, on occasions, after someone has required help to be transported to Switzerland where euthanasia is not allowed but no one has been prosecuted. In 2009, a multiple sclerosis sufferer successfully took her appeal to the Law Lords to demand legislative guidance as to whether her partner would be prosecuted under the Suicide Act 1961 quoting Article 8 of the Human Rights Act 1998. The Law Lords ruled that:

'Everyone has the right to respect for their private life and the way that Ms P determines to spend the closing moments of her life is part of the act of living. Ms P wishes to avoid an undignified and distressing end to her life. She is entitled that this too must be respected.'

Physician-assisted suicide

This occurs when a person is assisted by a doctor to commit suicide. It generally occurs in the setting of a painful terminal illness such as cancer or a degenerative neurological disease and it contravenes Section 2(1) of the Suicide Act 1961.

It is argued more and more that the law relating to doctor-assisted suicide should be changed and there is a lot of feeling that people should not be denied control over their own deaths.

There have been landmark cases testing this hypothesis in the western world such as *Rodriquez* v. *British Columbia (A-G)* (1993) *82 BCLR (2d) 273 (Can Sc)*, in which a patient suffering from amyotrophic lateral sclerosis wished to avoid choking to death. She wanted to have an intravenous line installed, which contained a substance that she could choose to use when she decided to end her life. Her appeal was dismissed.

A suffragette who had been force-fed sought damages against the Home Secretary. At that time, suicide was still an illegal act and the people attending her would have been guilty of a crime. The woman was not successful in her claim, and the verdict was qualified by a statement that it was a time of 'dramatic conflict'.

In the UK, 'Dignity in Dying' had sought for clarification in the law as to what factors are likely to influence prosecution of assisted suicide under the Suicide Act 1961. In February 2010, Keith Starmer QC stated:

'Following this clarification, and because of some important developments in care over recent decades, the case for a change in the law is now weaker ...'

The law – together with the values and standards of our caring professions – supports good care, including palliative care for the most difficult of conditions, and also protects the most vulnerable in our society.

For, let us be clear; death is an option and an entitlement, via whatever bureaucratic processes a change in the law might devise, would fundamentally change the way we think about mortality.'

He went on to add that there were no guarantees against prosecution. And he outlined the factors which would determine a prosecution:

- Whether a person stands to benefit financially from assisting at a suicide or if they were acting out of compassion.
- If the individual wanting to die was deemed competent enough and had a clear and settled wish to make such a decision. Particular attention would be paid to such issues as being under 18 and having a mental illness.
- Whether the person was persuaded or pressured into committing suicide, or if it was their own decision.

The then Prime Minister, Gordon Brown, pointed out in a letter in the *Daily Telegraph* that the case for a change in the law to liberalise assisted suicide was now weaker.

In Switzerland, where the law is different to the UK, euthanasia is illegal but assisted suicide is legally condoned and can be performed by non-physicians. This situation has given rise to conditions for the formation of the Dignitas clinic founded by Lugwig Minelli. The clinic charges a fee to provide accommodation for a person to commit suicide and 115 plus people from Britain have availed themselves of this service and no one who has assisted them to get there has been charged under the Suicide Act.

Palliative care

Palliative care is medical care of people who are terminally ill. It has in part of its philosophy the administration of drugs designed for pain control in dosages that are designed for pain control but may hasten the death of the patient.

The distinction between palliative care and assisted suicide or euthanasia is that the former is to ease pain and the latter is to cause death. The term 'double effect' has been used to describe medication being used for pain relief also speeding up death. In places where assisted suicide is legal such as Oregon, the Netherlands etc., there is a tendency to develop less palliative care.

Suicide prevention

Suicide prevention is a major public health challenge and there have been several research projects to look at suicide in the setting of mental health problems and also in other groups such as offenders.

One of these prevention agencies is the **National Confidential Inquiry into Suicide and Homicide by People with Mental Illness NCI/NCISH** and is funded largely by the National Patients Safety Agency (NPSA) and the Scottish Government, DHSS and Public Safety in Northern Ireland. It examines all incidences of suicide and homicide by people in contact with mental health services in the UK. It also examines cases of sudden death in psychiatric in-patient populations.

Research with Offenders (RwO) examines the incidence of suicide in current and recently released prisoners in England and Wales.

The **Manchester Self-Harm (MaSH)** project is an audit and research project established at the University of Manchester in April 1997.

The **National Patient Safety Agency** announced in May 2010 plans to reduce levels of harm in 10 areas. One of these is suicide prevention within Health in the Community. It says that 95 per cent of all suicides take place in the community and that 74 per cent are not in touch with mental health services in the previous 12 months. It aims:

- to raise awareness of suicide prevention programmes. It aims and intends to lead to changes in behaviour and practice that involve leadership and multidisciplinary working in the prevention of suicide;
- to maintain the suicide prevention working group and introduce representation from primary and secondary care networks for sharing and learning and multidisciplinary working;
- to involve service-users, carers, families as a key partner in all elements of the suicide prevention programme.

There is also the National Clinical Survey published in 2006 which aimed to describe social and clinical characteristics of a comprehensive sample of in-patients and post-discharge patients with mental health problems.

A four-year national clinical survey (1996–2000) sampled cases of suicide in England and Wales who had been in contact with mental health services (*n*=4859).

The results showed that nearly one quarter of in-patient deaths occurred in the first seven days of admission and the majority were caused by hanging. Post-discharge, suicide was most frequent in the first two weeks of life in the community after leaving hospital and the highest number occurred on a Friday.

National Service Framework for Mental Health

This is a minimum set of standards for promoting mental health and care for all. There are similar standards for diabetes and paediatrics. Standard 7 – Preventing Suicide looks at the epidemiology of suicide and then focuses on service models and good practice, with emphasis on care management and operational issues.

Conclusion

Suicide is a complex issue that gives rise to strong feelings and causes acute distress. It is influenced by religious and cultural aspects of life, and there are large variations from country to country. It is not necessarily a consequence of mental ill health. Society has a strong sense of preservation of life and tries to reduce the number of people killing themselves, but there have always been a significant number of people for whom suicide is very seductive.

Reference

Appleby, L (2006) The National Clinical Survey on Rates of Mental Disorder in People Convicted of Homocide. *British Journal of Psychiatry*. **188**: 143–7.

27 Assessment of risk of violence

Violence has multifactorial causes and is a biopsychosocial, environmental, political phenomenon. Clearly, all behaviour has a biochemical basis, but while biochemical abnormalities can cause psychological symptoms, including aggression, there is also increasing evidence that psychological events, for example, severe abuse in childhood or severe psychological trauma in adulthood, may cause neurobiological abnormalities, e.g. in serotonin (5-hydroxytryptamine, 5-HT) metabolism in adults. Models of violence are shown in Table 27.1. No model can adequately explain all violence, and some models are more appropriate than others for different situations.

Table 27.1 Models of and factors in violence

Biological factors	
	Fight or flight response
	Males and young people more violent
	Testosterone levels
	Reduced serotonin levels in brain
Alcohol, drugs	
	50 % of violent offences follow alcohol abuse in the UK
	Disinhibition
Psychological models	
Instrumental aggression	Learn to achieve ends by violence
Cognitive model	Look at world aggressively
Behavioural model	Inconsistent, erratic parental punishment
Social learning	Peer pressure/modelling
Status	Status of being violent
Psychodynamic models	
Freudian	Primary drive due to frustration; later primary drive libido and aggression secondary drive
Kleinian	Annihilation anxiety
Kohut	Secondary to developmental insults or deprivations
Object relation school (Winnicott)	Creative of another
Attachment theory	An insecurely attached infant, e.g. deprived or abused, later relates to others with hostility
Family factors	
	Physical abuse as child
	Parental discord and violence
	Parental irritability, usually due to depression
Social models	
	Subcultural norm, e.g. Hell's Angels, pub brawls
	Sporting, political and industrial violence
	Relative poverty and inequality
	Comparative anthropology, e.g. Margaret Mead's studies
Environmental factors	
	Avoidance of frustration by well-structured and staffed milieu and non-provocative regime

Aggression

Aggression, using the biological definition, is intraspecific fighting. Normal aggression is seen in all members of a species, while pathological aggression or violence is either excessive in degree and/or arises from mental disorder. Almost all forms of mental disorder can be associated with pathological aggression and violence (Table 27.2), although anyone can become violent. There has been debate about whether aggression is instinct, that is, determined genetically but called out by the environment, or learned. Probably there is a normal inborn assertiveness, with aggression being secondary to early developmental deprivation and insults and/or mental disorder, rather than a primary drive. Aggression often follows frustration and threat, for example, to a low self-esteem, and increasing tension. Aggression may, of course, be displaced from the original object on to a symbolic representation of it, for example, arson, or to another person, e.g. anger towards the person's mother displaced on to women in general. Aggression can also be a social phenomena, for example, in altruistic aggression and war.

Table 27.2 Violence and psychiatric disorder

Non-psychiatric causes	
	Criminal, e.g. drug-dealing
	Cultural, e.g. subcultures
Psychiatric causes	
	Violence or threats of violence in 40 % pre-admission
	Schizophrenia – paranoid and non-paranoid
	Mania, hypomania, also depression
	Alcohol abuse/withdrawal
	Drug abuse/withdrawal, e.g. hallucinogens, PCP, benzodiazepine withdrawal
	Organic mental disorder and brain damage, epilepsy (especially TLE), dementia
	Personality disorder, particularly antisocial, impulsive and borderline
	Learning disability
	Child and adolescent behaviour disorder
	Dissociative states
Intrafamilial	
	Spousal abuse
	Child abuse
	Elder abuse

PCP, phencyclidine; TLE, temporal lobe epilepsy.

Violence, dangerousness and risk

Violence is action; dangerousness is a potential and a matter of opinion. The term 'risk' is now used in professional practice in preference to the term 'dangerousness'. Risk is, ideally, a matter of statistical fact. It emphasises a continuum of levels of risk, varying not only with the individual but also with the context, i.e. it is multidimensional. It may change over time and with circumstances and, in principle, should be based on objective assessment. Dangerousness tends to imply an all-or-nothing phenomenon and a static intrinsic characteristic of an individual. However, clearly risk assessment is less important than risk management, although risk management does not imply risk elimination.

Risk assessed as low, medium, high or very high is often arbitrary. The meaning of risk can include:

- *Likelihood of offending:* risk measures are often over periods of up to 20 years.

- *Imminence of offending:* risk instruments say little about this. It can sometimes be associated with substance abuse and an acute breakdown in a relationship.
- *Frequency of offending:* sadistic murderers rarely kill again.
- *Consequences of offending:* exhibitionists are at high-risk but have low consequences.

For instance, what does an 80 per cent chance of offending mean? Is it eight out of ten individuals like this person will offend, or, given the same circumstances, that this person will offend eight out of ten times? Is 80 per cent merely a measure of subjective belief?

Background to risk assessment

Risk assessment developed from observations on released prisoners, empirical associations with reconviction and its extension to forensic psychiatric patients. In England, the Ritchie report of the inquiry into the care and treatment of Christopher Clunis (Ritchie et al., 1994), who 'avoidably' killed Jonathan Zito, identified failures in risk assessment and risk management and inadequacies in communication and service provision. Christopher Clunis was given 20 different clinical diagnoses, was placed in about 20 different accommodations, and was seen by about 35 different professionals in the period before the offence. This report led to increased emphasis on risk assessment.

In response to increasing public concern that something needed to be done to improve the management of people, albeit few in number, who are deemed at serious risk to others, for example, predatory paedophiles, legislation has been introduced to improve the risk management of such individuals. This includes the Sex Offenders Act 1997, the Crime Sentences Act 1997, the Criminal Justice and Court Services Act 2000 and Multi-Agency Public Protection Panels (MAPPAs) in 2001.

Ethics of risk assessment

Ethical issues in risk assessment include whether it can be done adequately and, if so, whether it should be undertaken if no treatment is available, whereupon it may merely result in an increase in the length of a custodial sentence. There can be a conflict between, on the one hand, the ethical principle of autonomy of individuals and the associated assumption of their safety and, on the other, the duty of care of professionals and the rights and safety of others. Further questions include whether it should be undertaken on every psychiatric patient or at least every forensic psychiatric patient seen. Risk assessment can be stigmatising, but one should also be cognisant of the negative consequences, including emotional, for an individual who behaves dangerously. For psychiatry, key issues are what the risk is and whether it can be modified. However, evaluating whether residual risk is acceptable may also be a multidisciplinary, political, or multi-agency matter, for example, involving the probation service, MAPPA, the Ministry of Justice in cases of Sections 41 or 49 restricted patients, First Tier Tribunals (Mental Health), potential victims and society in general.

Violence and mental illness

For most of the last 20 years, there has been no evidence of increasing rates of homicide by mentally ill people in the UK (Bennett 1996), in spite of this being the media and public's perception, which probably reflects only increasing awareness.

Such homicides by mentally ill people have a negligible effect on public safety compared with other factors, such as road-traffic accidents. In the past, factors associated with violence were said to be the same, regardless of whether the offender was mentally ill, for example, personality disorder, impulsivity, anger, violent family background and substance abuse. However, since 1992, studies have shown that having a diagnosis of mental illness is associated weakly with violence due to a subgroup with specific types of symptoms, such as paranoid (persecutory) delusions (false beliefs) and delusions of passivity (being under external control). It is thus certain symptoms, and not a particular psychiatric diagnosis alone, that are associated with violence. Nevertheless, the risk of violence is still better predicted by being a young male than by having a diagnosis of schizophrenia (Swanson et al., 1990).

Psychiatrists are better than chance or laypeople in predicting violence and better still at assessing situations where there is no risk. However, they tend to underestimate the risk of violence in females (Lidz et al., 1993). Professionals also underestimate the high background base rates of violence in the community in general, for example, up to 40 per cent of males may have been seriously violent by the age of 32 years (Farrington, 1995). The majority of violence never results in criminal charges. This also applies to in-patients who are violent, where formal charges may often be seen as serving little purpose if the patient is to remain in hospital.

Among individuals with mental illness, affective disorders are underrepresented in forensic psychiatric facilities. Violence is, however, increased in people with schizophrenia, especially those who have drifted out of treatment, and in young males with acute schizophrenia compared with those with chronic schizophrenia. Violence may arise directly from positive psychotic symptoms of mental illness, such as delusions (false beliefs) and hallucinations (for example, voices). Mental illness, especially schizophrenia, may, however, lead indirectly to violence through associated deterioration in social functioning and personality, so that such individuals become more antisocial, impulsive and unpredictable and develop a lower tolerance to stress. This sometimes leads to disputes in court about the disposal of such individuals with few or no positive psychotic symptoms, with such individuals sometimes being given, wrongly, an additional diagnosis of personality disorder to explain their violence. A mentally ill individual may also behave violently for 'normal' emotional reasons, such as fear and anger, and then experience accompanying corresponding positive psychotic symptoms, for example, hallucinations of aggressive content. Violence, law involvement and imprisonment may themselves precipitate mental illness. Violent offenders in general have often committed non-violent offences. However, some non-violent offenders may only commit violent offences when mentally ill.

For a mentally ill person, a key issue is whether the individual has a delusion of a content on which he or she might act dangerously, for example, of persecution or infidelity, but even then not all morbidly jealous individuals, for instance, assault their spouse. Twenty per cent of people presenting to hospital with their first episode of schizophrenia have threatened the lives of others, but among these half have already been ill for a year (Humphreys et al., 1992). Overall, however, it is unusual for a person with schizophrenia to present for the first time with serious violence. One established period of higher risk is within a few months of discharge from hospital (Taylor, 1993). People with both schizophrenia and substance abuse have higher rates of violence than those with substance abuse alone, who, in turn, have higher rates than those with schizophrenia alone (Swanson et al., 1990).

In countries with high homicide rates, such as the USA, this is usually due to high numbers of non-mentally ill offenders, their violence being related to criminal activities, drug dealing and cultural and economic factors, and there is a corresponding lower proportion of mentally ill homicide offenders. Rates of mentally ill homicide offenders may be fairly constant across countries.

Research has generally, but not universally, shown a consistent association between violence and delusions, particularly of threat/control override (TCO) content, for example, persecutory delusions, passivity delusions and thought insertion (Link and Stueve, 1994) which doubles the risk, although most with such TCO symptoms will not be violent. These findings are in keeping with the social psychology theory that violence in general is associated with an individual feeling under threat or losing control of his or her situation.

Based particularly on the work of Steadman and Monahan's group (for example, the subsequent publication of Steadman et al., 1998) in the USA (the McArthur Foundation Violence Risk Assessment Study), the Royal College of Psychiatrists in 1996, in their booklet *Assessment and Clinical Management of Risk of Harm to Other People*, detailed 'warning signs' that professionals should be aware of; these were:

- beliefs of persecution, or control by external forces
- previous violence or suicide attempts
- social restlessness
- poor compliance with medication or treatment
- substance abuse
- hostility, suspiciousness and anger
- threats.

Steadman and colleagues (2000) have developed a computer algorithm of largely actuarial factors for risk assessment of violence (not homicide) (the Monahan/Steadman iterative classification tree).

Psychiatric patients tend to peak for violent offending at a later age than the general population. It is important to be aware that the oft-quoted 'best predictor of future behaviour is past behaviour' (after Kvaraceus, 1954) is based on non-psychiatric populations and, in any case, accounts for only five per cent of the variance. A history of previous violence is, of course, required for this to be relevant in any case. Among severely psychotic mentally ill people, delusions of threat/control override, for example, respectively delusions of paranoid content or passivity, are better predictors than past behaviour, though clearly even for the mentally ill, if present circumstances match past circumstances when the individual behaved violently, this would clearly be very relevant, for example conditions when the individual's mental illness was not controlled.

Among all individuals, including mentally ill people, a history of expressed threats (as opposed to generalised anger), substance misuse and a history of personal deprivation and/or abuse are all associated with violence. Law-breaking behaviour in general and violence in particular usually decrease when the basic needs of an individual are met. This is reflected in the current greatly reduced rate of homicide in England and Wales (around 30 times less) compared to Victorian times. For instance, an individual with schizophrenia who is violent often has a characteristic history of not only non-compliance with medication, leading to relapse of his or her mental illness, but also of being in a situation of social isolation and poor home conditions. Some individuals may even offend to remove themselves from their situation in the community to the security of prison or hospital. The risk of self-harm or suicide is greater for people with schizophrenia, even if they have behaved seriously violently, than homicide or serious harm to others. Compulsory admission under the Mental Health Act for reasons of a patient's health is clearly better than at a later time for the protection of others as a last resort after someone has been hurt.

In summary, the existing evidence suggests that there is a link between mental illness and violence. Mental illness is a risk factor, but not a great one, and the risk is increased by substance abuse.

Risk assessment

This can be only a probability assessment. Dangerous behaviour is rare and sporadic, so most of our worries about individuals never materialise. This can lull professionals into a false sense of security and to underestimate the risk. Risk assessment can be difficult, e.g. predicting how an individual in conditions of security will behave outside such conditions with the availability of alcohol and illicit drugs and potential victims, or predicting intrafamilial violence among those with personality disorder.

When undertaking a risk assessment, it is necessary to look at factors not only in the individual but also in his or her victims or potential victims and the environment, including the security of interview rooms and procedures for assessing an individual in the community, that is, an offence is a function of the offender, the victim and the environment.

Dangerousness is often associated with repetition, failure to respond to the counter-measures of society, unpredictability and untreatability. Truly dangerous people are, by definition, unpredictable. People labelled at risk of serious harm to others include those previously convicted of dangerous offences, those who use firearms and other weapons and, by definition, people subject to restrictions under Section 41 of the Mental Health Act 1983 in England and Wales and those in special hospitals. A legal offence category may not reflect the current risk. Short-term prediction is better than long-term prediction; the risk of serious harm itself is often long-term and not obvious on short-term follow-up. False-positive assessments of risk are made more often than false-negative assessments. Prediction, for example, of an absence of risk of violence, may be accurate, but does not preclude an otherwise negative outcome, for example, fire-raising. Professionals tend to err on the side of caution, but they may be reluctant to take on individuals considered at serious risk of harming others due to negative counter-transference feelings, for example, related to shock at past offences, or from fear of being held professionally responsible for the individual's actions and feeling overwhelmed by this. This, in turn, can lead to overestimating risks and inappropriate precipitate actions to cover oneself and displace responsibility on to others. The courts, however, expect professionals to give an opinion on dangerousness. On occasions, professionals inappropriately attempt to 'rescue' dangerous untreatable individuals who they feel have been managed badly by others. Professionals must guard against overidentifying with the subject, denying what they do not wish to hear and not acting on threats and behaviour giving rise to concern, especially among those in the community who, if they had been in-patients and behaved in such a fashion, would cause great concern. Professionals must ask directly what thoughts, fantasies, impulses and/or plans to be violent an individual has, for example, of homicide, in a similar manner to the way in which they would question directly in a suicide assessment.

Risk factors include dispositional factors, such as demographic and historical factors, including past violence, constitutional factors, stress and lack of social support, and clinical factors, including diagnoses, symptoms and substance abuse. A summary of variables often sought in risk assessment includes the following:

- Demographic factors, e.g. previous violence, age, sex. Such variables can be documented easily. Among mentally ill people, age under 35 years and male predominance are less predictive. Risk in females is underrated (Lidz et al. 1993). The relationship of violence to when the person is mentally unwell is of importance.
- Environmental factors: these are harder to document and include family support, poor social network, lack of intimate relationships, unemployment, poverty, homelessness, and availability of weapons.
- Substance abuse: alcohol and cannabis abuse are most common.
- Current context: recent major life events, e.g. of loss.
- Dispositional factors, e.g. impulsivity, irritability, suspiciousness.
- Interests, e.g. cruelty, fantasies, weapons.
- Social functioning.
- Attitudes, e.g. to violence and previous and future victims.
- Poor engagement and compliance with services.
- Mental state, e.g. feelings, emotions, thinking, perceptions, behaviour. Violence is associated with fear, anger, humiliation and jealousy. Note should be made of tension, depression, paranoid ideas, delusions, hallucinations, including command hallucinations, clouding of consciousness and confusion, and anger and threats. Data on command hallucinations are equivocal but more positive for threat/control override delusional symptoms (Link and Stueve 1994), e.g. paranoid delusions and delusions of passivity.

Table 27.3 shows the factors to be considered in a risk assessment with special reference to an offender. Table 27.4 summarises those factors.

Table 27.3 Risk assessment

The aim is to get an understanding of the risk from a detailed historical longitudinal overview, obtaining information not only from the patient, who may minimise his or her past history, but also from informants. Ideally, it should not be a one-off single interview assessment.

1	Reconstruct in detail what happened at the time of the offence or behaviour causing concern. Independent information from statements of victims or witnesses or police records should be obtained where available. Do not rely on what the offender tells you or the legal offence category, e.g. arson may be of a wastepaper bin in a busy ward or with an intent to kill. Possession of an offensive weapon may have been a prelude to homicide. Offence = Offender × Victim × Circumstances/Environment (i) Offender: • alone or in group, e.g. gang (less inhibition in groups); • planned or impulsive (beware rationalisation of behaviour post-offence); • triggers, e.g. behavioural, emotional, physiological or situational; • provoked; • displaced aggression, e.g. mother kills baby to spite father; • recent discontinuation of medication; • disruption of therapeutic alliance, e.g. professional holidays; • during other criminal behaviour or deliberate self-harm. • Mental state at time of offence: link specific symptoms, e.g. delusions, or emotional state, e.g. overarousal, anxiety, fear, irritability, anger or suspiciousness, or disinhibition, to violence.

- Degree and quality of violence: overall more violent, more risk. Bizarre violence seen in mental illness and severe psychopathic disorder. Is there satisfaction from inflicting pain? The more precarious the psychological defences, the more violence. More often not predictive of repetition, but reflects relationship with victim, e.g. resistance of victim to dying and arousal of offender. Paradoxically, less violence in general if victim fights back, except in rape and sexual assaults, where violence may increase.
- Alcohol/drugs facilitating or precipitating aggression.
- Use or possession of weapons, i.e. carrying means of destruction, if only for self-protection, e.g. knife, if loses temper.

(ii) Victim:
- Victim may be consciously or unconsciously provocative, e.g. if drunk, due to their own background, or if not aware of effect of own behaviour on offender.
- Is violence against a particular named individual for specific reason e.g. relative, therapist, or victim blamed in homosexual panic, against a particular type of victim, or against staff with whom in clinical contact or of an institution, or against the world in general?
- Is victim merely an object of displaced aggression to others, e.g. from mother, society?
- Is victim the real intended victim? If not, risk of repetition.

(iii) Circumstances/environment:
- Current stresses, particularly recent loss or threat of loss.
- Circumstances, e.g. both offender and victim intoxicated in a public house.
- Precipitating factors in social environment. Now removed? Can they be modified?
- Culture: inhibiting or sensitising? Varies over time.

(iv) Type of offence behaviour:

Was offence behaviour without warning or could it have been predicted? What caused it to cease?

Some behaviours are predictive of future dangerousness, including:
- morbid jealousy;
- sadistic murder;
- sexual offender overwhelmed with aggression;
- at least two offences of serious violence or sexual assault.

---

2 Behaviour after offence:
- did the offender summon help for victim?
- freezing;
- regression: associated with future dangerousness;
- manner of talking about the offence, e.g. dispassionate, guilt-free manner or capacity for sympathetic identification. Any 'unfinished business'?
- admission of guilt and transparency;
- beware of protective psychological defence mechanisms, e.g. after homicide, leading to appearance of callous indifference.

---

3 Progress in custody and/or hospital:
- capacity for self-control or explosiveness;
- no relationships;
- feelings of professionals, especially females, in cases of psychopaths and sex offenders;
- reaction of other inmates/patients;
- do his or her pets survive?

---

4 At interview (ideally, interview and mental state examination should take place on more than one occasion and should be repeated over time):
- threats of violence (verbal anger is a poor predictor of violence);
- expressed intent;
- feeling of fear in interviewer;
- impulsive: cannot delay gratification;
- paucity of feeling for victim/indifference;
- over- or undercontrolled;
- depression;

- morbid jealousy;
- content of delusions, hallucinations etc., e.g. threat/control override, i.e. of paranoid or passivity content;
- insight into mental disorder and offending: is violence regarded as unacceptable?
- attempting to self-control? Help requested?

---

5 Assessment of personality traits:

- informants and historical information important, especially when offender mentally ill;
- impulsive, antisocial, lack of guilt, affectionless;
- deceptive/lying (e.g. due to learned strategy to deal with overdominant or aggressive parents) compared with transparent;
- inadequate personalities overall commit more serious offences than aggressive psychopaths;
- jealous/paranoid: does he or she feel continually threatened?
- poor self-image, low self-esteem;
- over-/undercontrolled;
- features of Brittain's sadistic murderer syndrome (Work in positions of power over people and animals, e.g. a butcher, interests in Naziism, torture and weapons; collectors and with room contents of weapons, Nazi gear) ;
- how does he or she handle stress, e.g. if by violence, is this egosyntonic or egodystonic?
- formal psychometric testing of personality and intelligence may assist.

---

6 Life history:

Age: younger more dangerous than older (dangerousness generally decreases with age, except for sadists and offences of retaliation against women).

Sex: male more than female, except in psychiatric hospitals, where rates are similar.

Family history: deprived, neglect, physical and/or sexual parental abuse, alcoholic father, domineering mother, parental discord and violence.

Childhood: classic dangerous triad of enuresis, cruelty to animals and fire setting, although only cruelty to animals proven to be predictive of future violence. Conduct disorder. A bully or bullied.

Employment: butchering, work in abattoir or for veterinary surgery, e.g. animals die in their care. Inability to sustain employment, e.g. due to problems of impulsivity or with authority or routine.

Sexual history: if sexual offence and no previous relationships with women, assume attacks will go on. Previous victimisation. Sadistic or violent sexual thoughts, fantasies, impulses or behaviour.

Social restlessness: for example, frequent change of address or employment. Few relationships. Among groups where increased violence, e.g. homelessness.

Previous medical history: head injury, brain damage (even minimal), temporal lobe epilepsy, extra Y chromosome. Abnormalities of electroencephalogram (EEG) or brain scans.

Substance abuse history.

Previous psychiatric history: diagnosis of psychopathy. Alcoholism or drug dependency. Low intelligence level. Previous suicidal behaviour, especially if impulsive and/or violent and/or associated with risk to others.

Relationship of offending to mental illness and its control by medication, etc.

Compliance with treatment, especially medication.

Attitudes to treatment.

Previous forensic history:

- violent/non-violent;
- worse if early-onset, persistent and serious;
- ask how close to violence he or she comes and his or her most violent act in the past;
- when is violence most likely to happen? Learn from 'near-misses';
- any evidence of escalation?

Current support systems.

Table 27.4 Risk factors for violence

Demographic factors	
	• Male
	• Young age
	• Socially disadvantaged neighbourhoods
	• Lack of social support
	• Employment problems
	• Criminal peer group
Background history	
	• Childhood maltreatment
	• History of violence
	• First violent at young age
	• History of childhood conduct disorder
	• History of non-violent criminality
Clinical history	
	• Psychopathy
	• Substance abuse
	• Personality disorder
	• Schizophrenia
	• Executive dysfunction
	• Non-compliance with treatment
Psychological and psychosocial factors	
	• Anger
	• Impulsivity
	• Suspiciousness
	• Morbid jealousy
	• Criminal/violent attitudes
	• Command hallucinations
	• Lack of insight
Current 'context'	
	• Threats of violence
	• Interpersonal discord/instability
	• Availability of weapons

Reference: National Mental Health Risk Management Programme (2007). Best Practice in Managing Risk. DoH: London. Appendix 2

Risk may change rapidly over time. If risk is identified, then it must be managed and the management plans documented. However, concern may arise before a non-cooperative patient is detainable under the Mental Health Act. Interventions may also increase the risk temporarily, for example, following detention in hospital or enforced medication treatment. Whatever is done may not remove the entire risk. There is also the question of how many false positives of those deemed at risk are acceptable compared, for instance, with the price of one homicide. Serious harm often follows a sequence of decisions by professionals rather than one major error of judgement. There is also not much relationship between in-patient and out-patient violence.

Clinical or practical risk assessment

Risk assessment requires information gathering, including by a full history from the subject, examination of past records and/or statements when available in Crown Court criminal cases, and from informants, including arresting police officers. Risk assessment should ideally be a continuous process rather than based on a single interview, during which an individual may be reluctant to discuss emotive issues or otherwise not willing to be transparent due to mental state abnormalities such as over-sensitivity. As a minimum, a risk assessment and management plan should include the following:

- Ask informants about history of violence.
- Request previous summaries, e.g. of in-patient care, and past psychiatric and probation reports.
- Document the above, and keep and use proper records.
- Make plans to manage the risk, and document this.
- Be particularly cautious in cases where treatment is refused, is reduced or is being withheld.

Clinical risk assessment, however, lacks an evidence base, is unstructured, is usually biased by a few factors, is subject to subjective bias, sometimes is based on the last case seen that went wrong, shows poor consistency, is difficult to quantify, and is inductive, i.e. based on previous cases. There is no evidence that countertransference is predictive.

Standardised structured risk assessment instruments

Increasingly, clinical or practical risk assessment, involving consideration of the history, mental state and environment, is being supplemented by standardised actuarial and/or dynamic risk assessment instruments, the former alone often being considered insufficient. However, standardised structured risk-assessment instruments may add little to a good clinical risk assessment by an experienced professional. Thus, risk assessment = clinical assessment + standardised instrument assessment.

Structured risk assessments can be used merely as aide-memoires and reference points rather than being scored numerically. The lack of standardised assessments has been cited as a factor in the excess of females and people of Afro-Caribbean origin in special hospitals.

Structured risk assessments are more useful at high levels of risk but are not very useful in predicting isolated dangerous acts such as homicide. They are more useful in cases of those with personality disorders rather than with psychoses and are also useful in predicting sex offending. Reliability is better with static rather than dynamic variables and hence such instruments are less helpful in deciding on discharge. Some structured assessments may, however, record risk factors that are otherwise explainable clinically, e.g. lack of emotional expression may result from antipsychotic medication treatment. There also appears to be a glass ceiling to prediction of risk which cannot be improved beyond 0.7, whether using single or even multiple such structured risk assessments.

Actuarial or standardised risk assessment instruments

Actuarial risk assessment instruments tend to measure static factors. Examples include the Violence Risk Appraisal Guide (VRAG) (Harris et al., 1993; Quinsey et al., 1998) and, for sex offenders, from the work of Hanson and Thornton (1999, 2000), Static 99 and the Risk Matrix 2000. Police use the Risk Matrix 2000 as a screen for cases referred to MAPPAs. Risk factors in this latter instrument include being male, younger age groups, and number of times in court for violent or sexual offences. The risk identified, however, is over a prolonged period. Actuarial risk assessment instruments are objective, unbiased and deductive. While good at identifying low-risk, they tend to overjudge high-risk cases. Problems with actuarial risk assessment instruments include the facts that first-time offenders score low, they are poor predictors of young and female offenders, they are blind to current circumstances, for example, a paedophile married to a female with children, and they provide a lifetime rather than an immediate assessment of risk.

Dynamic risk assessment instruments

Dynamic risk assessment instruments look not only at dynamic factors but frequently also actuarial factors. Structured (professional judgement) clinical assessments of risk have the advantages of actuarial risk assessments and also of an unstructured clinical assessment that can emphasise risk factors specific to an individual.

The **Historical–Clinical–Risk-Management 20-Item instrument (HCR-20)** (Webster et al., 1977) includes ten historical (H) factors, five present clinical (C) factors and five risk-management (R) factors. These are listed in Table 27.5. It thus covers both dynamic and actuarial risk factors. Those with high H scores, which reflects base risk, are more likely to be, or perhaps should be, under forensic psychiatric services. This instrument can be used as an enquiry guide and prompt rather than as a numerical rating scale. Clinical (C) factors reflect current risk and are best to concentrate on if time precludes completing the full twenty items. In some countries, its use is becoming mandatory for particular groups of serious offenders.

Table 27.5 The 20 Items of the HCR-20 (Webster et al, 1997)

Historical items	
	H1: Previous violence
	H2: Young age at first violent incident
	H3: Relationship instability
	H4: Employment problems
	H5: Substance abuse problems
	H6: Major mental illness
	H7: Psychopathy
	H8: Early maladjustment
	H9: Personality disorder
	H10: Prior supervision failure
Clinical items	
	C1: Lack of insight
	C2: Negative attitudes
	C3: Active symptoms of major mental illness
	C4: Impulsivity
	C5: Unresponsive to treatment
Risk management items	
	R1: Plans lack feasibility
	R2: Exposure to destabilisers
	R3: Lack of personal support
	R4: Non-compliance with remediation attempts
	R5: Stress

NB: The best validity is for items H2, 5, 8, 10; C2, 4; and R2 and 4

Apart from assisting in a formulation of risk, a second stage in using HCR-20 is the development of feared risk scenarios and their management. This approach originated from military planning exercises ('War Games'). Factors that increase risk are identified, as are protective factors. Interventions and their priority are developed to manage the risk.

However, such scenario planning lacks established validity compared to the scoring of the twenty items. Increased levels of psychopathy also reduce the HCR-20 predictiveness.

Hare's Psychopathy Checklist – Revised (PCL-R) (Hare 1991) has two main components: (i) emotional/interpersonal traits (Factor 1), such as callousness, selfishness, and lack of remorse, and manipulative use of others, which are mainly static traits, and (ii) social deviance (Factor 2), i.e. chronically unstable and antisocial lifestyle, which has some dynamic elements and may vary between countries. It involves a structured interview and an expert rating form. It is for use in people aged 18 years or older. Items are scored on a three-point scale. Scores range from zero to 40. Only one-third of people with antisocial personality disorder reach the scale's criteria for psychopathy (i.e. score over 30). Some argue that such tools are superior to clinical risk assessment in people with personality disorder, while the reverse may be the case for people who are mentally ill. Candidates for dangerous severe personality disorder (DSPD) units in prisons and special hospitals are defined as having more than a 50 per cent risk of committing a serious offence due to a severe personality disorder, and the PCL-R is usually used pre-admission, including to establish this risk.

The PCL-R has been supplemented by a 12-item screening version (PCL-SV) (Hart et al., 1995). Scores on this range from zero to 24 (cut-off 18) and have been found to have good predictive validity for violence (Monahan et al., 2000).

The most recent revision to the PCL-R is the PCL-R™ second edition (Hare 2003). This has a 20-item symptom–construct rating scale with a Quickscore Form to record and profile results. It subdivides both Factors 1 and 2 into two valid subscales. Factor 1 has been divided into Factor 1a Interpersonal (four items) and Factor 1b Affective (four items); Factor 2 is divided into Factor 2a Impulsive Lifestyle (five items) and Factor 2b Antisocial Behaviour (five items).

The Violence Risk Scale (VRS) was developed by Wong and Gordon (2000). This has been found to be particularly useful in the assessment of violent but also sex offenders, and it can measure change. It includes six static variables, including age and age at first conviction, and 20 dynamic variables, including violent lifestyle, criminal personality, mental disorder, substance misuse, community relationships, community supervision, release to a high-risk situation and anger and violence.

Other dynamic risk-assessment instruments include the Sexual Violence Risk (SVR-20) Scale (Boer et al., 1997), the Spousal Assault Risk Assessment Guide (SARA) (Kropp et al., 1995) and the Sex Offender Risk Appraisal Guide (SORAG) (Quinsey et al., 1995, 1998), a variation on the VRAG. The Structured Risk Assessment (SRA) framework developed by Hanson and Thornton (2000) for sex offenders now uses both the Risk Matrix 2000, based on static actuarial factors, and dynamic risk factors.

A summary of risk assessment tools is shown in Table 27.6

Table 27.6 Risk assessment tools

1. Risk assessment of violence	
(a) Structured clinical	HCR-20 (Historic-clinical-risk management 20 item instrument): 20 fields combining static and dynamic risk factors. Supports development of risk management plan Violence Risk Scale (VRS): strong dynamic element. Supports measurement of change and formulation of treatment plans Offender Assessment System (OASys): Used by UK National Offender Management Service, e.g. Probation officers Risk Assessment Guidance Framework (RAGF) Risk Assessment, Management and Audit Systems (RAMAS) Short-Term Assessment of Risk and Treatability (START): Seven risk-related domains. Informs decision-making regarding risk to self as well as to others
(b) Actuarial	Violence Risk Appraisal Guide (VRAG) Offender Group Reconviction Scale (OGRS): Used by National Offender Management Service Risk of Reconviction (ROR) Score Reconviction Prediction Score (RPS)
2. Psychopathic checklist: PCL-R and PCL-SV	
	Measures presence and level of psychopathy. Proven predictor of risk. Short-version (SV) can be used in non-forensic populations
3. Risk matrix 2000 (Previously Structured Anchored Clinical Judgement (SACJ))	
	Actuarial. Categorises sexual and violent offenders from low to very high risk
4. Spousal Assault Risk Assessment (SARA)	
	Structured clinical assessment of spousal abuse
5. Sexual offending	
(a) Structured clinical	• Structured Assessment of Risk and Need (SARN): Dynamic tool for working with sex offenders. Useful in developing treatment plans and measuring change • Risk of Sexual Violence Protocol (RSV) (previously SVR-20)
(b) Actuarial	• Static 99: Actuarial tool for measuring risk in sex offenders • Sex Offending Risk Appraisal Guide (SORAG) • Rapid Risk Assessment of Sex Offender (RRSOR) • Sex Offender Need Assessment Rating (SONAR)

Actuarial variables should not override clinical variables, as the latter are more likely to determine when and how a person may behave dangerously. Specific individual risk factors may be of more importance than those listed in a tick box checklist. Uncertainty in risk assessment is due to the many variables involved, randomness, and the effects of human interaction and intervention. Dynamic variables are, by definition, subject to change and may be subject to interaction with other factors, such as other people, which actuarial risk assessments are generally less helpful in predicting. Risk assessment is comparable to weather forecasting, which may be accurate in the short-term and also, broadly, in the longer term, e.g. winter compared with summer, but not specific enough to indicate where it might rain in a few days' time. Structured risk assessments may provide evidence for institutionalising a person, but they are less useful in getting a person out of an institution. Indeed, even in secure psychiatric units, increased length of stays may have more to do with the persistence of positive psychotic symptoms than reflect actual current risk.

Other problems in risk assessment include the following:

- The low base rate problem. For example, a rate of less than one per cent for serious violence makes it difficult to predict such a rare event.
- Risk valuation following risk assessment estimation. For example, what action is warranted by a particular risk of violence? What is an acceptable false-positive rate, e.g. for detaining patients?
- The quality of a professional's relationship with a patient determines the accuracy of a risk assessment, but admission to secure forensic psychiatric facilities often depends on bed availability. In addition, mental state examination may be of little use in assessing risk of sex offending.
- Assessment scales have not always been developed in the populations to which they are applied, for example, scales developed for non-psychiatric prison populations are used for psychiatric cases.

Risk assessment allows for a longitudinal formulation of the individual, assessment of whether any risk is associated with particular victims, family members or the public in general, and whether it is unconditional or conditional on particular factors, and assessment of whether these factors are amenable to change. Conditional risk factors can include mental state deterioration, non-compliance, disengagement from supervision and treatment, substance abuse and life events, especially of loss, for example, of relationships, accommodation, financial and employment. The aim should be to produce a person-specific biography of the individual, allowing the individual to tell his or her own story, and then to negotiate a plan of action with the individual and other parties. Risk assessment for violence has many parallels with suicide risk assessment.

Risk management

Once a risk assessment is made, it is essential to develop and document a risk management plan. This is not dependent on any mental disorder present being treatable. Other risk factors may still be manageable, for example, substance misuse. In the community, careful supervision by well-briefed professionals is required. It is important not to ignore threats and to avoid provoking violence by appearing to precipitously reject requests for help. For an individual who has offended dangerously, a restriction order, such as a Mental Health Act 1983 Section 41 Restriction Order in England and Wales, may need to be recommended to a Crown Court judge, for the judge to add this to a hospital order, such as a Section 37 Hospital Order in England and Wales, to 'protect the public from serious harm' and to facilitate long-term psychiatric management, including in the community, particularly with regard to compliance with treatment there, but also by specifying a suitable place of residence. Special hospital placement, for example, in Broadmoor Hospital in England, may be required if an individual suffers from a mental disorder and is a 'grave and immediate danger' to others, especially if the person is also at risk of determined absconding and cannot be managed in lesser conditions of security. A medium secure unit may be indicated if a mentally disordered individual needs conditions of security that are less than those of a special hospital but are more than those of an ordinary locked intensive or low secure unit.

Avoidable deaths: The National Confidential Inquiry into Suicide and Homicide by People with Mental Illness, University of Manchester, England

This Inquiry for England and Wales was set up in 1996 to collect detailed clinical information on homicides and suicides by individuals in contact with mental health services. About nine per cent of mentally abnormal homicide offenders (about 50 per year) were in such contact.

The typical perpetrator of stranger homicides in England and Wales remains a young male who has been drinking alcohol or abusing drugs.

People with schizophrenia are responsible for about 30 out of the 50 patient homicides each year. Half are current or recent patients, but one-third had no previous contact with services.

People with personality disorder and a history of current or previous contact with psychiatric services are responsible for about ten cases per year.

Rates of mental disorder found in all perpetrators of homicide are as follows:

- Lifetime mental disorder: 30 per cent
- Lifetime history of schizophrenia: 5 per cent
- Contact with mental health services: 18 per cent
- Contact within past twelve months: 9 per cent
- Mental illness at time of offence: 10 per cent
- Convicted of manslaughter on grounds of diminished responsibility (Section 2 Homicide Act 1957): 4 per cent
- Hospital order: 6 per cent

The Inquiry has indicated that about 14 per cent of homicides (7 per year) can be considered 'most preventable' due to service failures, for example, lack of adequate supervision or poor compliance.

The resulting recommendations have included the following:

- *Insure high-risk patients receive enhanced care planning, backed by peer review:* lack of this was considered the cause of 53 per cent of the most preventable homicides.
- *Respond robustly when a care plan breaks down:* Lack of response was considered to have caused 18 per cent of the most preventable homicides. Twenty-five per cent of patient homicides were preceded by non-compliance.
- *Develop services for dual diagnosis patients:* 36 per cent of homicide cases had dual diagnoses, i.e. mental disorder and substance abuse. Drug induced psychosis can be just as dangerous as a functional psychosis such as schizophrenia.

Inquiries into homicides by psychiatric patients

These are mandatory and have emphasised failures in care due to poor communication between professionals and agencies, downgrading of previous violence, failure to recognise and manage social restlessness and escalating

problems, lack of contact of subjects with consultant psychiatrists, rigid catchment area practice, lack of resources, e.g. lack of acute beds and trained staff, failure to use the Mental Health Act appropriately to detain for reasons of health before violence, and lack of carer involvement, although the latter may raise issues of patient confidentiality. Non-compliance with treatment in the community has been the most common major factor characterising these cases. However, there can, of course, be no real 'supervision' in the community in the sense of continual observation. Overall, such inquiries have highlighted not the limitations of risk assessment, as real as these are, but failure to communicate or manage a known risk. Improving community psychiatric care may thus be more useful in reducing the risk of violence than attempts at perfecting risk assessment instruments. Certainly, the use of standardised structured risk assessment instruments would not alone prevent most homicides by psychiatric patients.

Government responses to inquiry findings

The political pressure of 'something must be done' has led to the following in England and Wales:

- Care Programme Approach (CPA) (Department of Health 1990).
- Supervision Registers (NHS Management Executive 1994a).
- Guidance on discharge of mentally disordered people (NHS Management Executive 1994b).
- Mental Health (Patients in the Community) Act 1995 (supervised discharge order).
- Mental Health Act 2007. This amended the Mental Health Act 1983 and placed more emphasis on risk assessment and management as key to detention, including by the introduction of a broader single definition of mental disorder, the removal of some exclusion criteria for mental disorder, such as sexual deviancy, and the introduction of Community Treatment Orders.

The usefulness of the above measures remains open to question. The CPA is a process rather than a treatment; individuals may be unable or unwilling to comply, and families may or may not wish to be involved. On the positive side, the CPA is a needs-led multidisciplinary approach to developing a care plan, which has to be monitored and should always include a risk assessment. Drawbacks to the CPA include lack of resources, large caseloads, increase in time required for meetings and documentation, and it leading to defensive practice.

These government responses also occured against a background of a general decline in psychiatric hospital beds, for example, from 152 000 in 1954 to 53 700 in 1993. Those psychiatric patients who have been violent in the community, however, tend not to be those who might previously have been on long-stay wards. However, if 100 long-term hospital beds are closed, then there is an additional need for about ten new acute beds to cope with resulting revolving door admissions, and this can lead to a lack of acute beds for the emergency admission of violent patients. Increasing the number of hospital beds alone is not the whole solution, as there is also a need for other measures, such as short-term crisis community facilities. While inquiries emphasise the need for direct face-to-face contact between professionals and patients, an average inner-city caseload for a social worker is 20 and for a consultant psychiatrist up to 450–500, with 300 new patients a year. However, CPA arrangements technically are required for all patients, and a legal duty of care applies to any patient to whom a professional talks. Funding has also been unrelated to epidemiology, for example, in urban areas, where there is an excess of schizophrenia due to social drift, and where drug abuse and a younger population are also more evident. There has otherwise been increased identification of cases, including via court and prison diversion schemes. One response by clinicians in England and Wales has been to increase the rates of detention under the Mental Health Act 1983, which has been most pronounced for Section 3 and for mental illness. While there has been no significant change in the number of Section 37 Hospital Orders, there has been an increase in Section 41 Restriction Orders. Another response has been the development of assertive outreach programmes.

Proactive measures to manage violence include adequate training of community mental health teams and the development of protocols for potential violent scenarios in hospital and in the community, for example, for home visits. Risk assessment should also lead to the identification of warning signs indicating early signs of relapse or increased risk. The importance of communication between a general practitioner (GP), hospital and social services, housing, police and probation is paramount. Clearly, the better a patient is known, the more likely the accuracy of the risk assessment. If in doubt about the safety of continued community care of an individual prone to violence, admission should be considered.

The Royal College of Psychiatrists (1998) has produced clinical practice guidelines for the management of imminent violence. These cover ward design and organisation, the need for adequate space, comfort and privacy, the anticipation and prevention of violence, including by fostering open communication with patients, anticipating risk and avoiding confrontation in a crisis, and training for staff to recognise warning signs of violence and to self-monitor verbal and non-verbal behaviour, and the appropriate use of medication. However, the guidelines acknowledge the lack of funding available for training, the shortage of qualified staff, and the levels of stress currently reported among those who work in the mental health field and deal with violence.

Conclusion

Aim to determine how serious the risk for a given individual is, that is, what are the nature and the magnitude of the risk? Is it specific or general, conditional or unconditional, immediate, long-term or volatile? Have the person's or the situation's risk factors changed? Who might be at risk?

From such a risk assessment, a risk-management plan should be developed to modify the risk factors and specify response triggers. This should, ideally, be agreed with the individual. Is there a need for more frequent follow-up appointments, an urgent CAP meeting or admission to hospital, detention under the Mental Health Act, physical security, increased observation and/or medication? If the optimum plan cannot be undertaken, then reasons for this should be documented and a back-up plan specified.

Risk assessments and risk-management plans should be communicated to others on a 'need-to-know' basis. On occasions, patient confidentiality will have to be breached if there is an immediate grave danger to others. The police can often do little, unless there has been a specific threat to an individual or an offence, whereupon they may warn or charge the subject. Law involvement rarely produces a long-term solution where there have been threats of violence or minor violent offences, as these rarely result in long prison sentences. Very careful consideration needs to be given before informing potential victims to this themselves to avoid their unnecessary anxiety. Their safety is often best ensured by management of those who present the risk. If a potential victim needs to be informed, the police prefer to do this themselves.

References

Bennett, D (1996). Homicide, inquiries and scapegoating. *Psychiatric Bulletin* **20**, 298–300.

Boer, DP, Hart, SD, Kropp, PR, Webster, CD (1997). *Manual for the Sexual Violence Risk. Vol. 20: Professional Guidelines for Assessing Risk of Sexual Violence*. Vancouver: British Columbia Institute on Family Violence.

Department of Health (1990). *Health Circular: HC (90)23/LASSL(90)11 (The Care Programme Approach)*. London: HMSO.

Farrington, DP (1995). The Twelfth Jack Tizard Memorial Lecture: the development of offending and antisocial behaviour from childhood: Key findings from the Cambridge Study in Delinquent Development. *Journal of Child Psychology and Psychiatry and Allied Disciplines* **36**, 929–64.

Hanson, RK, Thornton, D (1999). *Static 99: Improving Actuarial Risk Assessments for Sex Offenders. User Report 99-02*. Ottawa: Department of the Solicitor General of Canada.

Hanson, RK, Thornton, D (2000). Improving risk assessments for sex offenders: a comparison of three actuarial scales. *Law and Human Behaviour* **24**, 119–36.

Hare, RD (1991). *Manual for the Hare Psychopathy Checklist: Revised*. Toronto: Multi-Health Systems.

Hare, RD (2003). *Manual for the Hare Psychopathy Checklist: Revised (PCL-R™)*, 2nd edn. Toronto: Multi-Health Systems.

Harris, GT, Rice, ME, Quinsey, VL (1993). Violent recidivism of mentally disordered offenders: the development of a statistical prediction instrument. *Criminal Justice and Behaviour* **20**, 315–335.

Hart, SD, Cox, DN, Hare, RD (1995). *The Hare Psychopathy Checklist: Revised Screening Version (PCL-SV)*. Toronto: Multi-Health Systems.

Humphreys, MS, Martin, S, Johnstone, EC, Macmillan, JF, Taylor, P (1992). Dangerous behaviour preceding first admission for schizophrenia. *British Journal of Psychiatry* **161**, 501–5.

Kropp, PR, Hart, SD, Webster, CW, Eaves, D (1995). *Manual for the Spousal Assault Risk Assessment Guide*, 2nd edn. Vancouver: British Columbia Institute on Family Violence.

Kvaraceus, WC (1954) *The Community and the Delinquent*. World Book: Yonkers-on-Hudson.

Lidz, CW, Mulvey, EP, Gardner, W (1993). The accuracy of predictions of violence to others. *Journal of the American Medical Association* **269**, 1007–11.

Link, BG, Stueve, A (1994). Psychotic symptoms and violent/illegal behaviour of mental patients compared to community controls. In: Monahan, J, Steadman,

J (eds). *Violence in Mental Disorder: Developments in Risk Assessment.* Chicago: University of Chicago Press.

Monaham, J, Steadman, HJ, Applebaum, PS, et al. (2000). Developing a clinically useful actuarial tool for assessing violence risk. *British Journal of Psychiatry* **176**, 312–20.

NHS Management Executive (1994a). *Introduction of Supervision Registers for Mentally Ill People from 1 April 1994: Health Service Guidelines HSG, (94)5.* London: Department of Health.

NHS Management Executive (1994b) *Guidance on the Discharge of Mentally Disordered People and Their Continuing Care in the Community: Health Service Guidelines HSG, (94) 27.* London: Department of Health.

Quinsey, VL, Rice, ME, Harris, GT (1995). Actuarial prediction of sexual recidivism. *Journal of Interpersonal Violence* **10**, 85–105.

Quinsey, VL, Harris, GT, Rice, ME, Cormier, CA (1998). *Violent Offenders: Appraising and Managing Risk.* Washington, DC: American Psychological Association.

Ritchie, J, Dick, D, Lingham, R (1994). *Report of the Inquiry into the Care and Treatment of Christopher Clunis.* London: HMSO.

Royal College of Psychiatrists Special Working Party on Clinical Assessment and Management of Risk (1996). *Assessment and Clinical Management of Risk of Harm to Other People. Council Report CR53.* London: Royal College of Psychiatrists.

Royal College of Psychiatrists (1998). *Management of Imminent Violence. Clinical Practice Guidelines: Quick Reference Guide.* London: Royal College of Psychiatrists.

Steadman, HJ, Mulvey, EP, Monahan, J, Robbins, PC, Appelbaum, PS, Grisso T, et al. (1998). Violence by people discharged from acute psychiatric inpatient facilities and others in the same neighbourhoods. *Archives of General Psychiatry* **55**, 393–401.

Steadman, HJ, Silver, E, Monahan, J, Appelbaum, PS, Robbins, PC, Mulvey EP, et al. (2000). Classification tree approach to the development of actuarial violence risk assessment tools. *Law and Human Behaviour* **24**, 83–100.

Swanson, JW, Holzer, CE, 3rd, Ganju, VK, Jono, RT (1990). Violence and psychiatric disorder in the community: evidence from epidemiologic catchment area survey. *Hospital and Community Psychiatry* **41**, 761–70.

Taylor, PJ (1993). Schizophrenia and crime: distinctive patterns in association. In Hodgins, S. (ed.). *Crime and Mental Disorder.* Beverly Hills, CA: Sage, pp. 63–85.

Taylor, PJ, Gunn, J (1999). Homicides by people with mental illness: myth and reality. *British Journal of Psychiatry* **174**, 9–14.

Webster, CD, Douglas, KS, Eaves, D, Hart, SD (1997). *HCR-20: Assessing Risk for Violence, Version 2.* Vancouver: Simon Fraser University Mental Health, Law and Policy Institute.

Wong, S, Gordon, A (2000). *Violence Risk Scale (VRS).* Saskatchewan: Department of Psychology and Research. Regional Psychiatric Centre: Solicitor General of Canada.

28 International comparison of mental health legislation

Comparison of legislation in the UK and Ireland

Table 28.1 compares civil detention under mental health legislation in the UK and the Republic of Ireland.

Table 28.1 Comparison of civil detention under mental health legislation in the UK and the Republic of Ireland

	Legislation	Not in hospital	In-patient
England and Wales	Mental Health Act 1983	Section 2 or 3 should be used rather than Section 4	Section 5(2) immediately or Sections 2 or 3
Scotland	Mental Health (Scotland) Act 1984	Section 24	Section 25(1)
	Mental Health (Care and Treatment) (Scotland) Act 2003	Part 5, if arranging Part 6 would involve undesirable delay (Requires approved doctor)	Part 5, if arranging Part 6 would involve undesirable delay (Requires approved doctor)
Northern Ireland	Mental Health (Northern Ireland) Order 1986	a. 4	a. 7(2) may be detained under a. 4
Republic of Ireland	Mental Treatment Act 1945	Section 184	Section 184
	Mental Health Act 2001	Sections 9 and 10	Section 2

Table 28.2 compares the legal provisions for mentally disordered offenders in the UK and the Republic of Ireland.

Table 28.2 Comparison of legal provisions for mentally disordered offenders in the UK and the Republic of Ireland

	England & Wales	Scotland	Northern Ireland	Republic of Ireland
	Mental Health Act 1983	**Mental Health (Care and Treatment) (Scotland) Act 2003**	**Mental Health (Northern Ireland) Order 1986**	**Mental Health Act 2003**
Police				
Detention of mentally disordered person found in public place	Section 136	Section 297	a130	Section 12
Detention of mentally disordered person in private premises	Section 135	Section 293	a129	Section 12
Pre-trial				
		Criminal Procedure (Scotland) Act 1995		
Remand to hospital for treatment	Section 35	Section 52B–J	a42	–
Remand to hospital for assessment	Section 36	Section 52K–S	a43	–
Transfer of untried prisoner to hospital	Section 48	Section 52K-S	a54	–
Trial				
Criteria for fitness to plead	*R* v. *Prichard* 1836 Test of decision-making capacity	*HMA* v. *Wilson* *Stewart* v. *HMA* (1942)	*R* v. *Prichard*	*R* v. *Prichard*
Procedure relating to a finding of unfitness to plead	Sections 2–3 and sch 1–2 CP(IUP) A1991	Sections 54–57 CP(S) A 1995	a49 and 50A	Lunacy (Ireland) Act 1821, Juries Act 1976
Criteria for insanity at the time of the offence	McNaughten Rules 1843	*HMA* v. *Kidd* (1960)	CJ(NI)A 1966	*Doyle* v. *Wicklow County Council 1974*
Procedure relating to a finding of insanity at the time of the offence	Sections 1&3 sch 1–2 CP(IUP)A 1991	Sections 54 and 57	a50 and 50A CJ(NI)O 1996	Trial of Lunatics Act 1883
Criteria for diminished responsibility	Section 2 Homicide Act 1957 as amended by Coroners and Justice Act 2004	*Galbraith* v. *HMA* (2001) Culpable Homocide	CJ(NI)O 1996	–
Post-conviction but pre-sentence	**Mental Health Act 1983**	**Criminal Procedures (Scotland) Act 1995**	**Mental Health (Northern Ireland) Order 1986**	**Mental Health Act 2003**
Remand to hospital for assessment	Section 35	Section 52B–J Section 200	a42	–
Remand to hospital for treatment	Section 36	Section 52K–S	a43	–
Interim hospital/ compulsion order	Section 38	Section 53	–	–
Transfer of untried prisoner to hospital	Section 48	Section 52B–J Section 52K–S	a54	Previous legislation applies
Sentence				
Compulsory treatment in hospital under MHA	Section 37	Section 57A	a44	–
Restriction order	Section 41	Section 59	a47	–
Hybrid order (hospital disposal with prison sentence)	Section 45A	Section 59A	–	–

	England & Wales	Scotland	Northern Ireland	Republic of Ireland
Compulsory treatment in community under MHA	–	Section 57A	–	–
Guardianship	Section 37	Section 58(1A)	a44	–
Intervention order for incapable adult	–	Section 60B	–	–
Psychiatric probation order	sch 2 (p5) Powers of Criminal Courts (Sentencing) Act 2000	Section 230	sch 1 (p4) CJ(NI)O 1996	–
Post-sentence				
		Mental Health (Care and Treatment) (Scotland) Act 2003		–
Transfer of sentenced prisoners to hospital	Section 47	Section 136	a53	Previous legislation applies
Restriction direction for transferred prisoner	Section 49	All	a55	–

Mental Health (Scotland) Act 2003

Section 328 defines mental disorder as any mental illness, personality disorder or learning disability. Sexual orientation, sexual deviancy, transsexualism, transvestism and dependency on or use of alcohol or drugs is excluded from this definition. Under the Act, provisions exist for an RMO, an Approved Medical Practitioner (AMP) (Section 22), a Mental Health Officer (MHO) (in practice a social worker), designated Medical Practitioners (DMPs), the Mental Welfare Commission and Mental Health Tribunals. All patients have a right to advocacy (Section 259). Advanced statements are possible under Sections 275 and 276.

Part 5 of the Act details emergency detention orders, Part 6 details short-term admission orders and Part 7 community treatment orders for hospital or community.

Mental Health Act (Northern Ireland) Order 1986

Mental illness is defined in the Act as a state of mind that affects a person's thinking, perceiving, emotion or judgement, to the extent that they require care or medical treatment in their own interests or in the interests of other people. Medical treatment is defined as including nursing and also care and treatment under medical supervision.

There are definitions in the Act for mental handicap, severe mental handicap and severe mental impairment. To be placed in the severe mental handicap category, there must be associated 'abnormally aggressive or seriously irresponsible conduct'.

It is stated that no person should be treated as having a mental disorder by reason of only a personality disorder, promiscuity or other immoral conduct, sexual deviancy or dependence on alcohol and drugs.

Part II of the Order allows compulsory admission for assessment for up to 14 days before being admitted for treatment. For the purposes of application for detention in Northern Ireland, the nearest relative can be someone living in the Republic of Ireland or the UK. Temporary holding powers are available for voluntary patients already in hospital, as with the English and Scottish Acts. These holding powers are for 6 hours by a professionally registered charge nurse and 48 hours by a doctor on the staff of a hospital concerned, which also includes a general hospital.

If the patient is not well enough to become a voluntary patient or to be discharged before the end of the 14-day assessment period, they may in the first instance be detained for up to 6 months if they are diagnosed as having mental illness or severe mental impairment and they remain at high risk of serious physical harm to themselves or others. The period of detention is renewable for a further 6 months and then annually, subject to approval, following an examination by a doctor from another hospital appointed by the Mental Health Commission.

Provisions for consent to treatment and guardianship are similar to those set out in the English Act.

Provisions exist similar to those in the 1983 English Act for individuals involved in criminal proceedings; for example, the courts have the power to remand for examination or treatment, and interim hospital orders are also available. Hospital orders may be made regardless of the apparent availability of places, unlike in the rest of the UK, and a court may also impose a restriction order on the patient's discharge. In all hospital order cases, psychiatrists are expected to give oral evidence in the court.

Individuals detained for 2 years are automatically referred to an MHRT.

The Mental Health Commission, unlike the English equivalent, covers voluntary patients, people in guardianship and people in residential accommodation or, indeed, anybody with a mental disorder. Where it upholds complaints, it has the power to hold a formal inquiry in order to establish the facts.

At any one time, Northern Ireland has fewer than ten patients in Britain's mainland maximum security hospitals, mainly Ashworth Hospital in Liverpool, England. Northern Ireland has no maximum-security hospital itself.

NB: *Therapeutic abortion* is allowed in Northern Ireland only where there is undoubted grave risk to the continuing physical or mental health of the pregnant woman. This leads to women crossing from Northern Ireland to the British mainland each year to have abortions.

Mental health legislation in the Republic of Ireland

The Central Mental Hospital Dundrum, which opened in 1850, is the only maximum security hospital in the country. Section 39 of the Mental Treatment Act 1961 refers to this hospital. It accepts many prison transfers (remand and sentenced) and also the majority of people found 'guilty but insane' and people judged 'unfit to plead'.

The Mental Treatment Act 1945 remained the main mental health legislation in Eire until 2001.

Mental Health Act 2001

This was to replace the Mental Treatment Act 1945 and other Acts passed in 1953, 1961 and 1981. However, its implementation has been gradual. Section 4 details the principles underlying the Act, including the best interests of the person but with due regard to the interests of others who may be at serious harm.

Definition of mental disorder

Section 3 defines mental disorder as 'mental illness, severe dementia or significant intellectual impairment'. Compulsory detention should be as a result of (i) mental disorder causing immediate and serious harm to the patient or to other people; or (ii) because of the severity of the mental disorder, the judgement of the person is so impaired that, if the patient is not admitted to an approved centre, it would lead to a serious deterioration; or (iii) because detention in an approved centre is likely to benefit or alleviate the condition.

Mental illness means a state of mind affecting thinking, perceiving, emotion or judgement. Significant intellectual disability means a state of arrested or incomplete development of mind, including significant impairment of intelligence and social functioning and abnormally aggressive or seriously irresponsible conduct.

Other official terms

Approved centres include in-patient facilities, hospitals and other facilities registered with the Mental Health Commission (MHC). There are review tribunals and an inspector of mental health services who is a consultant psychiatrist appointed by the MHC.

Important sections of the Mental Health Act 2001

These include the following:

- Application for involuntary admission (Section 9)
- Medical assessment (Section 10)
- Power of the Garda to detain and apply for involuntary admission (Section 12)
- Removal to an approved centre (Section 13)
- Admission to an approved centre (Sections 14 and 15).

Part IV of the Act concerns consent to treatment for patients subject to compulsion.

Guernsey

The current mental health law in Guernsey dates back to 1939 and has its roots in the 1890 Lunacy Act. Contrary to many people's belief, the Channel Isles are not part of the UK though they do form part of the British Islands. The Bailiwick of Guernsey covers Alderney and Sark as well as Guernsey and, after many years of reviewing its mental health law, is on the brink of new law which is expected to come into effect in 2012. It draws heavily on the Mental Health Act 1983 as is in force in England and Wales, but there are some significant differences. The patient will be able to nominate someone who will act as their nearest relative (a measure that many had pressed for unsuccessfully in England). The controversial Community Treatment Orders from the English model are included but with some differences in the law concerning compulsory medical treatment. Approved Social

Workers, Mental Health Tribunals, Consent to Treatment rules and various other safeguards will be introduced. However, there is no sign of any change in the law concerning mental capacity, so practitioners will still rely on customary law in many cases.

Jersey

Jersey law is separate from that in Guernsey. Currently the Mental Health (Jersey) Law 1969 applies. This has had a few amendments to reflect the requirements of the European Convention of Human Rights to which Jersey subscribes. The Human Rights Law came into effect in 2006 which, as with equivalent law in the UK, requires courts to construe law as far as possible in a way which is compatible with Convention rights; allows courts to make a Declaration of Incompatibility regarding principle legislation which may lead to a remedial order; and makes it unlawful for a public authority to act in a way which is incompatible with a Convention right.

The definition of mental disorder is 'mental illness, arrested or incomplete development of mind and any other disability or disorder of mind' and so equates well with the law in England and Wales. In practice, most applications for detention are made by officers whose role parallels that of the Approved Mental Health Professional in England and Wales.

There are discussions on possible law reform and it is possible that this might result in four separate new pieces of law covering: mental illness, learning disability, mentally disordered offenders and finally mental incapacity.

Isle of Man

The Isle of Man also has its own mental health legislation, which differs from that of England and Wales.

Mental health legislation in Canada

The courts are under provincial jurisdiction. The ten provinces and two territories also have a court of appeal. The highest court, the supreme court of Canada, is situated in Ottawa, the national capital. There is a criminal code that covers mentally abnormal offenders, but their management varies between provinces due to their respective mental health legislations. The criminal code does, however, allow a trial judge to remand an offender for psychiatric assessment under Section 543(2), and the court of appeal has similar provision under Section 608.2(1).

There are two maximum security hospitals in Canada, the Mental Health Centre at Penetanguishene, Ontario, and the Institut Philip Pinel in Montreal.

The maximum security hospital at the Oak Ridge Division of the Mental Health Centre at Penetanguishene has around 200 patients. The majority are warrants of the lieutenant governor patients, having been found not guilty by reason of insanity, or involuntary patients under the Ontario Mental Health Act. Patients who have been stabilised are referred to long term medium security units. When fit for rehabilitation in the community, such patients may be referred to local forensic services, such as the university based Clarke Institute of Psychiatry in Toronto.

The Metropolitan Toronto Forensic Service (METFORS) is well known for its provision of psychiatric services to the courts and prisons. METFORS has a brief assessment unit and otherwise undertakes standard forensic psychiatric pre-trial assessments and treatments. In Ottawa there is a well-developed clinic for the treatment of and research into sexual offenders, and it has a close relationship with the probation service.

With the provinces and territories having differing mental health legislation, definitions of mental disorder vary between them. The criteria for involuntary civil committal are wide in all the provinces, except Ontario, where objective evidence of potential dangerousness to self or others is required. Provinces other than Ontario have less stringent admission criteria regarding general health, welfare and safety. Most provinces require certification by two physicians before involuntary admission of a patient to a psychiatric facility. Periods of detention vary with the various mental health acts of the provinces. Most provinces have provision for police officers to take a person for a psychiatric examination and for judges to order that an individual charged with a criminal offence be examined, admitted and treated in a psychiatric facility.

Regarding consent to treatment, an incompetent involuntarily detained patient has the right to refuse all forms of psychiatric treatment in Nova Scotia and Ontario. If found incompetent, consent from the nearest relative is required; in the absence of the nearest relative, review board procedures exist to hear the case and issue treatment orders.

There is considerable variability in the roles and powers of the mental health tribunals of the various provinces and territories of Canada. People found not guilty by reason of insanity or found unfit to proceed with a trial and who are made subject to conditions of a warrant of the lieutenant governor of the province of Ontario are reviewed by an advisory board, appointed by the lieutenant governor in council on at least one occasion every 12 months.

There are provisions under sections of the Criminal Code of Canada to remand a mentally abnormal offender for a psychiatric assessment for fitness to proceed with trial, if that individual is mentally ill or the balance of the individual's mind is disturbed. The period of assessment is up to 30 days. If the person is deemed not fit to plead or stand trial, then a trial of fitness is ordered. If the person is found unfit, then the Court orders that the person be kept in custody until the pleasure of the lieutenant governor of the province is known. Similarly, if found not guilty by reason of insanity, the individual is also made subject to the terms of the lieutenant governor's warrant and kept in a place of custody. Custody is nearly always a psychiatric facility with either maximum or medium security.

If the offence committed is minor, then a probation order with a condition of psychiatric treatment may be ordered. Some correctional institutions have programmes for psychiatric treatment. If a prisoner becomes mentally ill while serving a sentence, there are provisions in the criminal code to transfer the patient to a psychiatric facility for treatment.

Mental health legislation in the USA

Most aspects of mental health law are delegated to the various states, so that they can enact legislation to suit local needs. Mental health legislation in the USA has been shaped by social and political forces and case law. The emphasis has always been on the least restrictive treatment. Involuntary psychiatric treatment has been considered in many ways out of keeping with the US constitution and philosophy of upholding the individual's rights of freedom, speech and behaviour.

In spite of the variation in mental health legislation from state to state in the USA, there have been certain common themes. In an important case in 1975 (*O'Connor* v. *Donaldson* (1975) Supreme Court), the Supreme Court ruled that states cannot constitutionally confine a person who is not dangerous and who can live on their own or with the help of others. Most states adopted the principle of seeking 'the least restrictive environment'. An example would be Missouri where the law was amended in 1978 to try to balance a person's rights with the ability to get services. There needed to be a physical threat or harm caused by the mental illness before a person could be detained. However, there are concerns over the numbers of untreated mentally ill people in the community. Other states have adopted a more rigorous approach to the idea of community treatment with financial benefits being linked with acceptance of medication and other treatment.

In the past 30 years, there has been a trend away from detention (certification) on grounds of need for treatment and towards increasing patients' rights and restricting involuntary treatment. This, together with a desire to reduce the number of in-patients and the cost of their care, has led to the general adoption as a criterion for detention of a standard of future or potential dangerousness to the patient or others, rather than grave disability, for reasons of health alone or the patient's need for treatment. Emergency hospitalisation can be initiated without prior judicial approval, but subsequent commitment needs to be ordered by a judge.

Involuntary patients have the right to refuse medication. Medication to control dangerous patients in an emergency has been sanctioned if the need to prevent violence outweighs the possibility of harm to the patient and all less restrictive alternatives have been ruled out. If the patient is not dangerous, then in many states the only way to enforce medication is to have the patient declared incompetent, whereupon treatment conditions can be made, often on the basis of what the patient would have decided were he or she competent to do so rather than what might be in the patient's best interests.

In keeping with the idea of the least restrictive treatment, orders allowing out-patient committal to psychiatric treatment have emerged in nearly all states. This assists the large number of patients who have been discharged from hospital in the USA and who are clearly incapable of coping with the outside world and meeting their own basic needs. Such community commitment orders have been legally challenged on the grounds that if an individual is well enough to live outside an institution, then it is hard to justify such a restriction of their constitutional liberty. American states are divided widely on this issue. Some have developed a new lower threshold for involuntary out-patient care.

The ruling in the case of *Tarasoff* v. *Regents of University of California* (a duty to warn in 1974 modified to a duty to protect in 1976) has led many American psychotherapists to acknowledge that patient confidentiality can be violated, in view of the court's assertion that 'protected privilege ends where community peril begins'.

Mental health legislation in Australia and New Zealand

Each of the six states of *Australia* and its territories has its own separate Mental Health Act and its own judicial system. Australian law is derived from, but is not identical to, the common law of England. Australian and UK mental health services and laws are, however, similar. Much Australian psychiatric care is privately based, with state provision concentrating on patients with severe (psychotic) mental illness. Mental health legislation in Australia has been under constant review over recent years, with new acts drafted and frequent amendments made to earlier Acts. The Mental Health Act 1986 of the State of Victoria included, for the first time, a Community Treatment Order. This Act, together with the Mental Health Act 1990 of New South Wales, had a significant influence on the development of legislation throughout Australia. Under the South Australia Mental Health Act 1993, it first became possible there to make Treatment Orders which allowed for compulsory treatment in the community. A Guardianship Board could make orders for set periods of up to one year. A Community Treatment Order required: that a person has a mental illness that is amenable to treatment; that a medical practitioner has authorised treatment which the person had refused or failed to undergo (or was likely to refuse or fail to accept); that the person should be given the treatment for the illness in the interests of his own health and safety or for the protection of others. Treatment could not include ECT. If a person did not comply with a Treatment Order, they could be conveyed to a treatment centre.

New Zealand has one Mental Health Act, which also has provisions for the compulsory treatment of patients in the community.

Singapore

Singapore is interesting in that it is an example of a country where doctors are given considerable powers to act for a significant period of time without reference to another body. This is still true despite the reforms that were included in the 2008 Mental Health (Care and Treatment) Act, which came into effect in 2010. A mentally disordered person is no longer someone of unsound mind who is incapable of managing him- or herself or his or her affairs, but who has a 'mental illness or any other disorder or disability of the mind' (Section 2).

This brings the law closer to current UK law and there is also a preference for informal admission rather than detention, contained in Section 6 which closely parallels Section 131 of the England and Wales Act. However, the absence of an applicant for civil detention leads to significant differences. The police or a doctor can initially require a patient to become an in-patient. An order for detention of a patient for up to 72 hours can then be made by a doctor in a psychiatric hospital. If another medical officer at the hospital sees the patient and signs an order, then the patient can be detained for up to one month. Within the month the person must be seen by two medical officers, who can sign an order of up to six months if 'it is necessary in the interests of the health or safety of the person or for the protection of other persons that the person should be so detained' (Section 10). Hospital visitors have specific powers and refer longer-term detained patients to magistrates, who can make further orders. Visitors also have a role in granting leave of absence and they can discharge patients.

Mental capacity law has also been reformed in Singapore. The Mental Capacity Act 2008 is very similar to the Mental Capacity Act 2005 that operates in England and Wales.

One major exception is with regard to advance decisions. There is a separate Advanced Medical Directives Act 1996 which covers terminal illnesses and excludes people with mental disorders. The dilemmas highlighted in England and Wales with patients who complete an advance decision to refuse life sustaining treatment and then take a potentially fatal overdose, would therefore be handled very differently in Singapore.

The other major difference from the English and Welsh Act is that there is no Deprivation of Liberty Safeguards, as there is obviously no impact of Article 5 of the European Convention on Human rights. However, an intriguing effect of the strong links with the 2005 Act is that many of the principles of the ECHR have been incorporated within Singapore law. This is because the English and Welsh Act applies to everyone making decisions in relation to those who lack capacity to make specific decisions. This will include people who are not public authorities and the Singapore Act deals with this in a number of instances by building in requirements that otherwise would have been found in the ECHR. The principles (Section 3 in the Singapore Act) are identical to those in the English Act. Section 4(3) also parallels the English Act when it states:

'A lack of capacity cannot be established merely by reference to:

(a) a person's age or appearance; or
(b) a condition of his, or an aspect of his behaviour, which might lead others to make unjustified assumptions about his capacity.'

Singapore is at the centre of a movement to develop an ASEAN Human Rights Convention in South East Asia and it will be intriguing to see how this affects mental health and mental capacity law.

China

At the time of writing, China still has no formal mental health act, but plans are now in place to develop a National Mental Health Law.

Appendices

- Appendix I Legal cases 248
- Appendix II Summary of civil treatment codes 263
- Appendix III Summary of civil compulsion sections 265
- Appendix IV Flowchart of decisions involving consent to treatment 266
- Appendix V Sample forms 267

Appendix I

Legal cases

RELEVANT MENTAL HEALTH CASES

(summarised by Paul Barber, Solicitor and Former Partner Bevan Brittan, Solicitors)

(a) *Winterwerp* v. *Netherlands* (1979) 2 EHHR 387
Deprivation of liberty under Article 5(1)(e) of the Convention in relation to a person of unsound mind must *inter alia* be 'lawful'. This case set down minimum criteria for this to be established:

1. There must be objective medical expertise establishing a true mental disorder, save in an emergency.
2. The mental disorder must be of a kind or degree which justifies detention.
3. To justify continued detention there must be a persistence of the mental disorder.

True mental disorder is to be distinguished from behaviour which merely deviates from society's norms. This may have implications for use of the compulsory powers to detain e.g. a paedophile.

It remains an open question whether Approved Clinicians who are not doctors will be held to have the necessary 'medical expertise' upon which lawfully to base the use of the compulsory powers in the MHA, in particular the renewal of a patient's detention under Section 20.

(b) *Gillick* v. *West Norfolk and Wisbech AHA* (1986) AC 112
The question that arose in this case was whether a child under the age of 16 can give a valid consent to medical treatment – in other words without the permission of someone with parental authority. The Court decided that she could if she had sufficient maturity to be able to understand the nature and effects of the proposed treatment.

While there may be little difference in practice between the test for inability to make a decision under the Mental Capacity Act Section 3 and the test of 'Gillick competence' it must be remembered that unlike for a 16/17 year old (or older) there is no presumption of capacity for someone under the age of 16.

In ***Re W (a minor)*** ((1992) 4 All ER 627) the Court of Appeal drew a distinction between a child consenting to and a child refusing treatment. 'No minor of whatever age has power by refusing consent to treatment to override a consent to treatment by someone who has parental responsibility...and...by the court'. This decision does not just apply to those under the age of 16. However in the light of more recent case law (e.g. ***Storck* v. *Germany***) and concerns that to rely on parental consent to override a child's competent refusal in such circumstances might in the future be held to amount to a breach of the child's Convention rights, the Mental Health Act Code of Practice advises against such reliance; instead it advises that the MHA should be considered if appropriate and if the criteria are met, or alternatively an application made to the court.

Even if a child's competent refusal may in theory be overridden, the child's wishes should carry very great weight. There is no requirement on the part of a doctor to rely on parental consent, merely the legal right to do so in appropriate circumstances.

(c) ***B* v. *Barking Havering etc. NHS Trust*** (1999) 1 FLR 106
This case marks the beginning of the use of 'long leash' Section 17 leave. In other words, is it lawful to renew a patient's detention under Section 20 while he is largely continuing on Section 17 leave? Here, the Court held that provided the patient's treatment as a whole involved treatment as an inpatient in a hospital, the fact that the patient was on Section 17 leave at the time of renewal did not invalidate it. The Court did not specify how much time in hospital as an inpatient was required.

In ***R (DR)* v. *Mersey Care NHS Trust*** ((2002) EWHC 1810 (Admin)) the judge took matters further stating that there was no requirement for any of the treatment to be delivered as an inpatient. What mattered was treatment **at** a hospital not **in** a hospital. That treatment must however be an essential part of the patient's overall care plan i.e. the requirement to attend a hospital ensures compliance by the patient with the overall care plan.

This principle has been applied in the context of an application to a Tribunal – *see* ***R (CS)* v. *Mental Health Review Tribunal*** ((2004) EWHC 2958 (Admin)) in which a decision of the Tribunal not to discharge a patient was upheld in circumstances in which, in the closing stages of treatment in hospital, the RC's grasp on the patient was 'gossamer thin', being engaged in a delicate balancing act by which she was, with as light a touch as she could, encouraging progress to discharge. The patient during this time had very limited contact with the hospital, but it remained an essential ingredient of the care plan.

The manner in which the courts have successively extended the reach of Section 17 leave means that the distinction between leave and the use of a CTO is far from clear, not to say artificial.

(d) ***R* v. *MHRT for South Thames Region,* Ex Parte *Smith*** (1999) COD 148
This case somewhat surprisingly raised the issue whether the words 'nature or degree' in the Mental Health Act meant 'nature *or* degree' or 'nature *and* degree'. The Court held that the former was the case and that 'nature' refers to the particular mental disorder from which the patient suffers. 'Degree' refers to its current manifestation.

The symptoms or manifestations of a patient's disorder may be largely in abeyance, and yet continued detention in hospital warranted where the underlying nature of the disorder is serious enough that if he ceases to take medication his history shows he is likely to relapse.

See also ***CM* v. *Derbyshire Healthcare NHS Foundation Trust et al.*** (2011) UKUT 129 (AAC) which confirmed earlier case law (***R* v. *London South & South West Regional MHRT,* Ex Parte *Moyle*** (2000) Lloyd's Rep 143) that a relapsing mental disorder may justify detention on the basis of its nature but only if the risk is of relapse in the *near* future.

Taken together with the cases on long leash Section 17 leave dealt with under ***B* v. *Barking Havering etc NHS Trust*** ((1999) 1 FLR 106) the consequences are that patients may remain liable to be detained for longer and this raises issues in relation to possible breach of Article 5. This may progressively lead to use of CTOs whose safeguards for patients make them less arbitrary than Section 17 leave, although concerns have been expressed that patients may be being kept on CTOs for longer than necessary rather than being discharged.

(e) ***Aerts* v. *Belgium*** (2000) 29 EHRR 50
The issue in this case was where a person detained on grounds of mental disorder must be held. The Court decided that although the Convention does not carry an entitlement to specific treatment for mental disorder, persons detained on this ground must be held in a therapeutic environment. The psychiatric wing of a prison did not qualify as such. Note that although the conditions in which a person was held might fail to reach the level of severity required to amount to inhuman or degrading treatment under Article 3 of the Convention, there could be a breach of Article 5(1) if he was not held in a 'hospital, clinic or other appropriate institution authorised for that purpose'.

(f) ***Re D (Mental Patient: Habeas Corpus) (Nearest Relative)*** (2000) 2 FLR 848
The daughter of a patient who did not reside with him and had provided more than minimal care was consulted by an AMHP as the nearest relative. The patient's detention was challenged as being unlawful on the grounds that his elder brother, rather than his daughter was the nearest relative. The Court of Appeal held that:-

(i) the correct question was whether the patient's daughter appeared to the AMHP to be the nearest relative, not whether the AMHP consulted with the nearest relative;
(ii) the word 'ordinarily' in Section 26(4) qualified 'resides with', but not 'is cared for' in the same section; and
(iii) there was no duty of reasonable enquiry on the part of the AMHP as to who was the nearest relative.

Consequently, since the daughter had provided more than minimal care, but did not reside with the patient, the AMHP was not wrong to consider her as the nearest relative.

(g) ***Re F (A Child)*** (2000) 1 FLR 192
The Court of Appeal held that the definition of mental impairment associated with seriously irresponsible conduct in Section 1(2) of the Mental Health Act 1983 should be given a restrictive construction and in so holding, the Court allowed a father's appeal against the Guardianship Order in respect of his daughter. The Judge had originally held that F suffered from mental impairment and that her desire to return home from the specialist children's home, constituted 'seriously irresponsible conduct'. The importance of this case is that it emphasises the difficulty placed in the way of Local Authorities and others in utilising Guardianship Orders in cases which might otherwise be thought to be appropriate.

(h) ***Re F (Adult Patient: Jurisdiction)*** (2000) 3 WLR 1740
A different point concerning the same patient came before the Court of Appeal again in June 2000. F had now reached the age of 18 and the question arose whether the Local Authority could apply for declarations that it would continue both to require that she remain in local authority accommodation and to restrict access on the part of her family.

The Court decided that such declarations could be made, following the ***Bournewood*** decision (before it reached the European Court of Human Rights), on grounds of necessity which was not limited to medical and similar short-term emergencies, nor to the statutory guardianship or other provisions of the Mental Health Act. Nor did this breach Article 5 of the Convention because it was a procedure prescribed by law, as was the requirement, and would not be overridden by any regard for the right to family life of F's mother or other relatives under Article 8.

(i)*R* v. ***London South & South West Regional MHRT,*** Ex Parte ***Moyle*** (2000) Lloyd's Rep 143
The applicant was subject to a Hospital Order and applied for discharge. Medical evidence showed that drugs controlled his illness and his condition was not such as would make it appropriate for him to be detained, but that if he were to stop taking his medication he would quickly relapse. The Tribunal was not satisfied that:

(i) he would continue to take his medication if discharged; nor that
(ii) his illness was not of a nature which made it appropriate for him to be detained.

Accordingly they rejected his application.

The Court held that the criteria for discharge were meant to be matching or mirror images equivalent to the admission criteria. Whether a patient's illness made it appropriate for him to be detained depended upon an assessment of the probability that he might relapse. If a Tribunal was not satisfied that there was no probability of relapse in the near future it would be unlikely to be able to conclude that the criterion for continued detention had not been satisfied, because the nature, if not the degree, of his disorder would warrant it. The refusal to discharge was remitted back to the Tribunal. This is an extension into English law of the principles developed in the Scottish case of ***Reid*** v. ***SOS*** for Scotland. As a result of that case the issue of treatability, which formerly was not a consideration on discharge (the ruling in Canon's Park) has become a relevant factor in relation to Section 72. A Tribunal must find that it would be appropriate or necessary for a patient to be liable to be detained in the hospital for medical treatment prior to deciding to reject an application for discharge.

(j) ***Epsom & St Helier NHS Trust*** v. ***MHRT(W)*** (2001) EWCA Admin 101
This case throws further light on the question what degree of continuing inpatient treatment is required to justify renewing a patient's Section 3 detention while the patient is on Section 17 leave. Since the decision in ***Re Barker*** it has been possible, provided that there is such an element of inpatient treatment, to renew a patient's detention while on leave, a situation which was previously regarded as having been outlawed by the case of ***R*** v. ***Hallstrom.*** In the Epsom case, the patient was on leave of absence to a nursing home which was not a registered mental nursing home. While ***Re Barker*** clarified the law it did not define the degree of inpatient treatment that would be required. In the Epsom case, there was no current in-patient treatment, simply the prospect or likelihood of treatment being required in the future during the period of detention under Section 3. That was held by the Court to be insufficient.

(k) ***Reed (Trainer)*** v. ***Bronglais Hospital etc.*** (2001) EWHC Admin 792
One of the two medical recommendations required to support an application for admission under Section 2 Mental Health Act must if practicable by Section 12(2) be from a practitioner who has 'previous acquaintance'. Here the doctor in question:

(i) attended a case conference which gave much background information on the patient and included the minutes of two previous case conferences.
(ii) following the case conference, saw the patient for about five minutes.

(iii) 'scanned' the medical records received from the Family Health Authority *(sic)*.

(iv) then saw the patient again to make his recommendation.

The Court held that the words should be given their ordinary meaning and that the reference in the Code of Practice to 'personal' knowledge did not import any greater requirement. The doctor had sufficient 'previous acquaintance', and any doctor would have who had some previous knowledge of the patient and was not coming to him or her 'cold'.

See also ***TTM* v. *Hackney BC et al.*** (below) which held that in the circumstances of that case the fact that it would have been practicable to have secured a recommendation from a doctor with previous acquaintance did not invalidate the subsequent detention.

(l) ***Keenan* v. *UK*** (2001) 33 EHRR 38)
Although the threshold for a breach of Article 3 of the European Convention is high, the Convention is a dynamic instrument which should be interpreted in the light of changing social attitudes and medical advances. There is the suggestion therefore that as a result the threshold might gradually be lowered. Support for this view is to be found in the recent case of ***Keenan* v. *UK***. Mr Keenan died in prison by hanging himself. He had longstanding psychiatric illness. The Court found that the lack of effective monitoring of his condition in prison and the lack of informed psychiatric input into his assessment and treatment disclosed significant defects in the medical care provided to a mentally ill person known to be a suicide risk. To add to this, he sustained a serious disciplinary punishment including segregation. This was held to be incompatible with the standard of treatment required in respect of a mentally ill person and, as such, breached Article 3. The comment by the Court that the lack of appropriate medical treatment could amount to treatment contrary to Article 3 is highly significant as was the comment that in the case of mentally ill persons, their vulnerability had to be taken into consideration in terms of how they might be affected by treatment, or the lack of it, or punishment.

(m) ***R (Ex Parte Wooder)* v. *Feggetter*** (2002) EWCA Civ 554; (2002) 3 WLR 591
A Second Opinion Appointed Doctor (SOAD) who certifies under Section 58 Mental Health Act that a detained patient should be given medication against his will should give his reasons in writing and these should be disclosed to the patient unless the SOAD or RC consider that this would be likely to cause serious harm to the physical or mental health of the patient or any other person.

(n) ***R (S)* v. *City of Plymouth*** (2002) 1 WLR 2583
The nearest relative of a patient lacking capacity applied for disclosure of the patient's (her daughter's) Social Services file so as to obtain advice as to whether an application (which she anticipated) to remove her as nearest relative under Section 29 Mental Health Act would be likely to succeed. The Local Authority refused on grounds of confidentiality, which they argued were not outweighed by other public interests. The mother failed before the High Court in her argument that this breached her rights under Article 6 of the European Convention on Human Rights ('the Convention'). She remained the patient's nearest relative with all the rights in respect of disclosure provided by the rules were an application to remove her under Section 29 in fact made. The matter went to the Court of Appeal by which time the Local Authority had altered its position so as to agree to disclosure of the information to the mother's experts but not directly to the

mother or her solicitors. The Court of Appeal reversed the earlier decision and ordered disclosure to the mother and her solicitors. A balance had to be struck between the protection of confidentiality and the right of an interested party to information. In this case, the balance came down in favour of disclosure. However in so deciding the Court emphasised the importance of preserving confidentiality, including for the Learning Disabled, and where disclosure was given this should be strictly limited to reports which would have to be placed before the Court and should not be more widely circulated; the information to be disclosed would not include Social Services files.

(o) ***R* v. *Tower Hamlets Healthcare NHS Trust (MHRT, Discharge)*** Ex Parte ***Von Brandenburg*** (2003) UKHL 58
The case concerns a patient detained under Section 2 whose Tribunal ordered his discharge, deferred for 7 days. Six days later, the patient was detained on Section 3. It was submitted that there should have been at least a change of circumstances between the decision of the Tribunal and the renewed detention to justify such an action.

The case reached the House of Lords which provided guidance on the powers and obligations of professionals faced with a Tribunal decision to discharge with which they disagree. In short the House of Lords confirmed:

(i) where a MHT has ordered discharge of a patient it is lawful to readmit him under Section 2 or Section 3 where it cannot be demonstrated that there has been a relevant change in circumstances. A conscientious doctor whose opinion has not been accepted by the Tribunal will ask whether his own opinion should be revised. But if he then adheres to his original opinion he cannot be obliged to suppress or alter it. His professional duty to his patient and his wider duty to the public require him to form and if called upon express, the best professional judgment he can, whether or not that coincides with the judgment of the Tribunal.

(ii) an AMHP may not lawfully apply for the admission of a patient whose discharge has been ordered by the decision of a MHRT of which the AMHP is aware unless the AMHP has formed the reasonable and *bona fide* opinion that he has information not known to the Tribunal which puts a significantly different complexion on the case as compared with that which was before the Tribunal. Three examples were given:

1. An AMHP learns after a Tribunal decision that the patient made an earlier serious attempt on his life, not known to the Tribunal and which significantly alters the risk as assessed by the Tribunal.
2. The Tribunal based a decision to discharge on the belief that the patient would take his medication (as he said he would). Before or after discharge he refuses to take his medication presenting a risk to himself or others.
3. After the Tribunal decision the patient's mental condition significantly deteriorates so as to present a degree of risk or to require treatment or supervision not evident at the hearing.

In such cases, the AMHP may properly apply for the admission of a patient, subject to the required medical support, notwithstanding a Tribunal decision to discharge.

(iii) Although the 'relevant change of circumstances' test is not the correct one, the principle that tribunal decisions should be respected for what they decide means that if an ASW is making a fresh application to detain, the reasons for departing from the earlier decision should be given, albeit in general terms.

The same requirement that where detention or continued detention is based on nature rather than degree the combination of risk of default and deterioration be such that there is risk of relapse in the *near* future was emphasised in **CM v. *Derbyshire et al.*** (2011) UKUT 129 (AAC).

(p) ***R (Ashworth SHA)* v. *MHRT W. Midlands*** and ***N.W. Region. R* v. *Oxfordshire MH Trust,* Ex Parte *H*** (2002) EWCA Civ 923; TLR 10/7/2002
The case of Von Brandenburg confirmed that a patient could lawfully be re-detained shortly after a Tribunal decision to discharge. The above two recent cases throw light on the circumstances in which in practice this can be done. In the Ashworth case, a Tribunal peremptorily discharged a patient after hearing that no aftercare arrangements had been made for him. He was therefore re-detained under the Mental Health Act. This was challenged by the patient but at first instance the Court held that it was sufficient if the AMHP and doctors were advised on substantial grounds, that the Tribunal's decision was unlawful and that proceedings to challenge it are at least imminent. They must act in accordance with their professional judgments and the patient's remedy is to apply to the Tribunal. The Tribunal should have adjourned for suitable aftercare provision to be arranged.

Thus to 'change in circumstances' or 'information not being available to the Tribunal' is added another example of where re-detention is lawful, even without a change in circumstances.

However this decision was reversed by the Court of Appeal which imposed tighter restrictions on re-sectioning in such circumstances.

(i) Faced with such a situation the Hospital should have applied for Judicial Review of the Tribunal's decision, coupled with a stay which would act to 'turn the clock back' (unless perhaps the patient had already left).
(ii) The Healthcare professionals must ask themselves whether the main grounds for re-sectioning have effectively been rejected by the Tribunal.
(iii) An application to resection would need to be founded on circumstances unknown to the Tribunal.

In ***Ex Parte*** **H** the patient deteriorated in the period between the Tribunal's decision to discharge and the date fixed for discharge, and was re-detained. The patient's application for judicial review was refused. Although the professionals were bound to take into account the Tribunal's decision when making their application and recommendations this was not a case of differing professional views of the same circumstances but a deterioration outside the contemplation of the Tribunal at the time of ordering discharge.

The **Von Brandenburg** case represents the current legal position. The suggestion that the correct procedure where there was disagreement with a Tribunal decision was to challenge it by judicial review coupled with an application for a stay is probably now best restricted to cases where the issue is whether the Tribunal has erred in law.

(q) ***R* v. *Doncaster MBC,* Ex Parte *W*** (2003) EWCA 192 Admin
This is another case, consistent with a line of recent cases concerning the extent of the obligation of the Health and Social Services Authorities to implement or comply with the conditions attached by a MHT to its decision to discharge a detained patient. Here one of the conditions was that the patient should reside in appropriate accommodation approved by named doctors and social workers. This proved impossible to fulfil and so the patient remained detained. However, the MBC had used its best endeavours to find suitable accommodation and accordingly its duty under Section 117 had not been breached and there had been no unlawful detention.

The problem with this line of cases is that unless a Tribunal can enforce its decision (including conditions attaching to discharge) there is a potential breach of the patient's rights under Article 5(4) to be able effectively to challenge his detention. On the other hand, Courts have been reluctant to compel Authorities or clinicians to adopt a particular course which conflicts with their own reasonably held professionally held views. This issue was clarified when the case of ***R (IH)* v. *Nottinghamshire Healthcare NHS Trust et al.*** (2003) UKHL 59 went to the House of Lords.

(r) ***R (IH)* v. *Nottinghamshire Healthcare NHS Trust*** (2003) UKHL 59
In ***R* v. *Camden and Islington Health Authority* Ex Parte *K*** a patient remained detained because of the inability of the Authority to find a psychiatrist willing to supervise the patient in the community on the conditions set by the Tribunal. Section 117 did not impose an absolute requirement to satisfy the Tribunal's conditions and the resulting continued detention would not be in breach of Article 5. In ***R (IH)*** a similar impasse arose, and the issue was whether the lack of power in the Tribunal to enforce compliance with its conditions meant that there was a breach of the effective, speedy review provision of Article 5(4). The Court held that the Tribunal retained a monitoring role in such circumstances and that this power was sufficient to prevent a breach of Article 5(4). If the Tribunal did not exercise that power then there could be a breach of both Article 5(1)(e) and 5(4).

This decision was upheld by the Court of Appeal which set out some guidance on how such an impasse was to be resolved. It confirmed that a Tribunal <u>does</u> have the power to revisit its decision before a patient's discharge where conditions it has set have proved impossible to fulfil. It had been thought that the Tribunal lacked that power which gave rise to the argument that this would lead inevitably to a delay which might breach Article 5(4) by leaving the patient in limbo.

The case reached the House of Lords which confirmed that the obligation in respect of conditions for discharge of a restricted patient set by a Tribunal is to use best endeavours, rather than absolute. A failure to use best endeavours or to act in good faith could lead to challenge. The fact that a Tribunal lacked the power to secure compliance with its conditions did not mean it lacked the necessary attributes of a court as required by Article 5(4). The Court of Appeal's new guidance was correct, from which it followed that Tribunals should reconsider conditions which turned out to be impracticable and if this led to the continued detention of the patient that would not be unlawful. The individual professional autonomy of the Consultant Psychiatrist has therefore been preserved. The House of Lords left open whether a Community RMO was a hybrid Public Authority and thus covered by the requirement of the HRA not to act in a way incompatible with an individual's Convention rights.

(s) ***HL* v. *UK*** (2004) 40 EHHR 761
This case, also known as **Bournewood**, raised the issue of the lawfulness of detention under the Common Law doctrine of necessity of a patient who lacked capacity to consent to admission to psychiatric hospital, but who did not resist being taken there and whether in particular there had been a breach of Article 5 of the Convention. The European Court decided that in the first place the patient had been deprived of his liberty; second that he could have been detained under the MHA; third that the patient's detention at Common Law was not in accordance with a procedure prescribed by law (there was a lack of procedural safeguards, rules and formal admission procedures) and was thus arbitrary and in breach of Article 5(1); fourth that the lack of an effective means of challenge to his detention (e.g. no possible Tribunal application) was in breach of the patient's rights under Article 5(4).

Article 5 does not prohibit restriction of movement and so a key question for health and social care professionals is whether the person is being deprived of his liberty or is being cared for in circumstances which fall short. This case confirmed that the distinction is one of degree and intensity not nature or substance. So no single factor is determinative of deprivation of liberty. All circumstances of a patient's care have to be considered in reaching a conclusion. Another important factor was stated to be that the healthcare professionals assumed 'complete and effective control' of the patient's movements, but in ***P and Q (aka MIG and MEG)* v. *Surrey CC et al.*** *((2011) EWCA Civ 190)* this was held to be not necessarily determinative of the issue.

Note: The Deprivation of Liberty Safeguards procedure (DOLS) is designed to permit lawful deprivation of liberty (within the meaning of Article 5) without use of the Mental Health Act or a Court of Protection order.

(t) ***R (AN)* v. *MHRT (Northern Region)*** (2005) EWCA Civ 1605
This case concerned the *standard* of proof required at a Tribunal hearing. The Court decided that the requirement is that the Tribunal be satisfied on the balance of probabilities, not on any higher criminal standard. Sections 72(1)(b)(i) and (ii) criteria are cumulative and the Tribunal must discharge if the detaining authority fails to satisfy as to either. The Court of Appeal held that 'the standard of proof will have a much more important part to play in the determination of disputed'.

Tribunals should be alert to the dangers of hearsay evidence and look to the medical records for contemporaneous evidence of assertions relied on.

The *burden* of proof before the Tribunal lies at all times on those arguing for the continued detention of the patient – *see* ***R (H)* v. *MHRT for NE London*** ((2001)3 WLR 512).

(u) ***R (E)* v. *Bristol City Council*** (2005) EWHC 74 (Admin)
In this case, the issue was the meaning of the words 'practicable' and 'reasonably practicable' in Sections 11(3) and (4) in relation to the requirement of the AMHP to inform or consult with the patient's Nearest Relative ('NR'). The Court held that guidance in the (now superceded) Code of Practice that the words meant that the duty to inform or consult with the NR arose if he was 'available' was wrong. The words could be construed as more akin to 'appropriate', so that if it was detrimental to the patient's well-being and in breach of his right to respect for privacy under Article 8 of the Convention, there was no need to inform or consult.

The case can be seen as an example of the requirement of a court under the Human Rights Act to construe a statutory provision if at all possible in a way that does not breach a person's Convention rights.

Because of the limited nature of the amendments to Section 29, which allow a patient in defined circumstances to apply to court for the displacement of his NR (but do not give him the right to choose who it should be) this case will continue to be relevant to the consideration by the AMHP of his obligations to consult or inform the patient's existing NR. This is particularly so given that the opportunity for applying to court will often occur for a patient when at his most vulnerable and least able to pursue it.

(v) ***R (Munjaz)*** **v.** ***Mersey Care NHS Trust*** (2005) UKHL 58

This is the leading case on the status to be accorded to the MHA Code of Practice, but it also raised questions about the nature of seclusion and its lawfulness. The House of Lords confirmed that the Code does not have statutory force: it is guidance which should be considered with great care and is more than advice which a person under an obligation to have regard to it is free to follow or not. The Code should only be departed from for cogent reasons.

Seclusion is not *per se* unlawful even at common law. Further (according to the Court of Appeal and not overturned by the House of Lords) it can constitute medical treatment for mental disorder under Section 63.

In a patient subject to the compulsory powers of the MHA it is not seclusion which constitutes a deprivation of liberty but the fact that he has been sectioned.

The question is less whether a patient is being managed in accordance with Code of Practice guidance, and more whether his treatment breaches his rights under the Convention: appropriate local policies and procedures in relation to seclusion can prevent a breach of the patient's rights under Articles 3 and 8, even if they allow for a departure from the Code's guidance.

The judgment is of general application, not just to the issue of seclusion.

(w) ***Storck*** **v.** ***Germany*** (2005) 43 EHRR 96

This far reaching case concerned the nature of the State's positive obligation under Article 1 to secure Convention rights for those within its jurisdiction, not merely to make them available. The Court held that the State had an obligation to ensure proper supervision and review of the deprivation of a person's liberty even if confined in a private institution. It could not delegate its responsibilities. The State's obligation extended to decisions to treat a patient against his will. The involvement of the State through the police in bringing a patient back to a private institution meant that it was implicated in the patient's detention and resultant breach of Articles 5 and 8 of the Convention. The State was under an obligation to consider the need for special safeguards for the vulnerable mentally ill.

It has been suggested that this case implies that the detention of a competent refusing child (or certainly young person) on the basis of parental authority might no longer be lawful. This is partly what has lead to the guidance in Chapter 36 of the MHA Code of Practice and the emphasis on the somewhat elusive concept of the 'zone of parental control'.

(x) ***JE*** **v.** ***DE and Surrey CC*** (2006) EWHC 3459 (Fam)

This case, again considering what constitutes deprivation of liberty as opposed to restriction of movement might be seen as having slightly muddied the waters after ***HL*** **v.** ***UK***. The judge drew a distinction between restrictions of a person's movements within an institution and his not being free to leave it and live where he chooses: not being free to leave the institution and live with his wife at home constituted a deprivation of person's liberty.

It is hard to reconcile this case with ***HL* v. *UK*** and other case law which had identified that no single factor was determinative of a deprivation of liberty: does this case elevate not being free to leave and live where he chooses above all other factors when deciding whether a person is deprived of his liberty? Is it no longer a question of degree and intensity? It also raises the issue of what weight should be attached to the apparent wishes of a person lacking capacity to make the relevant decision in determining whether he is deprived of his liberty? *See* ***LBH* v. *GP*** ((2009) FD08P01058) which suggests that even though the person lacked capacity to consent to where he was to reside his views had to be given considerable weight (as opposed to being decisive).

Does this decision mean that use of Guardianship under the Mental Health Act might constitute a deprivation of liberty?

(y) ***Wilkinson* v. *UK (Application 14659/02, Admissibility Decision Feb 06)***
An adult of sound mind is entitled to refuse medical treatment even if that decision is unwise or irrational. This principle is modified by the MHA for those detained patients to whom Part 4 applies. The question that therefore arose in this case is whether treatment forced on a capacitated detained patient under Section 58 breaches his Convention rights. The Court decided that the safeguards built into the MHA (such as the SOAD), and the remedy of Judicial Review prevented the high threshold for breach of Article 3 (prohibition against inhuman and degrading treatment) being reached. There was a breach of Article 8(1) (right to private and family life) but this was justified by Article 8(2) (for the protection of the patient's health).

One question is whether treatment with ECT would have lead to the same result. Perhaps it was concerns about this that lead to ECT in face of capacitated refusal now only being permitted under limited Section 62 exceptions.

For treatment under Section 58 against the wishes of capacitated patient to be lawful it must be convincingly shown to be a therapeutic necessity – *see* ***Herczegfalvy* v. *Austria*** ((1993) 15 EHRR 437), and ***R (N)* v. *Dr M et al.*** ((2003) 1 WLR 3284) in which the relevant factors were identified.

Note also the case of ***Keenan* v. *UK*** ((2001) 33 EHRR 38) which indicates that the failure to provide appropriate psychiatric input to a patient known to be seriously mentally disordered might constitute a breach of the prohibition under Article 3 against inhuman and degrading treatment. If that failure leads to the patient's death there might also be a breach of his right to life under Article 2.

(z) ***GJ* v. *The Foundation Trust et al.*** (2009) EWHC 2972 (Fam)
The complexity not to say near incomprehensibility of the DOLS scheme is nowhere more apparent than in applying the 'eligibility' assessment set out in Schedule 1A to the Mental Capacity Act which seeks to define the dividing line to be drawn between use of DOLS and detention under the MHA. The Court in this case identified three requirements:

1. Are the MHA criteria met? Assessors must assume that the medical recommendations have been given and that no alternative is available under MCA (MCA Schedule 1A para 12). The MHA has primacy.
2. Is the person to be accommodated in hospital for the purpose of medical treatment for mental disorder (or is real reason for hospital admission

treatment of a physical condition)? To decide this assessors must apply the 'but for' test – i.e. but for the need for treatment of the physical condition would detention in hospital be sought?

3. Does the person object to what is proposed to be authorised by DOLS (bearing in mind past and present behaviour, beliefs, wishes and feelings)? The Court set a low threshold set for objection.

The implication of the case is that where there is deprivation of liberty professional discretion is curtailed: 'It is not lawful for [decision makers under both the MHA and MCA] to proceed on the basis that they can pick and choose between the two statutory regimes as they think fit having regard to general considerations (e.g. the preservation or promotion of a therapeutic relationship with P) that they consider render one regime preferable to the other in the circumstances of the case.'

The decision also creates the possibility of a new 'gap': a person may object sufficiently to be ineligible for DOLS but not sufficiently to justify use of MHA compulsory powers. The Court implied that the MHA should be used in these circumstances under the 'primacy' principle.

As a result of this decision treatment of mental disorder in *hospital* under compulsion will, in most cases, be under MHA not DOLS where there is a deprivation of liberty.

(aa) *MD* v. *Nottingham Healthcare NHS Trust* (2010) UKUT 59 (AAC)

The new requirement for *inter alia* the admission of patients under Section 3, their being placed on a CTO and the renewal or extension of these powers is that there is appropriate medical treatment available. What is the meaning and scope of this new test?

The Upper Tribunal decided that merely benefitting from the ward 'milieu' meant that appropriate medical treatment was available. Detention without possibility of reduction of risk did not merely amount to containment. Treatment must be appropriate but not need to reduce risk. The argument that a theoretical capacity to engage with psychological therapy did not equate to a practical ability to benefit from treatment was 'untenable'.

This case reinforces the view that the threshold for meeting the test is low and that 'medical treatment' is to be very broadly construed. As a consequence, it is easier to justify use and renewal of (*inter alia*) the Section 3 compulsory powers than when the previous 'treatability' test had to be met. *See also* the case of ***DL-H* v. *Devon Partnershipship NHS Trust and S o S*** ((2010) UKUT 102 (AAC)).

(bb) *RM* v. *St Andrew's Healthcare* (2010) UKUT 119 (AAC)

This case dealt with the circumstances in which information (in this case that he was being covertly medicated) may be withheld from a patient in Tribunal proceedings.

The situation is now governed by Rule 14. There is discretion to prohibit disclosure of reports in Tribunal proceedings if disclosure would be likely to cause serious harm to the patient or another and if this would be proportionate with regard to interests of justice. A patient does not have an absolute or unqualified right to see every document, but in this case the Upper Tribunal concluded that if the information was withheld the patient would not be able effectively to challenge his detention because he did not know that he was being covertly medicated. Disclosure was therefore ordered in the interests of justice, even though such disclosure would be likely to cause serious harm to the patient's health. The requirement under Article 6 for a fair trial was considered to be of greater importance than the avoidance of likely serious harm to the patient and it may be increasingly difficult to justify withholding information from patients in future. It is interesting to speculate whether the same decision would have been reached if the prospect was of serious harm to someone other than the patient.

(cc) ***AH* v. *W London MHT*** (2011) UKUT 74 (AAC)
The issue in this case concerned the circumstances in which Tribunal proceedings should be held in public. The Court held that open justice is a right, which does not require justification on a case by case basis. On the contrary it is the exceptions which need to be justified. A 'threshold test' as to whether the hearing should be in public must be applied comprising four questions:

1. Is it consistent with the subjective and informed wishes of the applicant?
2. Will it have an adverse effect on the applicant's mental health in the short or long term?
3. Are there any other special factors for or against a public hearing?
4. Can practical arrangements be made for an open hearing without disproportionate burden on the authority?

A public hearing was directed despite the practical problems and expense involved.

Despite the decision in this case, compared to old Rule 21, new Rule 38 in fact appears curiously to reflect a shift from the wishes of a patient to the more general interests of justice in determining if hearing should be in public. It is likely that the costs would have to be considerably greater than the £150,000 annual anticipated sum for Broadmoor Hospital for its 170 tribunals before this would influence a court against ordering a public hearing.

(dd) ***C* v. *A LA et al.*** (2011) EWHC 1539 (Admin)
This case raised amongst many others the issue of the application of the MHA and MCA Codes of Practice to circumstances not directly within their remit. It involved an 18 year old. The Court stated that the LA should have referred the circumstances of his care and management to the Court of Protection when he was16 (as DOLS not applicable) – i.e. before any deprivation of liberty occurred in order to have obtained the necessary authority. The Court went on to state that the DOLS Code of Practice would be relevant even where DOLS was not possible (because no detention in hospital or care home); further that the MHA Code of Practice should be deemed to apply even if the patient is not detained under MHA, where *prima facie* his condition falls within MHA definition of mental disorder, and possibly even where it does not. This would for example apply to seclusion.

(ee) ***LBH* v. *Neary*** (2011) EWCH 1377
This is a potentially far reaching decision concerning the approach Local Authorities ('LA') should take towards use of DOLS in face of disputes with a person's family and generally. In particular, it deals with the issue of when reference should be made to the Court of Protection.

The Court decided that the LA's powers were strictly limited in face of a dispute with family carers (*see also* ***A LA* v. *A*** ((2010) EWHC 978). The LA's role is to support, not impose its own will. It must demonstrate its own arrangements are better than the family's. Faced with dispute with a person's family the LA should not impose its will by use of DOLS but refer to the Court of Protection.

There was held to be a breach of Article 8 as there had been no effective balanced assessment of the alternatives. The Supervisory Body must scrutinise assessments with care: perfunctory best interests assessments will be unlawful and a subsequent DOLS authorisation will not render it lawful (*see also* **A CC v. *MB*** ((2010) EWHC 2508).

The MCA Schedule A1 states that a DOLS authorisation must be given if the six assessments are positive but this only applies if the Supervisory Body is satisfied that the assessment is thorough and adequate.

There was also held to be a breach of Article 5(4) because no IMCA had been appointed in a timely manner, there had been no effective review of the DOLS authorisation and no speedy review by a *Court*. The positive obligation of the Supervisory Body was to enable and *ensure* a review by referring to court.

The case is an example of the Court attempting to make the DOLS safeguards a reality, rather than a mere procedure. *See also* **A CC v. *MB*** ((2010) EWHC 2508) and ***Cheshire and Chester* v. *P*** ((2011) EWCA Civ 1257). **Neary** involved a dispute between the LA and the family, but the judge did not specifically limit his conclusions to such cases and it is an open question whether (and if so when) in all cases of DOLS authorisations (even where no such dispute exists) a reference to the Court of Protection must be made to ensure the person has his Article 5(4) right to a speedy review of detention by a Court protected. The problem arises because unlike under the MHA there is no provision for eventual automatic referral to a Tribunal (which is a court for MHA purposes). This is particularly important where the person lacks capacity to make his own application to the Court.

There is a need to beware of potential for serious conflicts of interests where the DOLS assessor, decision maker and managing authority are the same.

(ff) *TTM* v. *Hackney BC et al.* (2011) EWCA Civ 4

What is the effect of an honest but mistaken belief that the Nearest Relative had no objection to a Section 3 application? Who is responsible for the legal consequence of such a mistake? What if neither doctor had 'previous acquaintance' with the patient?

It was held that the effect was that the detention was unlawful from the outset not merely from when a court so declared. The fact that the Hospital Trust did not act unlawfully within Section 6(3) in admitting and detaining the patient did not retrospectively render the detention itself lawful. Section 139 could not be interpreted so as to render lawful what was unlawful. Article 5(1) had been breached so the patient was entitled to compensation. The Local Authority was liable to pay the claim, not the hospital Trust (as detaining authority).

It was also held that there was no breach of MHA Section 6(3) by the Hospital Trust in admitting patient without either doctor having previous acquaintance. 'Practicable' was to be broadly construed. Even if it had been practicable this would not have invalidated the application.

A number of other useful comments were made by the Court in relation to the duties of the Managers:

1. The Managers' duties to check and scrutinise applications is limited: the first stage is to check that the documents appear to amount to an application that has been duly made; the second stage is to scrutinise for defects which fundamentally invalidate the application.
2. The Managers were entitled to rely on the AMHP's confirmation that there had been no objection by the nearest relative; when P's solicitors asserted post admission that the nearest relative had objected the Managers acted

sufficiently in checking with the AMHP who again assured them that this was not the case.

3. The Managers also acted correctly in treating solicitors' allegation as the nearest relative exercising his right to discharge P and so a barring order was correctly made.

Appendix II

Summary of civil treatment codes

Section number and purpose	Maximum duration	Can patient apply to Tribunal?	Can Nearest Relative (NR) apply to Tribunal?	Will there be an automatic Tribunal hearing?	*Do consent to treatment rules apply?
2 Admission for assessment	**28 days** Not renewable	Within first 14 days	No – Section 23 gives them power to discharge, but see Section 25 below	No	Yes
3 Admission for treatment	**6 months** May be renewed for 6 months & then yearly	Within first 6 months and then in each period	No – Section 23 gives them power to discharge, but see Section 25 below	If one has not been held Managers refer to Tribunal at 6 months and then every 3 years (annually if under 16)	Yes
4 Admission for assessment in an emergency	**72 hours** Not renewable but 2nd doctor can change to Section 2	Yes. But only relevant if Section 4 is converted to a Section 2	No	No	No
5(2) Doctor's holding power	**72 hours** Not renewable	No	No	No	No
5(4) Nurse's holding power	**6 hours** Not renewable but doctor can change to Section 5(2)	No	No	No	No
7 Reception into guardianship	**6 months** May be renewed for 6 months and then yearly	Within first 6 months and then in each period	No – Section 23 gives them power to discharge	No	No
17A Community treatment order (CTO)	**6 months** May be extended for 6 months and then yearly	Once in each period	No unless based on Section 37A. But has discharge powers	It CTO is revoked	Yes Part 4A
19 Transfer from guardianship to hospital	**6 months** May be renewed for 6 months and then yearly	In the first 6 months of detention and then in each period	No – Section 23 gives them power to discharge, but see Section 25 below	If one has not been held Managers refer to Tribunal at 6 months and then every 3 years (annually if under 16)	Yes
25 Restriction of discharge by Nearest Relative	Variable	No	Within 28 days of being informed (No appeal if Section 2.)	No	–
29 Appointment of acting Nearest Relative by court	Variable	No	Within one year and then yearly	No	–
135 Warrant to search for and remove patient	**72 hours** Not renewable	No	No	No	No
136 Police power in public places	**72 hours** Not renewable	No	No	No	No

Notes: Under Section 67 the Secretary of State can refer Part II patients to the TRIBUNAL at any time.

*Where consent to treatment rules do not apply, the patient is in the same position as an informal patient and should not be treated without their consent except in an emergency under Common Law.

Appendix III

Summary of civil compulsion sections

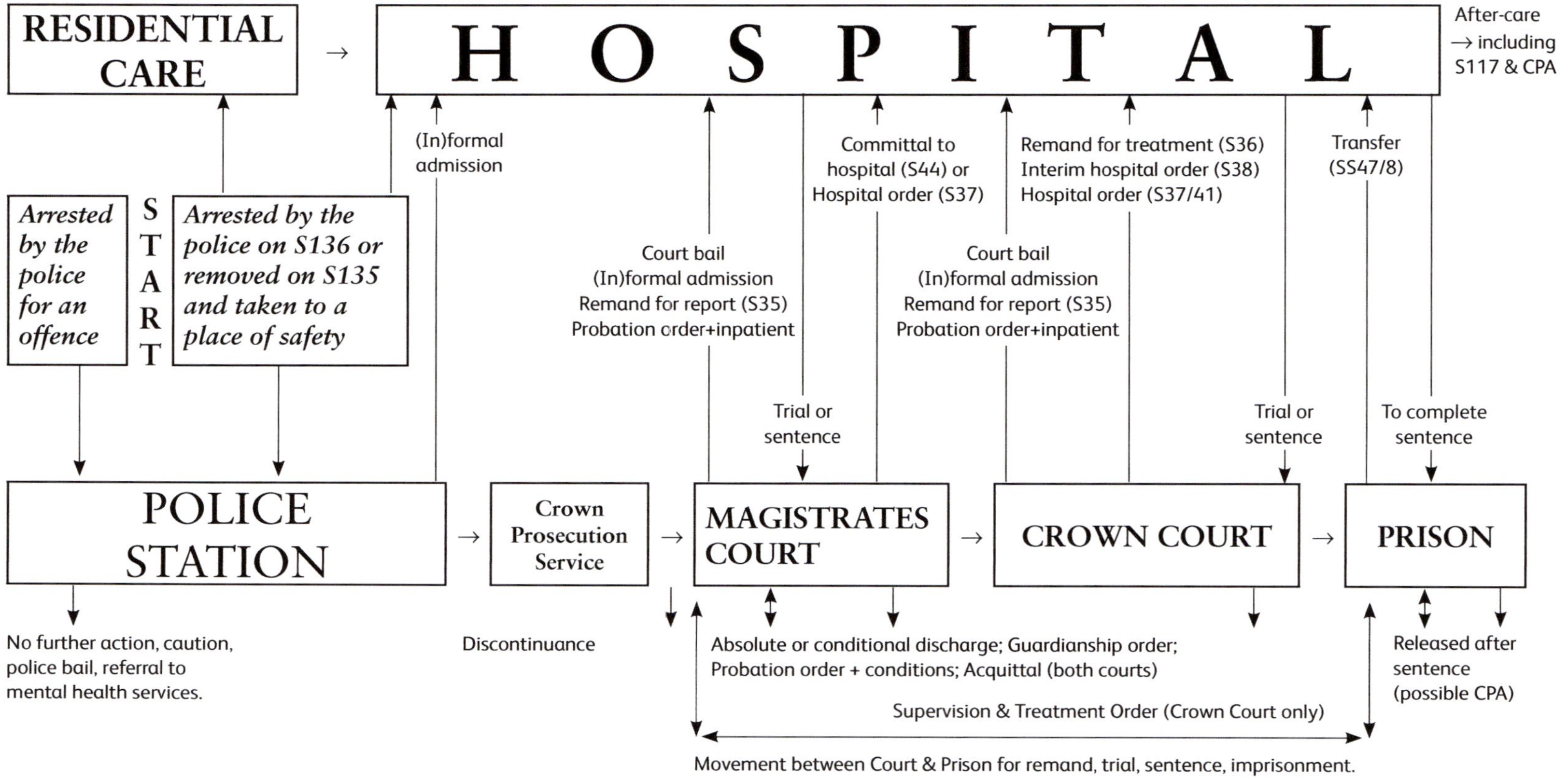

Note: *all section references are from the MH Act 1983.*
see earlier pages for fuller discussion of legislation and diversion

Appendix IV

Flowchart of decisions involving consent to treatment

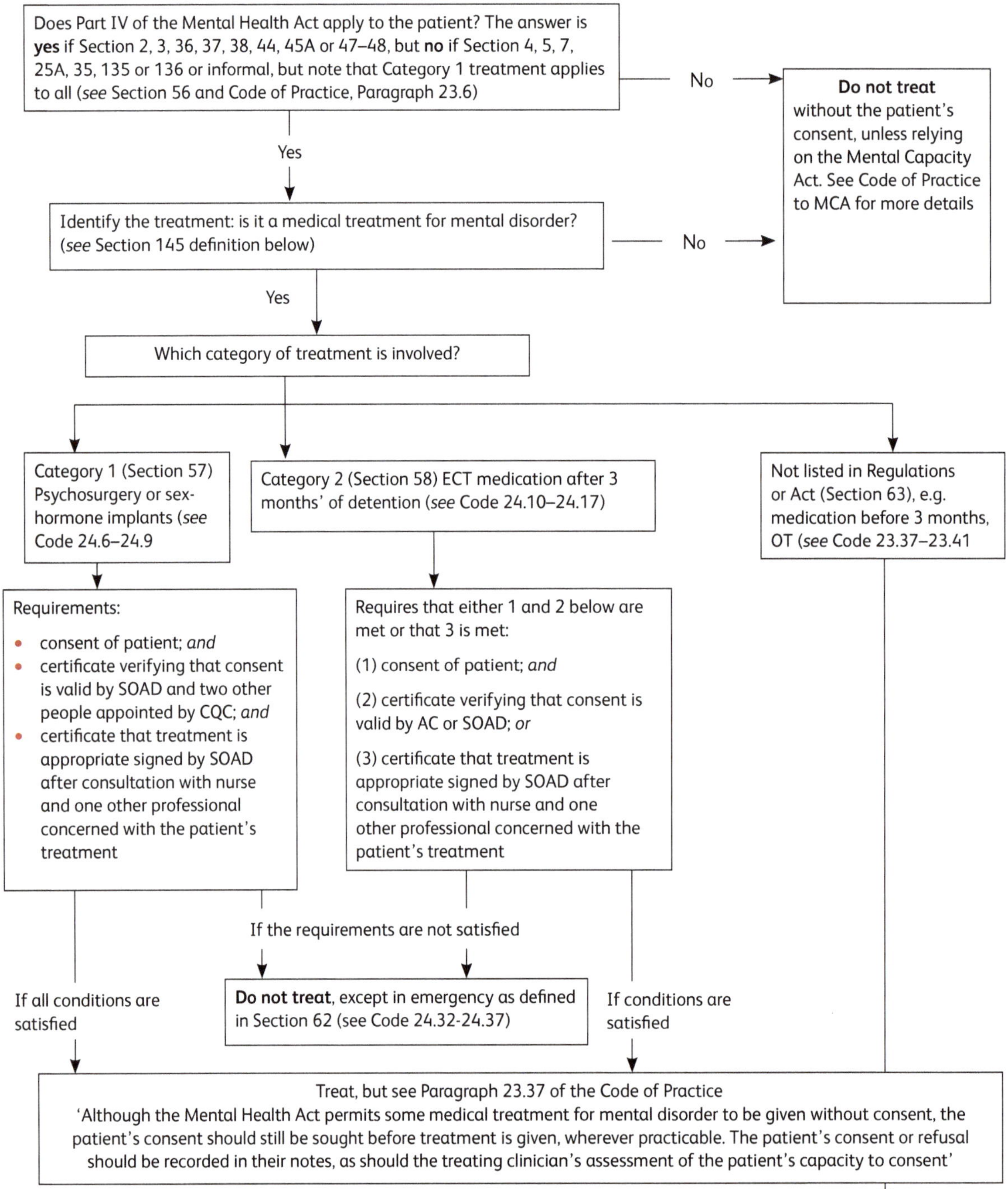

ECT is now dealt with separately under Section 58A see Code Paragraphs 24.18–24.24; CQC, Care Quality Commission; AC approved clinician; OT, occupational therapy; SOAD, second-opinion appointed doctor. Section 145 states 'medical treatment' includes nursing, psychological intervention and specialist mental health rehabilitation and care… the purpose of which is to alleviate, or prevent a worsening of the disorder or one of more of its symptoms or manifestations.'

Appendix V

Sample forms

Form A2 *Regulation 4(1)(a)(ii)* **Mental Health Act 1983**

Section 2 - application by an approved mental health professional for admission for assessment

To the managers of (*name and address of hospital*)

Royal Wessex Hospital, Wessex NHS Partnership Trust, Hipardi Avenue, Casterbridge, GG20 1RU

I (*PRINT your full name and address*)

MALCOLM PRACTICE,
ANGST HOUSE,
DECISION STREET, CASTERBRIDGE, GG1 2PT

apply for the admission of (*PRINT full name and address of patient*)

AGATHA ROYAL, 24 HARDY AVENUE,
CASTERBRIDGE, GG17 2BU

for assessment in accordance with Part 2 of the Mental Health Act 1983.

I am acting on behalf of (*PRINT name of local social services authority*)

WESSEX COUNTY COUNCIL

and am approved to act as an approved mental health professional for the purposes of the Act by *(delete as appropriate)*

that authority

~~*(name of local social services authority that approved you, if different)*~~

Complete the following if you know who the nearest relative is.
Complete (a) or (b) as applicable and delete the other.

(a) To the best of my knowledge and belief (*PRINT full name and address*)

Deborah Royal, 2 Cackle Row, Bank St. John,
Casterbridge, GG42 6RU

is the patient's nearest relative within the meaning of the Act.

~~(b) I understand that (*PRINT full name and address*)~~

~~has been authorised by a county court/the patient's nearest relative*~~
~~to exercise the functions under the Act of the patient's nearest relative. (**Delete the phrase which does not apply*)~~

I have/~~have not yet~~* informed that person that this application is to be made and of the nearest relative's power to order the discharge of the patient. (**Delete the phrase which does not apply*)

 continue overleaf

Complete the following if you do not know who the nearest relative is. *Delete (a) or (b).*

(a) I have been unable to ascertain who is the patient's nearest relative within the meaning of the Act.

(b) To the best of my knowledge and belief this patient has no nearest relative within the meaning of the Act.

The remainder of the form must be completed in all cases.

I last saw the patient on

20 / 07 / 2011 [date],

which was within the period of 14 days ending on the day this application is completed.

I have interviewed the patient and I am satisfied that detention in a hospital is in all the circumstances of the case the most appropriate way of providing the care and medical treatment of which the patient stands in need.

This application is founded on two medical recommendations in the prescribed form.

If neither of the medical practitioners had previous acquaintance with the patient before making their recommendations, please explain why you could not get a recommendation from a medical practitioner who did have previous acquaintance with the patient -

This is a first presentation of mental disorder and I have been unable to find a GP who has had any acquaintance with the patient.

(If you need to continue on a separate sheet please indicate here ( ) and attach that sheet to this form)

Signed [signature] Date 20 / 07 / 2011

Form A4 *Regulation 4(1)(b)(ii)* **Mental Health Act 1983**

Section 2 – medical recommendation for admission for assessment

I *(PRINT full name and address of practitioner)*

Denise Croimak
Royal Wessex Hospital, Hipardi Avenue,
Casterbridge , GG20 1RU

a registered medical practitioner, recommend that

(PRINT full name and address of patient)

Agatha Royal
24 Hardy Avenue
Casterbridge, GG17 2BU

be admitted to a hospital for assessment in accordance with Part 2 of the Mental Health Act 1983.

I last examined this patient on

20 / 07 /2011 (date).

* ~~I had previous acquaintance with the patient before I conducted that examination.~~

* I am approved under section 12 of the Act as having special experience in the diagnosis or treatment of mental disorder

(Delete if not applicable)*

In my opinion,

(a) this patient is suffering from mental disorder of a nature or degree which warrants the detention of the patient in hospital for assessment (or for assessment followed by medical treatment) for at least a limited period,

AND

(b) ought to be so detained
(i) in the interests of the patient's own health
~~(ii) in the interests of the patient's own safety~~
(iii) with a view to the protection of other persons.
(Delete the indents not applicable)

My reasons for these opinions are:

(Your reasons should cover both (a) and (b) above. As part of them: describe the patient's symptoms and behaviour and explain how those symptoms and behaviour lead you to your opinion; explain why the patient ought to be admitted to hospital and why informal admission is not appropriate.)

continue overleaf

The patient is very depressed but is refusing any help. She has been very low in mood for several weeks and is now refusing food and drink. Urgent intervention is necessary in the interests of her health and to protect her children (aged 5 and 3). Agatha has refused the offer a bed on the admission ward.

(If you need to continue on a separate sheet please indicate here ( ) and attach that sheet to this form)

Signed	Date
Denise Crooks	20 / 07 / 2011

Form A6 *Regulation 4(1)(c)(ii)* **Mental Health Act 1983**

Section 3 - application by an approved mental health professional for admission for treatment

To the managers of *(name and address of hospital)*

ROYAL WESSEX HOSPITAL
WESSEX NHS PARTNERSHIP TRUST
HIPARDI AVENUE, CASTERBRIDGE, GG20 1RU

I *(PRINT your full name and address)*

MALCOLM PRACTICE,
ANGST HOUSE,
DECISION STREET,
CASTERBRIDGE, GG1 2PT

apply for the admission of *(PRINT full name and address of patient)*

AGATHA ROYAL,
24 HARDY AVENUE,
CASTERBRIDGE.
GG17 2BU

for treatment in accordance with Part 2 of the Mental Health Act 1983.

I am acting on behalf of *(name of local social services authority)*

WESSEX COUNTY COUNCIL

and am approved to act as an approved mental health professional for the purposes of the Act by *(delete as appropriate)*

that authority

~~*(name of local social services authority that approved you, if different)*~~

Complete the following where consultation with the nearest relative has taken place.
Complete (a) or (b) and delete the other.

(a) I have consulted (PRINT full name and address)

DEBORAH ROYAL
2 CACKLE ROW
BANK ST. JOHN
CASTERBRIDGE, GG42 6RU

who to the best of my knowledge and belief is the patient's nearest relative within the meaning of the Act.

~~(b) I have consulted [PRINT full name and address]~~

~~who I understand has been authorised by a county court/the patient's nearest relative* to exercise the functions under the Act of the patient's nearest relative. *(*Delete the phrase which does not apply)*~~

That person has not notified me or the local social services authority on whose behalf I am acting that he or she objects to this application being made.

continue overleaf

Complete the following where the nearest relative has not been consulted.
Delete whichever two of (a), (b) and (c) do not apply.

(a) I have been unable to ascertain who is this patient's nearest relative within the meaning of the Act.

(b) To the best of my knowledge and belief this patient has no nearest relative within the meaning of the Act.

(c) I understand that *(PRINT full name and address)*

is

(i) this patient's nearest relative within the meaning of the Act,

(ii) authorised to exercise the functions of this patient's nearest relative under the Act,

(Delete either (i) or (ii))

but in my opinion it is not reasonably practicable/would involve unreasonable delay *(delete as appropriate)* to consult that person before making this application, because -

(If you need to continue on a separate sheet please indicate here ( ) and attach that sheet to this form)

The remainder of this form must be completed in all cases.

I saw the patient on

10 / 08 /2011 (date),

which was within the period of 14 days ending on the day this application is completed.

I have interviewed the patient and I am satisfied that detention in a hospital is in all the circumstances of the case the most appropriate way of providing the care and medical treatment of which the patient stands in need.

This application is founded on two medical recommendations in the prescribed form.

If neither of the medical practitioners had previous acquaintance with the patient before making their recommendations, please explain why you could not get a recommendation from a medical practitioner who did have previous acquaintance with the patient -

(If you need to continue on a separate sheet please indicate here ( ) and attach that sheet to this form)

Signed [signature] Date 10 /08 /2011

Form A8 *Regulation 4(1)(d)(ii)* **Mental Health Act 1983**

Section 3 – medical recommendation for admission for treatment

I *(PRINT full name and address of practitioner)*

Denise Croimak
Royal Wessex Hospital, Hipardi Avenue
Casterbridge, GG20 1RU

a registered medical practitioner, recommend that
(PRINT full name and address of patient)

Agatha Royal
24 Hardy Avenue
Casterbridge, GG17 2BV

be admitted to a hospital for treatment in accordance with Part 2 of the Mental Health Act 1983.

I last examined this patient on

10 / 08 /2011 (date),

* I had previous acquaintance with the patient before I conducted that examination.

* I am approved under section 12 of the Act as having special experience in the diagnosis or treatment of mental disorder

(Delete if not applicable)*

In my opinion,

(a) this patient is suffering from mental disorder of a nature or degree which makes it appropriate for the patient to receive medical treatment in a hospital,

AND

(b) it is necessary
(i) for the patient's own health
(ii) for the patient's own safety
(iii) for the protection of other persons
(delete the indents not applicable)

that this patient should receive treatment in hospital,

AND

(c) such treatment cannot be provided unless the patient is detained under section 3 of the Act,

because – (Your reasons should cover (a), (b) and (c) above. As part of them: describe the patient's symptoms and behaviour and explain how those symptoms and behaviour lead you to your opinion; say whether other methods of treatment or care (eg out-patient treatment or social services) are available and, if so, why they are not appropriate; indicate why informal admission is not appropriate.)

continue overleaf

Agatha is suffering from profound depression. Her mood is still very low and she is expressing nihilistic thoughts and a deep hopelessness. She only takes medication under duress and though not asking to leave hospital she sees no point in being here. Agatha needs to be deprived of her liberty while we treat her with anti-depressants. We intend to follow this with psycho-therapy when she is well enough to participate.

(If you need to continue on a separate sheet please indicate here ( ) and attach that sheet to this form)

I am also of the opinion that, taking into account the nature and degree of the mental disorder from which the patient is suffering and all the other circumstances of the case, appropriate medical treatment is available to the patient at the following hospital (or one of the following hospitals):-

(Enter name of hospital(s). If appropriate treatment is available only in a particular part of the hospital, say which part.)

Royal Wessex Hospital, Casterbridge

Signed Date

Dennis Cromack 10 / 08 / 2011

Index

Note: 'vs' indicated differential diagnosis.

'abnormality of mental functioning' and killing 82–3, 84
'abnormality of mind' and killing 82–3, 88
abortion, therapeutic, Northern Ireland 240
absent without leave 17
accommodation (provision)
  adults
    by local authority 163
    by NHS 162–3
  children, secure 194
Act for the Better Care and Maintenance of Pauper and Criminal Lunatics (1808) 3
Act for Regulating Private Madhouses (1774) 3
Act for the Safe Custody of Insane Persons Charged with Offences (1800) 3
actuarial risk assessments 227–8, 230
  sexual offending 230
actus rea 73
  involuntary manslaughter 87
  murder 87
admission
  alternatives to 27
  compulsory *see* compulsory admission
  duration, Section 2 44
  informal 119–20
  voluntary *see* voluntary admission
adolescents (and 16–17 year olds), consent and capacity 134, 201, 202–3
adoption 142, 174, 193, 194, 196, 197
Advance Decisions 144, 164, 169
  Singapore 246
advocates *see* independent mental health advocates
Aerts v. Belgium (2000) 179, 250
after-care 62, 154
age
  assessing/establishing
    in capacity assessment 155
    for deprivation of liberty 152, 153
    in risk assessment 225
  child's
    environment appropriate to 198–9
    services appropriate to 11
  suicide and 211
aggression 218
AH v. W London MHT (2011) 260
alcohol 88–9
  dependency 19
  violence 217
aliens, removal of 17, 112–14
allocation of responsible clinician 29
amnesia 88
applicability test, Advance Decisions 144
appropriate adult 74–5, 76
appropriate national authority 10, 28, 110
appropriate treatment 21
approved clinician 21, 28–30
  hospital managers and 105
approved mental health professionals 21, 25–7
  assessment and 26–7
  community service orders and 58, 59
  guardianship and 65
  in legal cases 250, 254, 255, 256, 257, 261–2
  nearest relative and 37–8
approved social worker, decision-making 27
Ashingdane v. United Kingdom 175, 176

assessment 26–7
of best interests (for deprivation of liberty) 151, 152, 153
of capacity *see* capacity
compulsory admission (Sections 2 and 4) *see* Sections
of consent 125
for detention/deprivation of liberty (incl. Section 2 and 3 compulsory admission) 45–9, 152, 153
Care Quality Commission and 125
forensic psychiatric 93
of mental state at time of offence, retrospective 84
risk (of violence) *see* risk
see also interviewing
assessment team, organising 26
assisted suicide 213–14, 214
authorization for deprivation of liberty 152–3, 169–70
lack of 170
automatism 85–6
autonomy 129–30

B v. Barking Havering etc NHS Trust (1999) 61, 249
bail 76, 77
Barbara v. Home Office (1984) 137
barbiturate 180
Barnes v. Crabtree (1955) 33
battery (in treatment without consent) 131
BB v. Cygnet Health Care and London Borough of Lewisham (2008) 116–17
belief(s)
reasonable 141–2
spiritual *see* religion
best interests 141, 168
assessment (for deprivation of liberty) 151, 152, 153
children 192, 195, 197, 199, 202, 203, 204, 205
treatment in 131–2
Bethlem Hospital 2, 3, 5, 133
Better Care and Maintenance of Pauper and Criminal Lunatics Act (1808) 3
biological factors causing violence 217
blanket security, unnecessary 126
blinding in clinical trial 183–4
BMA (British Medical Association) guidelines on assessing capacity 136
Bolam test 31–2, 131, 133
Bolitho v. Hackney Health Authority (1997) 133
Bournewood case (*HL v. UK* (2004)) 37, 41, 62, 70, 119, 120, 149–50, 203, 250, 256
brain, impairment or disturbance of *see* impairment or disturbance
British Medical Association guidelines on assessing capacity 136
business conflict 34
Butler Report 8

C v. A LA et al (2011) 260
Canada 242–3
cannabis and cannabis derivatives 180
capacity (mental) and competency 135–8, 139–71
assessment/testing 125, 136, 155–9
Advance Decisions and 144
recording 125
Care Quality Commission on 125, 125–6
children and young persons 134, 149, 155, 191–2, 201–3
Code of Practice 46, 120, 155, 161, 165, 167–71
informal and voluntary admission and 120
flow chart 156
scenarios 157–9
fluctuating 159
guardianship and 68
lack (incapacity/incompetence) 132, 134, 139, 140, 155
acting in best interests with *see* best interests
cause of/reasons for 137
child 202–3
decision-making with 136, 143, 202–3
definition 139–40
proving 159

research and 148, 164–5, 189
Singapore 246
urgent and emergency treatment with 178–9
legal principles 136
presumption 140, 155
Singapore 246
see also Mental Capacity Act
care
children and young persons in (and care orders) 23, 194, 195, 196, 197
duty of *see* duty
palliative 214
patient
involving patient 125
liability for 145–6
safety in 182
see also after-care
Care and Maintenance Lunacy Act (1815) 4
Care Programme Approach (CPA) 233, 234
Care Quality Commission (CQC) 39, 123–7
community treatment orders and 126–7
first annual (2010) report 124–6, 126–7
hospital managers and 103
race and 210
statutory basis 123–4
case law and legal cases 248–62
adoption 197
on consent and capacity
after Mental Capacity Act (2005) 138
before Mental Capacity Act (2005) 137, 248–9
certifying consent 29
Channel Islands 241–2
removal to and from 17, 111–12
childhood in risk assessment 225
children (minors) and young persons 191–206
adoption 142, 174, 193, 194, 196, 197
age-appropriate services 11
capacity issues 134, 149, 155, 191–2, 201–3
see also consent
in care/under care order 23, 194, 195, 196, 197
definition 192
legal frameworks applying to 192–5
in need 195
see also adolescents; family; infanticide
Children Act (1989) 191, 193–8
Mental Health Act (1983) or 199
China 246
Chronically Sick and Disabled Persons Act (1970) 8
civil partner 23
civil treatment codes 263–4
clinical trials of drugs 183–5
clinician *see* approved clinician; responsible clinician
close proximity (to patient), duty of care to those in 31
CM v. Derbyshire Healthcare NHS Foundation Trust et al (2011) 249
Code of Practice (Mental Capacity Act) 149, 152, 155, 158, 164, 165, 167–71
advanced decisions and 144
chapters/coverage
DOLS code 169–70
main code 168–9
checklists 171
civil treatment codes 263–4
independent mental health advocates and 161–2, 169
research and 165
status 167–8
Code of Practice (Mental Health Act) 40–1, 115–21, 149
capacity and 46, 120, 155, 161, 165, 167–71
children and 192, 197, 199, 202, 204
Community Treatment Orders and 57
court procedure and 77
detention and 45, 46, 47, 49
discharge and 44
guardianship and 65, 68, 68–9, 70
guiding (5) principles 117–18
historical developments 9, 10, 11

Code of Practice (Mental Health Act) – *contd*
hospital managers and 38, 104, 105
and information for victims 104
leave and 60
legal cases and 248, 252, 256, 257, 260
police custody and 74
policy agreements 117
purpose 115–16
risk assessment and 26
status 116–17
tribunals and 101–2
urgent neccesity and 34
coercion and duress
to consent 132, 137
false confessions under 76
common law 1–2
suicide 212
communication
of decision, inability 159
by professionals *see* consultation; liaison
community patient 24
definition 21
removal to Northern Ireland 111
treatment *see* community treatment
community treatment (and orders/CTOs) 54, 55, 57–60, 100–1, 126–7, 263
Australia and New Zealand 245
Care Quality Commission and 126–7
conditions 58–9
discharge *see* discharge
grounds 57–8
guardianship compared with CTOs 71
hospital element 61–2, 92–3
legal cases 249, 259
race and 127, 210
recall to hospital *see* hospital
removal to Scotland 110
revocation 59–60
supervised (SCT) 11, 29, 30, 35, 106, 126, 178
time periods/duration 59, 263
USA 244
virtual 61
competency *see* capacity
compulsory admission (detention; deprivation of liberty/DOL for treatment)
assessment for *see* assessment
Canada 243
Care Quality Commission and 125
involving patients in their care and treatment 125
community treatment order with compulsion element 61–2, 92–3
comparisons within British Isles 237–9
Northern Ireland 237–9, 240
criteria (Mental Health Act 2007) 10, 43–51
definition (of DOL) 169
historical aspects 2, 4, 6, 8, 9, 10, 11
Human Rights Act Article 8 and 176
leave of absence *see* leave
mechanisms 152–3
patient concerned in criminal proceedings or under sentence 14
responsible clinicians and 30
revocation (of community treatment order) resulting in readmission 59–60
Section 2/3/4 *see* Sections of Mental Health Act
Singapore 245
USA 244
conditional discharge of offenders 91
confessions, false 76
confidentiality 30–2, 33
children and 191–2
duty of *see* duty
see also disclosure
conflicts of interest 33–5, 120
conscience, right to freedom of 174
consent to treatment 15, 39, 54–6, 129–38, 201–3
Canada 243
capacity to *see* capacity
Care Quality Commission on 125
assessment and recording 125
certifying 29

children and 191–2, 201–3
Gillick competence 134, 191, 203–5, 248–9
civil treatment codes and 263
definition 130
English Law 133–4
exceptions to usual requirement for 135
express 131
flowchart of decisions involving 266
implied 130, 135
informed 129, 131, 132–3, 135, 136, 138
lack/absence of 132, 179
children 201, 205
treatment with 131–2, 205
legal considerations 132–8
principles of 145
refusal 28, 129, 130, 132
advance decisions *see* Advance Decisions
attempted suicide followed by 136
case law 137, 138, 248, 253, 258
children and 205
USA 244
in research studies 189
situations requiring 132
types 130–1
voluntary 132
constructive manslaughter 87
consultation requirement for research on persons lacking capacity 165
continuation of treatment 29
contractual liability for service provision 30–1
control, recording of episodes of 125
controlled drugs 180–1
conveyance 27
Coroners and Justice Act (2009) 82, 87
County Asylums Act (1808) 3
court(s)
Mental Capacity Act Code of Practice and 168
police/criminal 74–6, 263
children 199–201
defence of mental abnormality 78–89
psychiatric reports 94–6
Court of Protection 143, 144, 146–7, 148, 168, 170
deputies appointed by 143, 146, 147
Crime (Sentences) Act (1997) 92
Criminal Justice Act (Northern Ireland) (1966) 82
Criminal Lunatic Asylum Act (1860) 5
criminal offences 73–89, 237–8, 263
assisted suicide 213–14, 214
Canada 242–3
children 199–201
comparing legislation within British Isles 237–8
Northern Ireland 237–8, 240
of ill-treatment or neglect 148, 164
by patients
accused patients 14–15, 73–89
removal from Channel Islands and Isle of Man 112
by professionals 18, 40
with lack of consent 131
research on persons convicted of 187
violent *see* risk
see also courts; sentencing
Criminal Procedure (Insanity and Unfitness to Plead) Act (1991) 79–81
criminal responsibility 73–4
cross-border transfer *see* transfer
culture *see* race and culture
custody, police 74–6

dangerousness 218–19, 222
deaths, avoidable 232
see also homicide; murder; suicide
decision-making 143–8, 263
children and 191, 197–8, 201–5
designated decision-makers 143
flowchart 266
Mental Capacity Act (2005) and 143–8, 201–3
patients' abilities 140
children 201–4
criteria 140
lack (incompetency) 136, 143, 202–3

decision-making – *contd*
patients' abilities – *contd*
maximising 140
scenarios in assessing and assisting 157–9
unwise decisions 140, 202
professionals 27
see also Advance Decisions
defence of insanity *see* insanity
see also plea
definitions/meanings (in law)
historical (1913) of mental disorders 10
modern times 13–22
children 192
consent 130
deprivation of liberty 169, 175
incapacity 139–40
of mental disorders *see* mental disorders
race discrimination 208
treatment 22, 130
degrading treatment, freedom from 173, 174
delusions and violence 220
demographic risk factors for violence 223, 226
dependency, alcohol or drugs 19
deprivation of liberty 13–14, 23–4, 43–51
definition 169, 175
legal cases 248, 256, 258–61
for treatment *see* compulsory admission
deprivation of liberty safeguards (DOLS) 70, 149–55, 169–70
children 203
legal cases 248, 256, 258, 259, 260, 261
Mental Capacity Act Code of Practice and 169–70, 171
monitoring 170
deputies, court-appointed 143, 146, 147
designated decision-makers 143
designated individual or persons (research institution) 188
detention *see* compulsory admission
'difficult' patient 48–9
diminished responsibility 81–4, 87
points in favour and against 84–5
direct proximity (to patient), duty of care to those in 31
discharge 100–1
from community treatment order 60, 100–1
hospital managers' powers 105, 106
Section 2 44
Section 3 45
Section 4 50
from guardianship 68, 101
from hospital 100, 120–1
deferred 100
hospital managers and 105–6, 120–1
legal cases 249, 251, 253, 254, 255, 256, 262
Reference Guide 121
tribunals and 16, 100–1, 251, 253, 254, 255, 256
of offenders 91–2
disclosure of information 33
children 205–6
justified 31
see also confidentiality
dispensing errors with drugs 181–2, 182
disturbance of mind or brain *see* impairment or disturbance; mental disorders/disturbances
diversion schemes (courts) 75, 76
doctors *see* medical practitioners
doli incapax 73
Domestic Violence, Crime and Victims Act (2004) 10, 79, 79–80, 104
see also spouse
Donaldson (Lord) MR in Re T (1992) 137
double-blinded trials 184
drugs 88–9, 177–86
abuse (substance abuse) 88
violence related to 217, 220, 223, 232
clinical trials 183–5
controlled 180–1
dependency 19
licensed, unlicensed use 183
mental disorders due to 89, 232
therapeutic use (medication/pharmacotherapy) 177–86
errors in administration 181–2

historical developments 8
USA, refusal right 244
dual diagnosis patients, services for 232
duress *see* coercion and duress
duty
of care 31, 32–3
breach of 31–2
children and 205
of confidentiality 33
breach of 31–2
dynamic risk assessments 228–9

early diversion 75
ECT *see* electroconvulsive therapy
education, right to 193, 198
'effectiveness, efficiency and equity principle' principle of Code of Practice 118
Egypt, ancient 1
elderly/old-age
capacity 135
assessment scenario 157–8
suicide 211
electroconvulsive therapy (ECT) 28
consent issues 54
historical aspects 7, 10
legal cases and 258
Mental Health Act 1983 and 178
eligibility requirement for deprivation of liberty 152, 153
embassy staff and alien repatriation 113–14
emergencies
assessment in, Section 4 detention for 49–50, 263
duty of care 32–3
treatment in, qualification criteria 178–9
see also entries under urgent
employment history in risk assessment 225
Enduring Power of Attorney 143, 145, 164
England
comparing legislation with rest of British Isles 237–9
removal to
from Channel Islands and Isle of Man 112
from Northern Ireland 111
from Scotland 110
environment
age-appropriate (child) 198–9
violence risk relating to 217, 223, 224
Epsom and St Helier NHS Trust v. MHRT(W) (2001) 251
equal consideration principle 157–8
Equality Act (2010) 208–9
errors
drug administration 181–2
policy on 122
ethics
consent and 129
research *see* research
risk assessment 219
ethnicity *see* race
European Court of (and Convention on) Human Rights (sometimes referred to as just 'European Court') 37, 41, 120, 149, 150, 173–4, 200, 250, 256
aliens and 113
race and 207
euthanasia 212, 214
expert evidence, psychiatric 93–4
express consent 131
expression, right to freedom of 174

fair trial *see* trial
false confessions 76
family
right to have a 174
right to respect family life 174, 176
Section 27 of Mental Capacity Act (2005) and the 142
violence causation relating to 217
family history
psychiatric court reporting 95
risk assessment 225
Family Law Reform Act (1969) 201
father, parental responsibilities of 196
feeble-minded, 1913 definition 6
females
suicide risk 211
violence risk 220, 223, 225
financial conflict 34
financial responsibility of local authorities 82

fitness
for interview by police 76
to plead *see* plea
to remain in police custody 76
forensic history
psychiatric court reporting 95
risk assessment 225
forensic psychiatry
assessment 93
capacity in 135
Forensic Treatment Orders 90
freedom (right to)
of expression 174
of thought/conscience/religion 174
from torture and inhuman or degrading treatment 173, 174
see also liberty
Freeman v. Home Office (1983) 137
Freud, Sigmund 6, 7

gender *see* sex
Gillick competence 134, 191, 203–4, 204, 248–9
GJ judgment (*GJ v. The Foundation Trust et al* (2009)) 120, 151–2, 258–9
global issues *see* international issues
good practice 50–1
development and monitoring 50
Goodwin v. United Kingdom (2002) 176
government response to homicide inquiry findings 233–4
guardian (of child), responsibilities 196
guardianship 13, 14, 24, 90, 263
community treatment orders compared with 71
discharge 68, 101
grounds 66–7
guardian's powers 67
nearest relatives and 65, 69
offenders 92
purpose 65
responsible clinicians and 24, 30
routes into 65–6
time limits/duration 67, 263
see also Special Guardianship Order
Guernsey 241–2

hallucinogenic drugs 180
Hare's Psychopathy Checklist – Revised (PCL-R) and further revisions (incl. PCL-SV) 229, 230
harm
risk of causing *see* risk
significant (children and the concept of) 195–6
see also dangerousness; self-harm
hazardous treatment 54
Health Inspectorate (Wales) 39
Health Secretary (of State) 78
hearings
hospital managers' 105–6
tribunal *see* tribunal
Historical–Clinical–Risk-Management 20-Item instrument (HCR-20) 228–9
historical perspectives
attitude to suicide 212
legislation 1–11
history, person/patient (and history-taking)
psychiatric court reporting 95
violence 221, 225
HL v. UK (2004) (Bournewood case) 37, 41, 62, 70, 119, 120, 149–50, 250, 256
homicide 81–9, 232, 232–4
amnesia claim 88
definition 86
diminished responsibility *see* diminished responsibility
epidemiology 86, 219–20
countries with high rates 221
inquiries into 232–3
government response to findings 233–4
legal classification 86–8
Homicide Act (1957) 81–2, 87, 232, 238
hospital 21
admission to *see* admission
children in 199
community treatment order with hospital element 61–2, 92–3
definition 21
discharge from *see* discharge
recall of community patients 59
patients not recalled, treatment 15–16
remands to 14, 76–8, 90

special 24, 231
transfer from prison to 15, 80, 90, 92, 93
hospital directions 15, 92, 99, 238
hospital managers 21, 38, 103–7, 121
duties 103–6, 121
legal case 261–2
tribunals and 98–9, 101–2, 103, 104, 105, 106
types 103
hospital orders 60, 78, 90
interim 90, 91, 92
Human Rights Act (1998) 10, 173–6, 179
alien repatriation and 113
children and 191, 192, 200
race and 207
see also European Court of (and Convention on) Human Rights
Human Tissue Act (2004) 188–9
husband 23
hybrid order (hospital directions) 15, 92, 99, 238

idiot, 1913 definition 6
Idiots Act (1886) 5
ill-treatment 148, 164
imbecile, 1913 definition 6
impairment or disturbance (of mind or brain) 157
in Mental Capacity Act (2005) 139
implied consent 130, 135
independent medical examination (for tribunals) 99
independent mental health advocates (IMHA) 10, 39–40, 147–8, 161–5, 169
children and 203
Independent Prescribers 185
infanticide 88
informal patient 119–20
information
in assessment of decision-making ability 157–9
for children (on care and treatment) 198
communicating (=informing) 27
disclosure *see* confidentiality; disclosure
gathering 26
for nearest relatives *see* nearest relatives
for patients 103
consent requiring 129, 131, 132–3, 135, 136, 138
hospital managers and 103
under guardianship 69
recording *see* recording
for victims 104
see also liaison
inhuman treatment, freedom from 173, 174
Insane Prisoners Act (1840) 4
insanity (defence of) 73–4, 81
and automatism 85
Integrated Research Application System (IRAS) 187, 188
interests
best *see* best interests
conflicts of 33–5, 120
public *see* public interest
interim care order 194
interim hospital order 90, 91, 92
international issues 237–46
alien repatriation 17, 112–14
race discrimination elimination 208
suicide rates 211
interviewing
by approved mental health professional 26–7
by police, fitness for 76
in psychiatric court reporting 95
in risk assessment 224–5
see also assessment
intoxication 88–9
involuntary intoxication 89
involuntary manslaughter 87
Ireland *see* Northern Ireland; Republic of Ireland
irreversible treatment 54
Isle of Man 242
removal to and from 17, 171–2
Israel, ancient 1

JE v. DE and Surrey CC (2006) 257–8
Jersey 242
Johnson v. United Kingdom (1999) 176
Judaic law 1

Justice Secretary (and Ministry of Justice) 78, 90, 187–8
justified disclosure of patient information 31

Keenan v. United Kingdom (2001) 174, 252, 258
killing *see* homicide; murder; suicide

Lasting Power of Attorney (LPA) 143, 144–5, 146, 164, 168, 203
Law Society guidelines on assessing capacity 136
lawful homicide 86
LBH v. GP (2009) 25, 260–1
LBH v. Neary (2011) 260–1
learning disability
  assisting understanding of a decision 157
  definition 19
least restriction principle (least restrictive intervention) 118, 141
leave (of absence) 60–1, 61
absent without 17
legal cases *see* case law
legal members of tribunals 97
liability 31
  for care or treatment (in Mental Capacity Act 2005) 145–6
  contractual, for service provision 30–1
  drug administration errors 181–2
  local research ethics committees 186
  professional 32–3
liaison (communication) with others 26
  by hospital managers with victims 104
  by psychiatrists with police and courts 75–6
  see also consultation; information
liaison psychiatry 136
liberty
  deprivation *see* deprivation of liberty
  right to 173–4
  see also freedom
licence holder (research institution) 188
licensed drugs, unlicensed use 183
life, right to 173, 174
life history in risk assessment 225
life-sustaining threshold 144
life-sustaining treatment 141, 144, 147, 151, 164
limitation directions 15, 92
line of duty of care 32
local authorities 17
  accommodation provision 163
    secure (for children) 194
  financial responsibility 62
  hospitalised children and 199
  parental responsibility for child under Care Order 196
  social services *see* social services
Local Authorities Social Services Act (1970) 8
local research ethics committees 185–6
Lord Chancellor 97, 147
Lord Donaldson MR in Re T (1992) 137
LSD 7, 180
Lunacy Asylum Enabling Act (1808) 3
Lunacy (Consolidation) Act (1890) 5
Lunatics Act (1853) 5
Lunatics Asylum Act (1845) 4–5
lysergic acid diethylamide (LSD) 7, 180

Macmillan Report (1926) 7
McNaughton Rules 4, 84
  criticisms 84
Madhouse Act (1828) 4
males
  suicide risk 211
  violence risk 220, 223, 225
malice aforethought 86
managers
  hospital *see* hospital
  registered establishment 22
Manchester Self-Harm Project (MaSH) 214
manslaughter 87
  murder charge reduced to, due to diminished responsibility *see* diminished responsibility
marry, right to 174
maximum security hospitals *see* special hospitals

Maynard v. West Midlands RHA (1985) 133
MB test for capacity 136, 137
MD v. Nottingham Healthcare NHS Trust (2010) 259
medical conditions
consent not obtained in testing for 134
recognised, homicide arising from 82
medical examination (for tribunals), independent 99
medical history (past/previous), psychiatric court reporting 95
medical practitioners/doctors
assisted suicide 213–14, 214
second opinion appointed doctors (SOADs) 39, 54, 55, 124, 125, 177, 178, 266
in tribunals 97
see also reasonable doctor medical test
Medical Registration Act (1858) 5
medical treatment *see* treatment
medication *see* drugs
men *see* males
mens rea 73
Mental Capacity Act (2005) 10, 46, 54, 120, 131, 132, 133, 134, 136, 139–54, 161–71
case law propositions on medical treatment prior to 137
children and 201–3
Code of Practice *see* Code of Practice (Mental Capacity Act)
guardianship or 68
informal and voluntary admission and 120
medication and 179
principles 139–42
provisions 143–54
see also capacity
Mental Deficiency Act (1927) 7
mental disorders/disturbances/abnormalities (and mental/psychiatric illness)
definitions 10, 19
Northern Ireland 239
Republic of Ireland 241
Scotland 239
drug or alcohol-induced 89, 232
homicide *see* homicide
police courts *see* courts
risk of violence 218, 219–22
see also impairment or disturbance
mental functioning, killing and abnormality of 82–3, 84
Mental Health Act (1959) 8
guardianship and 66
Mental Health Act (1983 and in general) 8–9
children and young persons 191, 197–8
adopted 197
Children Act (1989) or 199
young offenders 201
Code of Practice *see* Code of Practice
compared with rest of British Isles 237, 238–9
consent under 53–6
medications and 177–9
Mental Capacity Act relationship to 149
monitoring use 124
race and 210
safeguards *see* safeguards
structure 13–18
Parts and Sections *see* Parts; Sections
Mental Health Act (2001) (Republic of Ireland) 237, 238–9, 241
Mental Health Act (2007) 13–18
children 197–8
definitions *see* definitions
main changes from 1983 Act 10–11
risk assessment in 233
Mental Health Act (Care and Treatment) (Scotland) Act (2003) 109, 237
compared with rest of British Isles 238–9
Mental Health Act Commission(ers) 39, 123–4
monitoring use of Mental Health Act 124
Mental Health (Northern Ireland) Act (1961) 8
Mental Health (Northern Ireland) Order (1986) 111, 112, 237, 238–9, 239–40

Mental Health (Patients in the Community) Act (1995) 10
mental health professionals *see* professionals
Mental Health (Scotland) Act (1959) 8
Mental Health (Scotland) Act (1984) 9, 237
Mental Health (Scotland) Act (2003) 239
Mental Health Treatment Requirement and Youth Rehabilitation Order 201
mental state/condition
  remand to hospital for report on 77
  risk of violence 223
  at time of offence, retrospective assessment 84
  unanticipated with drug use 89
Mental Treatment Act (1930) 7
Mental Treatment Act (1945) (Republic of Ireland) 238, 240
Mental Treatment Act (1961) (Republic of Ireland) 240
Metropolitan Toronto Forensic Service (METFORS) 243
mind
  'abnormality of', killing and 82–3, 88
  disease of, killing and 84
  impairment or disturbance of *see* impairment or disturbance
Ministry of Health Act (1919) 7
Ministry of Justice and Justice Secretary 78, 90, 187–8
minority ethnic groups *see* race and culture
minors *see* children
Misuse of Drugs Act (2004) 180–1
modern times (Mental Health Act 2007 = amended 1983 Act) of mental disorders 10, 19
moral defectives, 1913 definition 6
mother, parental responsibilities of 196
Multi-Agency Public Protection Panels (MAPPAs) 219, 227
murder (charge) 86–7
  reduced to manslaughter due to diminished responsibility *see* diminished responsibility
National Assistance Act (1948) 7
National Clinical Survey 211, 215
National Confidential Inquiry into Suicide and Homicide by People with Mental Illness 211, 214, 232
National Health Service (NHS)
  accommodation provision 162–3
  independent mental health advocacy and the 147
National Health Service Act (1946) 7
National Health Service and Community Care Act (1990) 9
National Health Service (Wales) Act (2006) 21
National Patient Safety Agency 182, 214
National Service Framework for Mental Health 215
nearest relatives 10, 22–3, 37–8
  guardianship and 65, 69
  information for 69, 103
    hospital managers and 103
  in legal cases 250, 252, 256, 261–2
  tribunal applications and 263
  unsuitable 38, 120
needle phobia and MB test for capacity 136, 137
neglect 148, 164
negligence (in treatment)
  drug administration 181
  without consent 131
NHS *see* National Health Service
no-order principle 193
no-refusals requirement for deprivation of liberty 152, 153
non-insane automatism 85
Northern Ireland 8, 237–9, 239–40
  comparing legislation with rest of British Isles 237–9
  homicide 82
  removal to or from 110–11

objective prudent patient test 133
occupational (employment) history in risk assessment 225
O'Connor v. Donaldson (1975 – USA) 244
offences and offenders *see* criminal offences

old-age *see* elderly
open study (clinical trial) 183–4
Osman v. United Kingdom (2000) 174

P and Q (aka MIG and MEG) v. Surrey CC et al ((2011) 256
PACE (Police and Criminal Evidence Act 1984) 9, 74
palliative care 214
parental responsibilities 193, 196
  adoption and 197
  consent with non-Gillick competent children 204
participation principle of Code of Practice 117
Parts of Mental Health Act
  Part 1 (I) of MHA 13, 20, 22
  Part 2 (II) of MHA 13–14, 30
    tribunals and 98–9
  Part 3 (III) of MHA 14–15, 30
    tribunals and 99
  Part 4 (IV) of MHA 15, 53–4
    capacity and 137–8
  Part 4A (IVa) of MHA 15–16, 55–6, 178
  Part 5 (V) of MHA 16, 97
  Part 6 (VI) of MHA 16, 109
  Part 8 (VIII) of MHA 17
  Part 9 (IX) of MHA 18
  Part 10 (X) of MHA 18
pathological intoxication 89
patient(s)
  community *see* community patient
  definition 23
  'difficult' 48–9
  informal 119–20
  participation principle of Code of Practice 117
  voluntary 119, 240
Patient Group Directions 185
Percy Report (1957) 8
person designated (research institution) 188
Personal Welfare Lasting Power of Attorney 145
personality traits in risk assessment 225
pharmacotherapy *see* drugs
phase 1–4 trials 184–5
physicians *see* medical practitioners
plea
  fitness or unfitness to plead 79–80
    child 199–200
  of insanity 81
police 263
  comparing legislation with rest of British Isles 238
  courts *see* courts
  custody 74–6
Police and Criminal Evidence Act 1984 (PACE) (1984) 9, 74
Poor Law Act (1601) 2
post-marketing targeted studies 185
Power of Attorney
  Enduring 143, 145, 164
  Lasting (LPA) 143, 144–5, 146, 164, 168, 203
Powers of the Court (of Protection) 146–7
Powers of the Courts (Sentencing) Act (2000) 92
prescription (prescribing)
  controlled drugs 180–1
  errors 182
    on prescription sheet 181
  non-medical 185
primary care trust as hospital manager 103
prison
  alternatives to remand to 14, 76–8, 90
  suicide in/after 214
  transfer to hospital 15, 80, 90, 92, 93
Pritchard test/criteria 79, 80, 199
privacy, right to respect 174, 176
  child 192
private law orders 194
private prescriptions, controlled drugs 181
professionals (mental health)
  approved *see* approved mental health professionals
  conflicts of interest 34
  consent based on information given by 132
  liability 32–3
  offences by *see* criminal offences
  roles 10–11, 25–35
Property and Affairs Lasting Power of Attorney 145

provocation to kill 87
psychiatric court reporting 94–6
psychiatric disorders *see* mental disorders
psychiatric expert evidence 93–4
psychiatric history, past/previous
  psychiatric court reporting 95
  risk assessment 225
psychiatric research, ethical issues 189
psychodynamic models of violence 217
psychological models of violence 217
Psychopathy Checklist – Revised (PCL-R) and revisions (incl. PCL-SV) 229, 230
psychosis, drug-induced 232
Public Guardian 143, 147
public interest, disclosure in 33
  children and 205
purpose principle of Code of Practice 117

R (AN) v. MHRT (Northern Region) (2005) 256
R (Ashworth SHA) v. MHRT W. Midlands and N.W. Region (2002) 254
R (CS) v. Mental Health Review Tribunal (2004) 249
R (DR) v. Mersey Care NHS Trust (2002) 61, 249
R (E) v. Bristol City Council (2005) 256–7
R (Ex Parte Wooder) v. Feggetter (2002) 252
R (IH) v. Nottinghamshire Healthcare NHS Trust (2003) 255
R (Munjaz) v. Mersey Care NHS Trust (2005) 116, 257
R (S) v. City of Plymouth (2002) 252–3
R v. Byrne (1960) 83
R v. Camden and Islington Health Authority ex parte K (2001) 255
R v. Doncaster MBC, ex parte W (2003) 254–5
R v. Hallstrom (1986) 251
R v. London South West Regional MHRT, ex parte Moyle (2000) 249, 251
R v. Mental Health Review Tribunal London South and West Region (2001) 176
R v. MHRT North and East London Region (2001) 176, 249
R v. North and East Devon Health Authority Ex Parte Coughlan 176
R v. Oxfordshire MH Trust, ex parte H (2002) 254
R v. Pritchard (1836) and Pritchard test/criteria 79, 80, 199
R v. Secretary of State for Home Department (2001) 174–5
R v. Tower Hamlets Healthcare NHS Trust (MHRT, Discharge) Ex Parte Von Brandenburg (2003) 253–4, 254
race (ethnicity) and culture 207–10
  community treatment orders and 127, 210
Re Barker 251
Re D (Mental Patient: Habeas Corpus) (Nearest Relative) (2000) 250
Re F (A Child) (2000) 250–1
Re W (A Minor) (1992) 248
reasonable belief 141–2
reasonable doctor medical test 132
recall to hospital *see* hospital
reception order 5, 6
recording (of information) 27
  capacity and consent 125
  episodes of control and restraint 125
Reed (Trainer) v. Bronglais Hospital etc. (2001) 251–2
Reference Guide 121–2
referral to tribunals
  by hospital managers 98–9
  by Secretary of State 98
registered establishment, managers 22
Regulating Private Madhouses Act (1774) 3
relatives 14
  nearest 10, 22–3, 37–8
  persons other than 23
relevant person's representative 170
religion and spiritual beliefs 209–10
  right to freedom of 174
remand to hospital 14, 76–8, 90

removal of patients (cross-border) *see* transfer
repatriation of aliens 17, 112–14
reports 29
on mental condition of accused, remand to hospital for 77, 90
psychiatric court 94–6
social circumstances 125
for tribunals 102
Republic of Ireland 240–1
comparison with UK 237–9
research 187–90
ethics 187–90
local committees 185–6
lack of capacity and 148, 164–5, 189
offender suicides 214
Residence Order 196
respect
in Code of Practice 117
for family life, right to 174, 176
for privacy *see* privacy
responsible clinician (RC) 23–4, 28–30
allocation 29
functions/roles 30, 38
community service orders 58, 59, 59–60
granting leave of absence 60–1
guardianship 24, 30
hospital managers and 105
restraint, recording of episodes of 125
restriction (incl. restriction orders and directions) 15, 90, 91–2, 109–10, 175, 231
discharge 101
guardianships and 69–70
legal cases 256, 257
removal of patient
to Northern Ireland 111
to Scotland 109–10
unnecessary 126
see also least restriction principle
return of patients (cross-border) *see* transfer
review tribunals *see* tribunals
revocation of community treatment order 59–60
Richardson Report (1999) 10
risk (of violence or causing harm) 217–36
assessment 26, 48, 222–31, 234
background to 219
clinical or practical 226–7
ethics 219
instruments 227–31
USA 221
factors (causes of violence) 217, 223, 226, 227, 228, 230
mental/psychiatric illness as 218, 219–22
management 231, 234, 234–5
problems 230–1
Risk Matrix 2000 227, 229, 230
RM v. St Andrew's Healthcare (2010) 259–60
Rodriquez v. British Columbia (A-G) (1993) 213
Roman law 1
Royal College of Psychiatrists
research ethics and 189–90
risk management and 234
Royal Prerogative (1334) 2

Safe Custody of Insane Persons Charged with Offences Act (1800) 3
safeguards
ancient world 1
modern world (incl. Mental Health Acts) 37–41
children 185–6, 205
deprivation of liberty *see* deprivation of liberty safeguards
exemptions from applying 46
psychiatric research 189
safety in patient care 182
see also harm
Schedule 1–5 drugs 180
schizophrenia and violence 220, 221, 222, 232
Scotland
comparing legislation with rest of British Isles 237–9
Mental Health Acts *see* Mental Health (Scotland) Act
removal of patients to 16, 109–10
removal of patients to England and Wales from 110
unfitness to plead 80
seclusion 174, 257

second opinion 53–4
second opinion appointed doctors (SOADs) 39, 54, 55, 124, 125, 177, 178, 266
Secretary of State 17
Code of Practice and 116
tribunals and 98
Secretary of State for Justice (and the Ministry) 78, 90, 187–8
Sections of Mental Health Act
Section 2 detention (for assessment) 23–4, 43–4, 45–9, 263
assessment for 45–9
choosing between Section 3 and 47
discharge 44, 100
duration 44, 263
grounds 43–4
purpose 43
sample application forms 267–70
tribunals and 98, 99, 100, 102, 263
Section 3 detention (for treatment) 23–4, 44–5, 263
choosing between Section 2 and 47
discharge 45
duration 45, 263
grounds 44–5
purpose 44
sample application forms 271–4
tribunals and 98, 102, 105, 263
Section 4 detention (for emergency assessment) 24, 49–50, 141–2, 263
Section 4a 141–2
Section 5 53, 82, 119–20, 145–6, 179, 263
Section 7 37, 65, 66, 68, 71, 98, 263
Section 8 67, 175, 193, 194
Section 17 19–20, 21, 57–61, 101, 110, 195
legal cases 249, 251
Section 17A 19, 21, 57, 71, 98, 263
Section 19 98, 263
Section 20 98, 99, 105, 147, 248, 249
Section 25 105, 194, 263
Section 29 8, 98, 252, 257, 263
Section 35 30, 53, 60, 76, 77, 90, 147, 161–2, 163, 179, 238
Section 36 76, 77–8, 90, 238
Section 37 53, 60, 65, 66, 68, 80, 89, 90–1, 91, 92, 93, 148, 162, 238, 239
Section 38 90, 91, 238
Section 41 33, 90, 91–2, 238
Section 45A 92, 238
Section 47 90, 239
Section 48 76, 78, 90, 238
Section 49 90, 99, 239
Section 53 82, 209
Section 57 53, 177, 178, 266
Section 58 29, 54, 147, 177–8, 252, 258, 266
Section 58A 28, 29, 54, 177, 178
Section 62 28, 29, 54, 144, 266
Section 63 28, 138, 257, 266
Section 64G 55, 178
Section 72 100, 101
Section 73 53, 101, 176
Section 74 53, 101
Section 75 101
Section 80 109–10
Section 81 110–11
Section 83 111, 112
Section 84 111, 112
Section 85 111, 112
Section 86 112, 113
Section 117 62, 154, 255
Section 118 116, 117, 118
Section 120 123–4
Section 132 103
Section 133 104
Section 135 26, 48, 49, 53, 59, 179, 238, 263
Section 136 53, 75, 125, 179, 238, 263
Section 165 138, 266
secure accommodation order 194–5
secure unit 8, 33, 231
security
blanket, unnecessary 126
maximum *see* special hospitals
Seebohm report 8
self-harm 213, 214
sentencing 14–15, 89–96
after 93
comparing legislation within British Isles 239

comparing legislation within British Isles 238–9
services
child age-appropriate 11
contractual liability for provision 30–1
dual diagnosis patients 232
sex (gender)
suicide risk 211
violence risk 220, 223, 225
sexual history
psychiatric court reporting 95
risk assessment 225
sexual offences
professionals having sexual activity with patient 40
risk assessment (offenders) 229, 230
victims of 104
Shipman, Harold 86
Sidaway v. Board of Governors of Bethlem Royal and Maudsley Hospital (1985) 133, 137
significant harm (children and the concept of) 195–6
Singapore 245–6
single-blinded trials 183–4
social circumstances reports 125
social models of violence 217
social services (local authority) 8, 21, 35
after-care and 62
guardianship and 66, 68–9
tribunals and 101–2
social worker, approved, decision-making 27
Special Guardianship Order 196
special hospitals (incl. maximum security) 24, 231
Canada 242
historical aspects 5, 6, 8, 9
Republic of Ireland 240
spiritual beliefs *see* religion
spouse 23
Spousal Assault Risk Assessment Guide (SARA) 229, 230
Standardised Authorisation for deprivation of liberty 152, 153, 169–70
statutory basis/principles
Care Quality Commission (CQC) 123–4
Mental Capacity Act (2005) 140–2
statutory consultees, Care Quality Commission and carrying out of duties as 125
step parent responsibilities 196
Storck v. Germany (2005) 257
structured risk assessments 227–8
sexual offending 230
substance abuse *see* drugs
'substantially' impaired mental functioning, killing and 93
suicide 211–15, 232
at-risk patients 211–15
attempted, and subsequent refusal of treatment in accident and emergency 136
epidemiology 211–12
historical attitudes 212
pact 87
prevention 214–15
Suicide Act (1961) 212–13
summary reception order 5
supervised community treatment (SCT) 11, 29, 30, 35, 106, 178
Supplementary Prescribers 185
Supply of Goods and Services Act (1982) 31
Switzerland, euthanasia 214

Tarasoff v. Regents of University of California (1976) 244
Thorpe J, in Re C (1994) 137
thought, freedom of 174
threat/control override 221
torture, freedom from 173, 174
transfer
cross-border
alien repatriation 17, 112–14
in UK 109–12
from prison to hospital 15, 80, 90, 92, 93
transportation 27
treatment (medical treatment)
appropriate 21
children, decision-making 198, 202
civil treatment codes 263–4
community *see* community treatment
compulsory admission for (Section 3) *see* Sections
consent to/refusal of *see* consent

treatment (medical treatment) – *contd*
continuation 29
decisions *see* decision-making
definitions 22, 130
emergency, qualification criteria 178–9
Forensic Treatment Orders 90
hazardous 54
historical aspects 7
involving patients 125
irreversible 54
liability for (in Mental Capacity Act 2005) 145–6
life-sustaining 141, 144, 147, 151, 164
pharmacological *see* drugs
remand of accused to hospital for 77–8, 90
second opinion *see* second opinion
urgent 28, 29, 54, 54, 178
see also care; hospital; ill-treatment
trials (clinical) 183–5
trials (criminal)
comparing legislation within British Isles for before/at/after 238
rights with 174
children 200
tribunals
Mental Capacity Act Code of Practice and 168
mental health/review/first-tier 11, 16, 38, 97–102, 263
Canada 243
children 199
civil treatment codes and 263
Code of Practice and 101–2
constitution and related aspects 16, 97
discharge and 16, 100–1, 251, 253, 254, 255, 256
eligibility criteria for appeal to 90
hospital managers and 98–9, 101–2, 103, 104, 105, 106
in legal cases 249, 251, 253–6, 259, 260, 261
part II patients and 98–9
part III patients and 99
see also hearings
TTM v. Hackney BC et al (2011) 252, 261
UK *see* United Kingdom
unconditional discharge of offenders 91
unfitness to plead *see* plea
United Kingdom (legislation)
comparison within, and with Republic of Ireland 237–9
removal and return of patients within 16–17, 109–12
United Nations Convention on the Rights of the Child 191, 192–3, 199
United States of America (USA) 243–4
homicide rates 221
unlawful homicide 86
unlicensed use of licensed drugs 183
Urgent Authorisation for deprivation of liberty 152–3, 170
urgent necessity (for assessment) 34
urgent treatment 28, 29, 54, 178
see also emergencies
USA *see* United States of America

Vagrancy Acts (1713 and 1744) 2–3
validity test, Advance Decisions 144
victims
information for 104
of violence, in risk assessment 224
violence *see* Domestic Violence, Crime and Victims Act; risk
Violence Risk Appraisal Guide (VRAG) 227
Violence Risk Scale (VRS) 229
virtual community treatment order 61
voluntary admission
Code confusing informal admission with 119
historical aspects 7, 8
voluntary confessions, false 76
voluntary consent 132
voluntary intoxication 88, 89
voluntary manslaughter 87
voluntary patient 119, 240
see also informal patient
voting 149
vulnerable people, protection 143

W v. Egdell (1990) 33
Wales
Code of Practice 118

comparing legislation with rest of British Isles 237–9
Health Inspectorate 39
National Health Service (Wales) Act (2006) 21
removal to
from Channel Islands and Isle of Man 112
from Northern Ireland 111
from Scotland 110
Wardship Order 197
Welfare Checklist (children) 193–4
wife 23
Wilkinson v. UK (Application 14659/02, Admissibility Decision Feb 06) 258
Winterwerp v. Netherlands (1979) 175, 179, 248
women *see* females
world-wide issues *see* international issues

young persons *see* children and young persons
younger adults, suicide risk 211
Youth Rehabilitation Order 200–1